Clinical Research in Communicative Disorders

Clinical Research in Communicative Disorders

Principles and Strategies

◆◆◆◆◆◆◆◆◆◆◆◆◆◆◆

Third Edition

M. N. Hegde

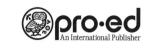
pro·ed
An International Publisher

8700 Shoal Creek Boulevard
Austin, Texas 78757-6897
800/897-3202 Fax 800/397-7633
www.proedinc.com

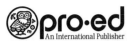

© 1987, 1994, 2003 by PRO-ED, Inc.
8700 Shoal Creek Boulevard
Austin, Texas 78757-6897
800/897-3202   Fax 800/397-7633
www.proedinc.com

Library of Congress Cataloging-in-Publication Data

Hegde, M. N. (Mahabalagiri N.),
     Clinical research in communicative disorders : principles and strategies / M. N. Hegde.—
3rd ed.
        p.   ;   cm.
     Includes bibliographical references and index.
     ISBN-13: 978-089079964-2
     ISBN-10: 0-89079-964-4
     1. Communicative disorders—Research—Methodology. 2. Research—Methodology. I.
Title.
     [DNLM: 1. Communication Disorders. 2. Research Design. WM 475 H462c 2003]
RC428 .H445   2003
616.85'5'0072—dc21

                                                              2002031908

This book is designed in Janson Text and Futura.

Printed in the United States of America

3 4 5 6 7 8 9 10 11 12 13 11 10 09

Contents

◆◆◆◆◆◆◆◆◆◆◆◆◆◆◆◆◆◆◆◆◆◆◆◆◆◆◆◆◆◆

Chapter 6

Observation and Measurement ◆ *183*

PART II:
Clinical Research Designs

Chapter 7

Research Designs: An Introduction ◆ *215*

Chapter 8

The Group Design Strategy ◆ *251*

Chapter 9

Single-Subject Designs ◆ 313

Chapter 10

Generality Through Replications ◆ 373

Chapter 11

Comparative Evaluation of Design Strategies ◆ 395

Chapter 12
Designs Versus Paradigms in Research ◆ 421

PART III:
Doing, Reporting, and Evaluating Research

Chapter 13
How To Formulate Research Questions ◆ 447

Chapter 14
How To Write Research Reports ◆ 467

Chapter 15

How To Evaluate Research Reports ◆ *509*

Chapter 16

Ethics of Research ◆ *531*

Preface to the First Edition

◆◆◆◆◆◆◆◆◆◆◆◆◆◆◆◆◆◆◆◆◆◆◆◆◆◆◆◆◆◆◆◆◆◆

I am a student and an instructor of philosophy and methodology of science and research. In my teaching of science and research, I have found it necessary to supplement information from a variety of sources. I knew that several of my colleagues who taught courses on research and science were doing the same to make their courses more relevant and useful to graduate students. To me, this meant that we did not have a comprehensive textbook on science and research. This book is an effort to fulfill that need.

My own teaching experience and discussions with many of my colleagues suggested that a book on science and research should address the following concerns. The first deals with the basic concepts of science and scientific methods. That is, the book should point out the need to study science and research methods and summarize the basic concepts of science and research. It should describe the true and lively process of research, not an idealized and frighteningly formalized process that typically discourages the beginning student from a further study of science and research. The book should give an adequate description of the different kinds of research that are conducted in communicative disorders. A discussion of observation and measurement, which are the basic tools of science, must be provided.

The second concern is clinical research designs. Most books on research designs tend to be statistically oriented. The enormously prestigious analysis of variance is constantly confused with experimental designs. A book on designs should present experimental designs, not methods of data analysis under the guise of research designs. Furthermore, the book should address both group and single-subject designs. Generally speaking, most books that offer information on research designs focus almost exclusively on group designs. Clinically more relevant single-subject designs are not well represented in those books. On the other hand, there are some books that focus exclusively on single-subject designs. There are not many books that present adequate information on both design strategies. Regardless of one's own methodologic preference and practice, a critical user and producer of research must have a knowledge of group as well as single-subject design approaches. It was thought that a single source that offered descriptions and comparative evaluations of both strategies would be useful to students and researchers alike.

The third concern is the discussion of some important philosophic issues that are an inexorable part of science and research. Research is based on methodology as well as philosophy. There is a tremendous lack of appreciation of the philosophic bases of research. Therefore, it was thought that this book should at least raise the issue of philosophy of research to stimulate further discussion in the discipline.

The fourth concern is the practical aspect of performing, writing, reporting, and evaluating research. Students need suggestions on where to find research questions, how to find current research trends, how to search the literature, how to refine research questions, and how to select designs that help answer those questions. They also need information on how to get started on theses and dissertations. A major problem instructors and students alike face is writing style and writing skills. It was thought that this book should offer basic information on principles of good writing.

The fifth concern is the ethics of research. Science and research are an ethical activity. From the beginning, science and research must be taught with due regard for the ethical principles that restrain research. A textbook on research should summarize ethical principles that govern research activities.

I have written this book with those five concerns as the guiding principles. An overall concern was to make a book on science and research especially relevant to clinical research in communicative disorders and write it in a less formal, and I would hope, more readable style. It is thought that such a style would also reflect the process of research more accurately than the typical style that formalizes research to an unnatural extent.

My wife Prema and my son Manu have been a part of all of my writings. This book, which I began to write soon after completing *Treatment Procedures in Communicative Disorders*, would not have been finished without their full support.

My students at both the undergraduate and graduate levels have been generous in their support and encouragement. My students have always tolerated and often appreciated my unlimited passion to teach science and research anytime and anywhere. Many students in my graduate seminar on research methods have offered excellent comments on earlier versions of several chapters in this book.

I am grateful to Dr. Raymond Kent for his review of the manuscript. His constructive criticisms and suggestions have helped me improve the quality of this book. Any limitations of the book, however, are entirely my own responsibility.

Preface to the Third Edition

◆◆◆◆◆◆◆◆◆◆◆◆◆◆◆◆◆◆◆◆◆◆◆◆◆◆◆◆◆◆◆◆◆◆◆

Since its first publication in 1987, many instructors have adopted this book as the main text in various courses on research methods and designs in communicative disorders. Most of these instructors have offered their gracious and positive comments on the book. The instructors have suggested that the comprehensive treatment of issues and methods of research is a strength of this book. I have retained that strength in revising it for this third edition.

I have added a new chapter on treatment research for this edition. This chapter provides an overview of special issues faced by treatment researchers. It also provides a review of randomized clinical trials and examines their usefulness in evaluating treatment procedures in communicative disorders.

The widespread use of this book as a text in classrooms across the country has strengthened my belief that instructors of research designs in communicative disorders would welcome a text that represents both the single-subject and group design strategies along with issues of measurement; philosophy of science; ethics of research; and planning, conducting, and reporting research. I wish to express my appreciation to all those instructors who have found this book an effective teaching device and have taken time to offer their thoughtful comments.

PART I

◆◆◆◆◆◆◆◆◆◆◆◆◆◆◆◆◆◆◆◆◆◆◆◆◆◆

Science and Scientific Methods

Chapter 1

◆◆◆◆◆◆◆◆◆◆◆◆◆◆◆◆◆◆◆◆◆◆◆◆◆◆◆◆◆◆◆◆◆◆◆◆

Why Study Science and Research Methods?

- The Need To Study Scientific Methods
- The Need To Produce In-House Knowledge
- Why Research by Clinicians Is Limited
- Problems Associated with Certain Research Practices
- Problems Associated with the Education and Training Models
- Evaluation of Research
- Summary
- Study Guide

ommunicative disorders is both an academic discipline and a clinical profession. As an academic discipline, communicative disorders seeks to study and understand normal and disordered communication. As a clinical profession, it is concerned with the methods of assessing and treating various disorders of hearing, speech, language, voice, and fluency. An academic discipline can research practical problems without applying the information it generates. For example, a biochemist who develops a new drug that can be used in treating a particular disease may not treat patients with that disease. In communicative disorders, researchers who develop new information or technology also may apply that information in the treatment of disordered communication. In this sense, communicative disorders is simultaneously concerned with both scientific and professional matters.

As the discipline of communicative disorders emerged and developed, the professional aspects, rather than the scientific bases, received greater attention. This is understandable because the starting point of our discipline was a professional concern to understand and treat speech problems, especially stuttering and articulation disorders. The profession had to begin providing clinical services without the benefit of a history of controlled experimental research to support clinical practice. Borrowing from several basic and applied disciplines, the speech–language pathologist of earlier days began to treat communicative disorders. Until recently, the emphasis has been on expanding clinical services rather than conducting experimental research to produce a scientific basis for those clinical services.

An unfortunate historical lesson of many human service professions, including that of communicative disorders, is that clinical services can continue to be offered without a strong experimental data base. Such services may be supported by subjectively solidified clinical experience, uncontrolled observations, anecdotes widely circulated by "authorities" in the field, descriptive research, and speculative theories. Systematic experimental evaluation of treatment techniques may be lacking. As a result, clinical services the profession offers may not be based on controlled research evidence. However, this may not deter a profession from offering services, partly because of practical exigencies and partly because something better is not available.

The problem with such a history is that the clinical practice does not change quickly when experimental research information begins to flow. The clinical practice of established clinicians may continue to be based on old and unverified assumptions. Typically, it takes several years to affect clinical practice on a wide scale because the research information must be incorporated into the training of new clinicians.

THE NEED TO STUDY SCIENTIFIC METHODS

It is now widely recognized that the profession of communicative disorders needs to strengthen the scientific bases of its clinical practice. The need to

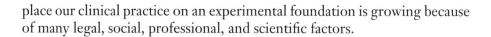

place our clinical practice on an experimental foundation is growing because of many legal, social, professional, and scientific factors.

Legal and Social Considerations

An increasing number of federal and state laws influence professional practices in communicative disorders. A major source of influence is a set of federal laws related to the education of children with disabilities. The original Education for All Handicapped Children Act of 1975 (P.L. 94-142) had a significant effect on public school special education services including those of communicative disorders. The law was amended in 1986 and reauthorized in 1990 under the new title Individuals with Disabilities Education Act (P.L. 101-476). The law was again reauthorized and amended in 1997. (Many federal laws are periodically reauthorized and amended to address new concerns; therefore, the reader should consult the latest versions of the laws of interest.)

Some of the most significant requirements under these laws are that special education services must be oriented to the individual child and his or her family and that service programs must have specific procedures, objectives, and evaluative criteria. The laws place considerable emphasis on clinician accountability in that the effects of treatment programs must be documented objectively so that they can be verified by independent observers. Such documentation requires that changes in client behaviors be measured systematically and continuously (Hegde, 1998a). As we shall see shortly, these and other requirements of the laws are in harmony with the requirements of scientific clinical practice.

Other kinds of legal concerns necessitate a more objective and scientific clinical practice. There has been a slow but steady increase in third-party payment for clinical speech, language, and hearing services. Various government agencies and private insurance firms that pay for the services are demanding more and more systematic documentation of the need, the procedures, and the outcome of such services. Uniform and objective means of evaluating treatment effects are being encouraged by agencies that pay for services.

Many social concerns are also leading us in the direction of clinical practice based on scientific methods. The profession continues to take steps to increase public awareness of speech and language problems and the services that are available to individuals with those problems. Consequently, an increasing number of individuals and families are seeking and paying for services in private clinics and hospitals. At the same time, many people who are seeking services are also inclined to question the effectiveness of those services. Inevitably, widespread social awareness of speech, language, and hearing problems combined with higher demands for services and increasing cost of service delivery will result in a thorough scrutiny of professional practices.

Professional and Scientific Considerations

Regardless of the legal and social requirements, there are professional reasons for developing a scientifically sound clinical discipline. Much concern surrounds the professional standing of communicative disorders in the community of clinical professions and scientific disciplines. There is a growing concern that the profession of communicative disorders does not have high social visibility. The profession may not be well recognized by other established or recently developed professions, such as medicine or clinical psychology.

A profession can try to draw attention to itself by various means. It may seek better legal recognition and protection by developing more effective lobbying efforts. Extensive public relations and public awareness campaigns may be launched. Services may be more aggressively publicized through advertisements in local and national media. Because all professions have a business side, most of these efforts are fiscally necessary. Indeed, all professions find it necessary to ethically market their services. Such efforts may yield somewhat quick results; however, to build a lasting and more solid reputation, the profession, in addition to taking all those steps, must put its practice on a scientific footing. In the long run, no amount of public relations can compensate for questionable and subjectively evaluated clinical practice. In fact, public awareness—which is generally beneficial—can expose the inherent and widespread weaknesses of a profession.

Scientifically based and technologically competent professions enjoy good reputations and higher visibility. A profession can make significant progress when its concepts are scientific and its methods are evaluated objectively. The ideal to strive for is a solid scientific discipline and a clinical profession with a single identity. This ideal, when achieved, will help assure the quality of speech and hearing services offered to persons with communicative disorders.

The typical argument supporting a more scientific orientation is made on the basis of the legal, social, and professional requirements described so far. Such requirements are compelling, and anything that forces a more scientific orientation is welcome. However, a profession need not be driven entirely by such requirements. Professionals need not face legal, social, and professional image-oriented reasons and requirements to strive to be more scientific. Although the statement may sound tautological, science itself is a good reason to be scientific. The logical beauty, methodological elegance, and practical benefits of science antecede the legal, social, and professional pressures.

Had the profession heeded the call of science from its inception, it is possible that most of the legal and social pressures would have become superfluous. Clinicians who by training and practice follow the methods of science do not need a push from public laws to write treatment targets in measurable terms. For such clinicians, the requirement that changes in client behaviors must be documented objectively will not come as news or as a legal nuisance. The clinicians' personal history of training and education will suffice for such purposes. Surely, social and legal demands can force clinicians to be systematic and objective in their clinical work, but those with a strong scientific background are inclined to be so regardless of such demands. The clinician who wishes to evaluate treatment effects under controlled conditions may not be driven by concerns regarding bad professional image. Such a clinician has better reasons, including science itself. Scientifically competent clinicians are unlikely to be overly concerned with image; nevertheless, they are probably better for the profession's image than those who are concerned with public reactions but continue to offer questionable services.

These comments should not be construed as a negative evaluation of legal, social, and professional reasons to be more scientific. In fact, governments, social groups, and professional bodies have an obligation to protect the rights of people who seek and then financially support professional services. Societal and regulatory forces are necessary for smooth and socially beneficial operations of professions as well as sciences. Such regulatory forces have helped all professions and sciences move in the right direction, as can be seen in Chapter 16. The comments are meant to underscore an additional and often neglected reason to be more systematic, responsible, and objective in clinical work: The philosophy and methodology of science that are capable of providing unsurpassed safeguards for both the profession and the public. Besides, science provides an unlimited and exciting opportunity to make significant advances in all areas of professional endeavor.

THE NEED TO PRODUCE IN-HOUSE KNOWLEDGE

During the time when service delivery, not scientific research, is the urgent business, the profession is dependent on other disciplines for a knowledge base. The profession of communicative disorders historically has depended on some nonclinical disciplines such as linguistics, experimental psychology, and child psychology. It also has depended on clinical professions such as medicine and basic sciences such as physiology and physics.

Communicative disorders has been a borrower for a long time, perhaps too much of a borrower and too little of an innovator. It borrowed not only basic or applied information but also conceptual frameworks, theories, paradigms, models, and methods of investigation and data analysis. Therefore, the slowly developing traditions of research in communicative disorders have been extensively influenced by other disciplines that have offered methods and theories of varying degrees of validity, reliability, relevancy, and applicability.

Unless a discipline quickly begins to produce its own experimental data base, it will continue to borrow theories and methods that may or may not be appropriate for studying its subject matter. The only way some professions can begin to generate their own data bases is to train their practitioners to do research. Professions such as medicine have the luxury of receiving a large and varied amount of custom-produced research information from outside their professions. Medicine has chemists, biochemists, physiologists, anatomists, biologists, geneticists, bioengineers, and a variety of technologists and technical product manufacturers (including global pharmaceutical companies) who do research and supply theoretical information and practical technology. There are not comparable bands of researchers and technicians supplying information and technology to the field of communicative disorders. Much of the information and technology the discipline borrows is not produced for it; its relevance may be incidental and in some unfortunate cases, mistaken.

Specialists in communicative disorders should produce their own knowledge base and technology, but this does not mean that they should not selectively borrow from other disciplines. Like other professions, communicative disorders will continue to borrow what is relevant and useful. Many fields of knowledge are interrelated. Therefore the fields benefit from each other's research. Nonetheless, what is urgently needed is a systematic effort to increase the in-house knowledge base and technology. A discipline cannot always expect other specialists to produce the basic scientific information necessary to understand its subject matter. A profession cannot always expect others to produce a relevant and effective technology. Kent (1983) stated that "a profession that provides its own research base is much more in charge of its own destiny than a profession that doesn't" (p. 76). Expressing a similar opinion, Flower (1983) said that "if we must rely on others both to achieve the scientific and technological advances and then to apply those advances within our field, we cannot pretend to be a mature and autonomous profession" (p. 13).

The most significant problem with increasing the amount of in-house knowledge is the scarcity of research institutions and sustained research programs in communicative disorders. Many university programs in communicative disorders are not research oriented, and large institutions that specialize in research are few or nonexistent. Producing a systematic body of reliable and valid scientific information is a slow process even under the best possible conditions. Therefore, under the existing conditions, the accumulation of valid knowledge in communicative disorders will be a prolonged process. There seems to be no easy or quick solution to this problem. Several steps are necessary to increase the amount of research; for example, the discipline can seek more government and private research funds, increase the number of theses produced by master's degree candidates, accelerate research efforts at existing research and teaching institutions, and establish new programmatic research.

Another tactic, which can be used in addition to all others, is to recruit practitioners into the kind of research that does not detract from clinical activities. That is, the field can make an effort to increase research by practicing clinicians. Because the majority of persons in the field are clinicians, even a slight increase in the number of clinicians doing research may have an appreciable effect. This is the kind of in-house knowledge base that can have immediate and simultaneous clinical and theoretical significance.

WHY RESEARCH BY CLINICIANS IS LIMITED

It is well known that a majority of clinicians do not do research. After all, they are busy serving their clients. There are many reasons why clinicians do not typically engage in research (Kent, 1983, 1985; Perkins, 1985). For example, most clinicians do not have the needed extra time for research. Besides, when research is thought of as something unrelated to clinical service, the clinicians obviously cannot do research. Also, the client scheduling may be good for clinical work but bad for research; when clients are seen twice weekly for a few minutes each time, collecting certain kinds of data may be difficult.

Most clinical settings do not emphasize research. Many public schools and hospitals do not require research from clinicians and may not encourage it. Much research, both good and bad, is done when research is required or valued in a given setting. It also may be noted that bad research can be done even when someone "wanted" to do research while it was not required to achieve promotions or pay raises. In many settings, research often is done over and above one's regular duties. When it is not required for professional advancement, the administration is unlikely to support research to any great extent.

It also is possible that clinicians themselves assume that (a) they are not well prepared to do research and (b) research does not necessarily help them, their colleagues, or their clients. Both of these assumptions may be valid to a degree. The first assumption may be due to many practitioners' limited training and experience in research methods. To do research, one should also maintain currency in the slowly-but-surely changing field of knowledge in the discipline. The pressures of day-to-day professional practice may not be conducive to spending the needed amount of time and energy on reading the literature. Though significant advances in communicative disorders have been few and far between, there has been an information explosion in recent years; it takes time just to keep up with published research. Because they do not have this time, many clinicians may think that they lack the technical knowledge of scientific procedures and current information needed to do research.

The second assumption—that research does not necessarily help clinical practice—may be based on experience. There is some question regarding the extent to which research affects day-to-day clinical practice (Attanasio, 1986; Barlow, Hayes, & Nelson, 1984; Siegel, 1987; Siegel & Spradlin, 1985). In treating clients, clinicians are likely to depend on their past training and clinical experience. Practitioners across professional settings do not automatically apply experimentally evaluated new techniques. Often, popular but unsupported theories and recent trends without substance have a greater influence on clinical practice than do technical research reports.

Workshops, presentations, discussions with colleagues, and lectures on the latest techniques may affect clinical practice more than experimental evidence does. However, even those who give frequent workshops often think that clinicians rarely apply exactly what the workshops offer. For example, some individuals who frequently attend workshops agree equally well with totally contradictory approaches, and most clinicians assimilate what they hear (or read) with their past experience and apply new techniques in modified ways. Such modifications are not bad. The only problem is that unspecified and varied modifications of published techniques make it difficult to identify successful techniques. In any case, the disturbing situation remains: Controlled and technical research does not affect clinical practice to the extent it should.

The belief that research does not necessarily help clinical practice is partially true. I am not referring just to basic research, which is not expected to give immediate solutions to practical problems; I am referring to the kinds of research that are expected to solve clinical problems. Purported clinical research on assessment or treatment of communicative disorders also may frustrate clinicians. Clinicians who read and evaluate such research to sharpen their clinical skills may be disillusioned about the usefulness of all kinds of clinical research. In essence, certain research practices may generate a justifiable skepticism regarding the relevance of research to clinical practice.

PROBLEMS ASSOCIATED WITH CERTAIN RESEARCH PRACTICES

There are multiple modes of clinical research, and not all of them are equally helpful to the clinician in solving current practical problems. In Chapters 4 and 5, I will describe different types of research in some detail. Here it may be noted that clinical–experimental research is likely to produce results that help solve immediate practical problems clinicians face. Many other types of research may lead to solutions to practical problems but only in the future.

Clinical usefulness is not the only criterion by which the value of research is determined. Basic research often does not have immediate practical significance. However, it is valuable because it might help explain a phenomenon, put unrelated observations in a single perspective, suggest new lines of experimental analysis, or produce a discovery with powerful applied potential. Thus, in the long run, basic research may produce data that can help solve practical problems. Every discipline needs basic research: Communicative disorders simply does not have enough of it.

The main problem with current research practices is that much of the research is neither basic nor experimentally clinical. Basic research can help secure the future of a discipline while experimental–clinical research can help solve current practical problems. Basic research creates a strong scientific base for a profession, and experimental–clinical research helps develop treatment techniques. When these two kinds of research are sparse, the profession can neither solve its clinical problems nor generate confidence that the problems will be solved in the future. In such a situation, skepticism regarding research is inevitable.

The clinical irrelevancy of "clinical research" is not the only reason why some clinicians have a negative approach to research in general; other factors contribute. First, if clinicians do not appreciate basic research, they may have received inadequate education and training in the philosophy and methodology of science. Second, if clinicians do not appreciate experimental–clinical research that shows better methods of treating disorders of communication, their education, again, may be to blame. A majority of clinicians neither use experimentally verified techniques nor demand such techniques from researchers. Third, if clinicians do not find a significant body of clinical research that can be applied in clinical work, then the research practices within the field must take the blame.

Education and training programs must address the first two factors, and research scientists and clinicians must address the third. To assess these problems, one must consider the type and quality of clinical research and the education and training of clinicians.

Possibly, clinicians who can evaluate current clinical research find very little that is applicable. This is because much research in the field is not concerned with evaluation and development of treatment procedures. Even clinical journals, expected to publish treatment research, may disappoint clinicians. A majority of papers published in journals in speech and hearing relate to description and assessment, not treatment. There is plenty of speculative, theoretical writing in the discipline, and much of the research is concerned with finding differences between "normal" and "disordered" groups of participants. For example, many studies attempt to establish norms of various communicative behaviors. In addition, classifying speech and language behaviors with no regard to their causal variables (structural analysis of language and speech) is very popular. This kind of research is typically justified because of its presumed clinical implications, but the research does not necessarily provide for more effective treatment procedures. Some clinicians who begin to read research reports of this kind may eventually stop reading them. Such clinicians decide to wait until the presumed implications are translated into procedures they can use.

A dominant research trend in communicative disorders is that many who suggest clinical implications of their nonclinical research do not take time to test those implications with clients. Many research specialists in communicative disorders seem to imply that to hypothesize is their job, but to verify is someone else's. Many researchers betray a striking lack of curiosity about the clinical validity of their own hypotheses. Consequently, they have created a new division of labor: Some researchers generate hypotheses, and other researchers verify them. Unfortunately, this division of labor has not worked well because many researchers are more interested in generating hypotheses than in verifying their own or anybody else's.

If studies of a different kind were to be frequently published in journals devoted to clinical practice, clinicians may find research to be valuable. This kind of research is experimental *and* clinical. It addresses issues of immediate practical significance. The strategy involves current clinical action, not a promise of some future clinical possibility. For example, research may be concerned with topics such as different target behaviors and their clinical relevance, experimental evaluation of treatment techniques, relative effects of multiple treatments, interaction between different treatment procedures, generality of treatment effects to clients of different ethnocultural backgrounds, different tactics of response maintenance after treatment, issues in the measurement or assessment of disorders and behaviors, and independent variables that may maintain normal as well as disordered speech and language behaviors, just to sample a few. These kinds of research topics generate data of immediate clinical significance. More important, efforts to investigate these topics are identical with clinical services.

The type of research in which the relevance of alternate target communicative behaviors and the techniques of teaching them are evaluated under controlled conditions will help illustrate how research and clinical practice may be integrated. Research on the relevance of target behaviors for clinical intervention is barely begun. This is the question of dependent variables; it often is thought that the only significant question is that of the independent variable. In other words, professionals may think that they know what the targets are, but they do not know how to teach them. Both are important questions, however. For example, in language disorders, what are the clinical targets: communicative competence, knowledge of the universal transformational grammar, grammatical features, grammatical rules, semantic notions, semantic rules, pragmatic notions, pragmatic rules, or empirical response classes? Similarly, what is (are) the dependent variable(s) in the treatment of stuttering: self-confidence, self-image, approach-avoidance conflict, anxiety reduction, correction of feedback problems, appropriate airflow, correct phonatory behaviors, fluent stuttering, negative attitudes, excessive parental concern for fluency, reduction in speech rate, or reduction in the dysfluency rates? Again, what are the dependent variables in the treatment of articulation disorders: individual phonemes, phonological processes, phonological knowledge, or phonemic awareness? It is clear that there are no generally accepted answers to these questions. These questions suggest that there is no agreement on the discipline's dependent variables.

Specification of a valid dependent variable is crucial to the development of a science. If biologists were as confused about their dependent variables as communicative disorders specialists are about theirs, biology's progress to date would be unthinkable. Because communicative disorders is a clinical science, it needs clearly defined dependent variables (communicative behaviors) that may be changed through manipulation of independent variables (treatment techniques). Therefore, research on the valid dependent variables that can be successfully taught to persons with communicative disabilities is useful. Besides, in the course of this kind of research, the clinician simultaneously provides clinical services.

Research on the effects of various treatment strategies also is synchronous with clinical service. The value of treatment research in communicative disorders is obvious but often is taken for granted. When a clinical researcher evaluates a given treatment in a controlled experiment, the clients who serve as subjects are exposed to one possible treatment. If the treatment is not effective, the clinician may evaluate another technique that may prove to be more successful. In more advanced stages of research, the clinician may evaluate the relative and interactive effects of more than one treatment technique or component. Except when control groups are used, the participants in research studies are the clients who receive treatment during the course of research.

The paucity of treatment-related research in communicative disorders supports the notion that research and clinical services are unrelated, and that training in research methods and philosophy of science is a waste of time. Contrary to this notion, research and clinical activities are more similar than different. As pointed out by Perkins (1985), "Each clinical encounter epitomizes the essence of experimental research" (p. 14). Basically, treatments are a manipulation of cause–effect relations. In treating clients, clinicians produce changes in communicative behaviors by rearranging certain variables (Hegde, 1998a). To be accountable, the changes must be demonstrated to be causally related to the treatment. Some other variable or someone else's treatment must not be responsible for the client's improved communicative behaviors. Such demonstrations are the essence of experimentation.

What is suggested here is that treatment-related research makes research immediately attractive to the practitioners, and therefore, they may be more likely to read, evaluate, and appreciate research. It is *not* suggested that basic research unrelated to immediate clinical concerns is less valuable or that there is no reason for clinicians to study basic research reports. Possibly, clinicians who do not understand or appreciate treatment research are less likely to understand or appreciate basic laboratory research. Therefore, one way of attracting clinicians to research of all kinds is to offer them treatment-related research that can make a difference in their day-to-day professional activities. Skills necessary to understand and evaluate treatment-related research, once mastered by clinicians, can help them understand basic research as well. In any case, the task of attracting clinicians to research is that of the clinical researcher, not that of the basic researcher.

PROBLEMS ASSOCIATED WITH THE EDUCATION AND TRAINING MODELS

As noted before, if at least a certain number of clinicians are involved in research, the amount of in-house knowledge can be increased in a fairly short time. However, when other conditions are favorable, clinicians can do research only if they are trained to do research that is synchronous with clinical services; it is impractical to expect a majority of clinicians to do basic research. It also is impractical for clinicians to engage in clinical research that does not involve direct assessment, treatment, or maintenance strategies. Even the clinical research of "implications" cannot fulfill the service requirements; that is, clinicians must investigate questions that can be answered while providing services to their clients. To accomplish this, communicative disorders must adopt an integrated model of education, training, and research.

If specialists in communicative disorders see their field as a clinical profession based on scientific knowledge and research, several much-debated pseudo issues—such as "Do we need to know scientific methods?" or "Do we need to engage in research?"—dissipate. The education of clinicians must include an understanding of existing knowledge and technology, methods of producing new knowledge and technology, and methods of evaluating all knowledge and technology.

An educational program cannot be limited to just imparting existing knowledge and training in extant technology to future practitioners. Future clinicians need also to know how new knowledge is produced and how any knowledge is critically evaluated before it is accepted or rejected. The methods of science and research are the methods of producing and evaluating empirical knowledge. Therefore, imparting knowledge of science and research is a part of training future practitioners who can evaluate new information and contribute new information to their chosen discipline. Most experts believe that such a training model gives scientific status and professional strength.

It is sometimes thought that education in the philosophy and methods of science takes time away from clinical training. Some may argue that training of professionals requires spending all the available time on clinical methods and service delivery models. That students in clinical programs should receive the best possible training in clinical methods is not controversial. Indeed, it is reasonable to state that during their education and training, future clinicians should not spend time studying science and research if that study is not expected to be useful. However, time spent on science and research in the training of practitioners is a waste only if clinical service and scientific work are conceptually and methodologically divorced. The argument that the study of science and research is a waste is irrelevant when communicative disorders is viewed as a scientific discipline and a clinical profession that adopts an integrated model of research and clinical service.

Unless clinicians are educated within an integrated model of research and clinical service, time spent training clinicians in research may not be as productive as it could be. But what is not so frequently recognized is that without the integrated model, even researchers are not likely to make a significant effect on the clinical issues of the profession. Therefore, the existing models of research in communicative disorders may need to be revised. If the same model is used to give more information on research at the master's level or at the doctoral level, there is no assurance that in-house treatment-related knowledge will increase. What is needed is an emphasis on, and training in, the concepts and methods of science as applied to clinical work. The clinician must have a thorough understanding of the experimental methodology used to develop and evaluate treatment techniques as well as scientific theories.

Historically, educators in the university departments of communicative disorders seem to have had the dual objectives of producing researchers and therapists, instead of developing a clinical science. Neither objective seems to have been achieved to a satisfactory degree because of a misunderstanding of the roles of clinicians and researchers. A productive interaction between clinicians, clinical researchers, and basic researchers is possible when the education and training model combines the logic and methods of science with the concerns of clinical description, assessment, and treatment evaluation. Such an education and training model will more successfully produce a clinical science.

Such a training model needs to be implemented from the very beginning. At increasing levels of complexity, students should learn various aspects of this model at appropriate levels of their education. This new model is needed in the training of clinicians as well as researchers and must be used in training undergraduates in addition to master's-level and doctoral-level graduate students.

Possibly, what little training most graduates receive in science and research may not be consistent with clinical work, and therefore, clinicians are not prepared to do research. Often, courses on research methods offer nothing but statistics (Kent, 1983). Concepts of science and designs of research may be presented inadequately or not at all. Information presented on research designs may be restricted to the traditional group designs. Clinicians quickly find that to do any kind of clinical research, they should be thorough in statistics, have access to a large population of clients who are willing to participate in a study, select a sample large enough to be justified statistically, select it randomly, assign participants to treatment groups randomly, and deny treatment to a control group.

Clinicians find that the research process as they understood it from an introductory course on statistics and group research designs is clinically formidable, unacceptable, or both when the immediate concern is professional service. First, most clinicians do not receive the depth of training in research methods needed to design clinically significant research. Second, in their everyday work, clinicians typically deal with a small number of clients, so they cannot find a population (a large group of persons with defined characteristics) of accessible, willing participants with specific communicative disorders; therefore, they cannot draw random samples as the theory says they should. Third, even if the clinicians did draw random samples, they find it ethically unattractive to have a control group to which treatment must be denied or postponed. In essence, what clinicians learn about research in most graduate schools is not easily applied in professional settings where the immediate concerns are assessment, treatment, maintenance, parent counseling, case conference, and other such clinical activities.

The popularity of traditional research philosophy and methodology based on statistics and probability theory is at least partly responsible for the paucity of treatment-related research, whether by practitioners or by clinical researchers. Students who are exposed to different traditions of research at all levels of their training may select strategies to suit the kind of problems they wish to investigate. For example, clinicians who know of a strategy that is useful in dealing with individual clients or clients in small groups and that is useful in conducting treatment-related research may be more likely to gather experimental evidence in their day-to-day work. Such a strategy, known as the single-subject strategy, is available, and it is eminently suitable for developing a clinical science. This strategy is described in Chapters 4 and 9. Unfortunately, this strategy is not well represented in the education of speech–language pathologists. An encouraging sign, however, is that the single-subject strategy is receiving increasing attention from educators, clinicians, and researchers (Olswang, Thompson, Warren, & Minghetti, 1990). Clinicians who are capable of using this approach may investigate questions while providing clinical services. This will also increase the amount of in-house knowledge, which may have the utmost clinical relevance.

EVALUATION OF RESEARCH

Evaluation of old and new research is about as important as the creation of new in-house knowledge. Professionals who cannot evaluate research data and theories also cannot make effective use of information. Critical evaluation of research should be a part of the clinician's repertoire. Critical evaluation of research data, however, requires the same knowledge needed to do meaningful research.

The process of evaluating research data follows the same logical steps as the process of designing experiments. Therefore, evaluation of research is possible only when clinicians understand how research is done. Clinicians who are not knowledgeable in science and methods of investigation in their field of study are likely to have difficulty in judging the relevance of the questions their colleagues research, the validity and reliability of observations, the relation between results and conclusions, the transition from evidence to theory, and the distinction between theory and speculation.

Furthermore, clinicians who are not sophisticated in the philosophy of science may not see logical and empirical mistakes in designs. In such cases, clinicians who read research uncritically accept the author's interpretations. However, bad interpretations are about as prevalent as bad designs, and clinicians who cannot detect inconsistent relations between interpretations and results cannot separate data from conclusions. Data that are based on sound methods are always more valuable and durable than the author's interpretations imposed on them. Future clinicians and researchers may keep the sound data while rejecting faulty interpretations.

Even when many practitioners are involved in treatment-related research, a majority of clinicians will read research papers mostly to improve their practice. The popular phrase "clinicians are consumers of research" has a ring of validity in that most clinicians will be users, not producers, of research. It is well known that naive consumers are victims of bad products. Similarly, clinicians who are naive in the methods and philosophy of science are likely victims of bad research; unfortunately, in this process the clients also become victims.

It is thus clear that clinicians who do not do research still need to understand science and research methods. Even if there is much research that cannot be applied, clinicians will have to keep reading and evaluating research because that is the only way they can find out what is useful and what is not. Those who avoid reading the research literature because some of it is irrelevant to clinical practice are sure to miss what is relevant to them. Meanwhile, when research practices improve and clinically relevant studies are routinely published, clinicians will be unaware of them and unprepared for them.

SUMMARY

- Communicative disorders is both an academic discipline and a clinical profession.

- Initially, communicative disorders developed more as a profession than as a scientific discipline. As a result, its scientific and technological base still needs to be strengthened.

- In recent years, the need to study scientific methods has been created by legal, social, professional, and scientific factors.

- Various state and federal legislation and agencies that pay for clinical services require the profession to be accountable through objective documentation of the effects of clinical services.

- The professional reasons to strengthen the scientific and technological bases include the need to gain better recognition and status and the advantages of a scientific orientation to professional practice.

- In the business of generating knowledge, communicative disorders needs to be as self-sufficient as possible.

- Many clinicians do not do clinical research for several reasons including inadequate training in research methods and the questionable relevance of published research to clinical practice.

- Much published research is theoretical, normative, and descriptive—not directly useful in clinical assessment and treatment (though this is slowly changing).

- Assessment- and treatment-related research can attract clinicians to research and improve treatment procedures.

- Future practitioners often receive training in statistics and group methods of research, which are difficult to use in treatment evaluation research.

- The historical notion that clinicians need not know much about science and research methods has created a dichotomy between researchers and therapists.

- Future practitioners should be trained in a model of science and research that is consistent with clinical service delivery and in methods of treatment evaluation that can be used while providing services to persons with communicative disorders.

- Clinicians who do not do research still need to understand the concepts and methods of science so they can critically evaluate technical information offered to them.

STUDY GUIDE _____

1. What were some of the early concerns of the discipline of communicative disorders? Did those concerns include experimental evaluation of treatment procedures?

2. What legal and social considerations are prompting the profession to be more scientific in its orientation and activities?

3. What are some of the reasons to develop a scientifically sound clinical practice?

4. How can a profession draw attention to itself? What is the most desirable method of drawing such attention?

5. What kinds of professions generally have better reputations and higher social visibility?

6. What are some of the problems of wholesale borrowing of knowledge and methods from other disciplines and professions?

7. What is meant by custom-produced information from outside a profession?

8. Why should specialists in communicative disorders produce their own data base?

9. What are some of the reasons many clinicians do not do research?

10. What are the two assumptions made by some clinicians regarding research?

11. What are some of the popular sources of influence on clinical practice?

12. What is the main problem with current research practice?

13. How is basic research distinguished from experimental–clinical research?

14. What are some of the reasons that many clinicians have a negative view of research?

15. What are the strengths of the experimental–clinical research strategy?

16. What are some of the problems associated with the education and training of clinicians?

17. Why were questions such as, "Do clinicians need to know scientific methods?" and "Why should clinicians do research?" described as "pseudo"?

18. What is the significance of single-subject designs in creating a science of clinical practice?

19. What is an integrated model of research and professional service?

20. From a clinician's standpoint, what are the problems of not being able to evaluate research?

Chapter 2

◆◆◆◆◆◆◆◆◆◆◆◆◆◆◆◆◆◆◆◆◆◆◆◆◆◆◆◆◆◆◆◆◆◆◆◆

An Introduction to Research: The Formal and Formative Approaches

- What Is Research?
- Why Do Scientists Do Research?
- How Is Research Done?
- Serendipity in Research
- Planning Is Still Important
- Summary
- Study Guide

The terms *science* and *research* have an air of extreme formality. Many students and professionals alike think that research is formidable, mechanistic, difficult, and somewhat boring. Some practitioners also think that research is an esoteric activity, irrelevant to clinical service. Graduate students who are not involved in research may look upon those who are doing theses or dissertations with admiration totally devoid of envy. Undergraduate students may consider research a mysterious activity that they will understand better in graduate school. In time, the mysterious activity may reveal itself to be both arduous and uninteresting.

To a certain extent, most of these stereotypic reactions to science and research are understandable. Textbooks on research methods are written in a formal and somewhat dull style. The books often are full of statistics in which many students and clinicians do not find much joy. Statistics are only one of several and by no means inevitable methods of analyzing data. Statistics is not the same as research, but many textbooks give an impression that it is. Typical textbooks also describe research as a highly organized, thoroughly planned, and mechanistically efficient activity. Most clinicians think they are not prepared for it. Clinicians and students may have heard or known of graduate students who have worked so hard on their theses or dissertations that those budding researchers "stopped living" until their project was complete. They may have seen professors and scientists who also seemed to have no fun doing research but went on with the drudgery for apparently no good reason. Finally, there is the reality of science and research itself: Science is restrictive and research can be hard work. There are formal aspects to science, and there is no way of getting around them.

These stereotypes and hard facts not withstanding, science can be provocative, even refreshing. The logic and the framework of science constitute one of the most elegant of the abstract structures human beings have ever built. Persons who understand the logic and structure of science will not find it too difficult to organize their work within the scope of science. The logic of science can prompt the most stimulating intellectual pursuits. Much of scientific creativity, though difficult, can be highly reinforcing. A scientist's immense reward comes when his or her work throws new light on a perplexing problem that suddenly becomes a little bit more understandable.

In our effort to gain a more favorable view of research, we can find encouragement in Bachrach's (1969) comment that "people don't usually do research the way people who write books about research say that people do research" (Preface, p. x). Though research can be hard work, it need not be a drudgery. Doing research can actually be fun, and there are rewards even when it is not much fun. Research is not as formal an activity as most textbooks make it appear to be. Research scientists are people, too, and they make mistakes like anyone else. Granted, there are people who do research not because they are especially good at it, but because they are required to. There are also people who love to do research—required or not. They may not be good researchers in the beginning, but soon they learn from their mistakes and improve the quality of their work. In this process, they have frustrations and pleasures.

A more balanced view describes both the pleasures and the hard work associated with research. When the research process is described the way it is typically implemented, a more realistic picture emerges. In a later section, we shall examine two ways of describing research activity.

WHAT IS RESEARCH?

Sometimes the terms *science* and *research* are used synonymously. The two terms have overlapping meanings but different connotations. Science is inclusive of research, but the term *research* may not capture all the nuances of science. In the next chapter, we shall consider in detail the different meanings of science. In its broadest sense, science is a certain philosophy, a viewpoint concerning the definition of natural phenomena and how such phenomena are interrelated. Science is also a set of methods designed to investigate research questions and thereby produce reliable and valid knowledge. Finally, science refers to the actions and behaviors of scientists.

Research is what scientists do in practicing science. While science is a description of certain philosophies, viewpoints, and activities, research mostly includes steps taken by scientists in their quest to more fully understand the order and uniformity of nature. Research is the process of investigating scientific questions. Research is science in action. According to various human subject protection guidelines, any systematic investigation designed to develop or contribute to generalizable knowledge is research. See Chapter 16 for legal and ethical implications of this definition.

It is only in the sense that science includes certain methods of investigations and actions of scientists that it is synonymous with research. Therefore, research refers to those activities by which science achieves its goals. Even as a set of methods, science is conceptual, whereas research is methodological. Science is the unifying theme and philosophy of research. It permeates all empirical research. Science gives the scientist both the conceptual and methodological means of doing research, but research refers to the behaviors of scientists in action.

It is probably not very useful to expand on the various definitions of research. Within the realm of science, different strategies of research have been devised. The full range of meaning of the term can be appreciated only when different types, strategies, and designs of research are understood along with the major reasons for doing research. In this sense, this entire book is about research. Therefore, we shall now turn to a discussion of some of the major reasons why research is done.

WHY DO SCIENTISTS DO RESEARCH?

Research is done for many reasons. For example, there are bureaucratic reasons for doing research although these reasons are not as important as other reasons. Bureaucratic reasons are those that require research from scientists as a matter of employment policy. For example, research is required of faculty members in many universities. Their tenure and promotion may depend upon the amount and quality of research they publish. When scientists are paid to do research for an organization, research becomes their duty. These are intermediate reasons for doing research, however. Even those who do research for bureaucratic reasons need to consider the more basic and universal reasons why research is done.

Curiosity About Natural Phenomena

Philosophers of science have long recognized that one of the classical reasons for doing research is people's curiosity about natural phenomena. Scientists tend to be curious, and once questions arise, they seek to satisfy that curiosity. In fact, Sidman (1960) has defined a scientist as a "person whose indulgence of his curiosity is also the means by which he earns his living" (p. 7).

Curiosity is not an exclusive characteristic of scientists. Most people are curious about various natural and social phenomena. People are curious about things they do not understand, causes that are hidden, and effects that are unknown. Often, everyday curiosity is satisfied when people find out why someone behaved in a certain way or why a certain event happened. Scientific curiosity is not that easily satisfied. To satisfy scientific curiosity, scientists use special methods to answer specific questions. Therefore, it often takes a long time to satisfy scientific curiosity because it seeks special answers to complex questions.

While everyday curiosity may be concerned with private events, scientific curiosity is almost always concerned with objective events. Even when subjective experiences such as feelings or emotions become its object, scientific curiosity treats them as objective events. Answers produced by scientific curiosity must be verified publicly, whereas those produced by private or personal curiosity need not be.

Private curiosity tends to produce answers with private implications, but scientific curiosity compels answers with public implications. Everyday curiosity may not necessarily lead to answers that have great social effect, but the answers sought by scientific curiosity can have significant social consequences. In this sense, the scope of scientific curiosity is larger than that of private curiosity. Also, scientific curiosity is always concerned with explaining natural phenomena, whereas private curiosity may be concerned with phenomena that cannot be investigated by scientific methods at all. For example, curiosity about why people have speech disorders can lead to empirical investigations using acceptable methods of science, whereas curiosity about supernatural phenomena may not lead to such investigations. However, interest in supernatural phenomena can itself be an object of scientific curiosity; a behavioral scientist may wonder why so many people exhibit certain kinds of behaviors toward supernatural phenomena and then proceed to investigate.

In many respects, scientific curiosity is insatiable. An answer to one question may contain the seeds of several more questions that need to be investigated. A curious scientist can go from one research activity to another because every piece of work satisfies some curiosity while arousing some other curiosity. In fact, good research typically raises important questions for further empirical investigations. Some investigations may not produce any answers at all; instead, they may raise important questions for research. Such investigations keep the proverbially curious scientist busy for a long time. It is this type of insatiable curiosity that sustains a chain of investigations and a lifetime of scientific research.

Research driven by curiosity is often not designed to test formal scientific hypothesis (Sidman, 1960). Scientists who wonder what causes an event may begin to arrange conditions under which that event can be systematically observed. A hypothesis is a tentative answer to a research question, but one may not have a tentative answer, only a desire to find out. After some observations, the scientist may manipulate some aspect of the situation under which the phenomenon occurs reliably. This is the stage of experimentation, which also can be devoid of formal hypotheses. The history of both natural and behavioral sciences is full of examples of research that was done to see what happens when some specific variable is introduced, increased, decreased, or withdrawn.

The contrasting features of everyday curiosity and scientific curiosity should not suggest that the two are unrelated. Everyday curiosity can be cultivated and modified into scientific curiosity. Furthermore, the fact that science is a human activity is illustrated by all research, but it is best illustrated by research done to satisfy one's own curiosity.

Explain Events

A well-recognized reason for doing research is to explain events and effects. Scientists wish to explain why certain events take place and why variables not yet identified seem to produce certain effects. It is often said that one of the goals of science is to explain natural phenomena. Therefore, a need to explain events is a significant reason for doing scientific research.

An explanation of an event specifies its causes. An event is scientifically explained when its cause or causes are experimentally demonstrated. For instance, when a clinical scientist shows that a certain treatment procedure can produce language in a client previously without language, one understands how language behaviors can be modified. Similarly, when animal experiments produce a certain disease by introducing a chemical into an animal's body, that disease is explained at some level of generality and confidence. Procedurally, experiments arrange certain conditions to see if a variable produces a measurable effect. If certain steps are taken, the influence of other potential variables is ruled out or controlled. In this manner, a cause–effect relationship between two events is established.

Research aimed at explaining events can follow one of two approaches. In one approach, the scientist first offers a comprehensive theory of an event and then tests it in a series of experiments. In other words, first the event is explained and then that explanation is verified; this explain-first-and-verify-later approach is called the deductive method. In the second approach, the investigator first conducts a series of experiments and then proposes a theory based on the results; this experiment-first-and-explain-later approach is known as the inductive method. These two approaches and their advantages and disadvantages are discussed in Chapter 3.

In science, a valid explanation of an event is worthwhile in and of itself. However, in many branches of science, a well-supported explanation suggests other possibilities. In most empirical sciences, a scientifically explained event may be changed. This means that scientists can gain some control over the events they explain. Typically, events not yet explained are difficult if not impossible to control or alter; that is, to change an event, one must manipulate the causes of that event. Only a valid explanation gives us the access to causes of events. The applied implications of a valid explanation, then, are self-evident: Valid explanations make it possible to control diseases, disorders, and undesirable social and personal conditions.

Research done to explain events poses several risks to scientists. Scientists who use the inductive method must constantly control their tendency to offer an explanation too soon. Scientists have to judge whether sufficient evidence has been gathered so that a reasonably valid explanation may be offered. Those who use the deductive method must promptly initiate a program of research to verify their explanations. Furthermore, scientists should modify the initial explanation to suit the data gathered through systematic experimentation.

It should be noted that the validity of scientific explanations is a matter of degree and that no explanation is 100% valid. This is because no scientist can claim to have made all possible observations of a phenomenon. There is always a possibility that some new observations will produce new data that may question the old explanation. Therefore, science treats all explanations as more or less tentative. Explanations with adequate support are sustained only until data indicate otherwise.

Solve Practical Problems

Another reason to do research is to solve practical problems. There are many varieties of practical problems that scientists try to solve, but they can be grouped into two broad kinds. The first kind of problems scientists try to solve is found in the physical, chemical, social, and behavioral realm of the scientists' milieu. These are the problems that people, including scientists, face in their day-to-day living. Much of applied research is designed to solve practical problems of this kind—for example, researching better ways of constructing houses; developing more effective fertilizers to improve crops; developing new methods of reducing energy consumption; reducing highway accidents; and treating cancer, stuttering, and language disorders. Obviously, this kind of research has the most immediate and highly visible social impact; therefore, it is the better known of the two kinds of research designed to solve practical problems.

Research done to solve practical problems is crucial for clinical sciences because this type of research includes research done to evaluate treatment procedures. The systematic experimental evaluation and modification of existing treatment procedures and the development of new and more effective procedures are important for any clinical profession. One would think that a significant part of research in communicative disorders is of this kind. Unfortunately, this is not the case. Other kinds of research dominate the field. There are many reasons why treatment evaluation research is not commonly done. Most of these reasons were discussed in Chapter 1.

When research done to solve practical problems is successful, it gives rise to technology. **Technology** is the application of the results of scientific research for further solving problems, improving living and working conditions, saving natural resources, enhancing the behavioral potential of people, treating various disorders and diseases, and so on.

The second kind of practical problems that scientists address are in-house problems. Scientists face many practical problems that impede or even prevent a scientific analysis of a problem under investigation. Most scientists cannot continue their research if effective methods of observation and measurement are not available. Before conducting a conditioning experiment involving rats, for example, early experimental psychologists had to build the needed experimental chambers themselves. When available methods of measuring a phenomenon are inadequate, new methods must be developed. When a phenomenon of interest cannot be directly observed, scientists first have to work on a means of observation. For example, the inventions of the microscope, the telescope, the physiograph, the audiometer, and the flexible fiberscope occurred in response to the need to solve the practical problems of observation. Such instruments extend the range, the power, or the precision of scientists' observations. New devices make it possible to observe events that were never directly observed before. For example, the laryngeal behaviors during stuttering were a matter of speculation for a long time, but the behaviors themselves were not directly observed until the fiberscope and cineradiography were developed and used.

Besides developing new instruments of observation and measurement, scientists also develop new methods of controlling phenomena. New experimental designs often are tried to see if they afford better control over the variables under study. When existing methods of arranging experimental conditions prove inefficient or in some ways unsatisfactory, new arrangements may be tested to find out if they help overcome the problems with the existing arrangements. Behavioral research contains many examples of new experimental arrangements developed to overcome some of the problems of the statistical approach to research. Skinner (1953), for example, found that the traditional method of superficially studying a large number of subjects was not suitable for an experimental analysis of behavior. He therefore devised the method of intensive study of individual subjects. When methods of averaging group performance to impose order on diverse behavior patterns were given up in favor of controlling conditions under which an individual organism could be studied, a true order and behavior patterning emerged. In essence, Skinner was able to gain better control over the behavior because he could then alter patterns of behavior by changing the conditions under which the organisms behaved.

The emergence of new experimental designs illustrates how scientists solve their methodological problems. In recent years, applied behavioral research has witnessed the development of many new experimental designs. For example, when it became evident that the single-subject *ABA* design (see Chapter 8) was undesirable for clinical research, the multiple-baseline design was developed as an alternative (Baer, Wolf, & Risley, 1968). In the *ABA* design, first a behavior is base-rated, then a variable that will change that behavior is introduced, and finally that variable is withdrawn. With these operations, the investigator hopes to show that the behavior changed from the baseline when the variable was introduced and that the change was nullified when the variable was withdrawn. However, the design that served well in laboratory experiments proved undesirable in treatment evaluation because the experiment would end with a no-treatment condition, and the clients would be where they were before the treatment was started.

The multiple baseline, which was designed to overcome the problems of the *ABA* design, afforded an opportunity to demonstrate the effect of treatment without neutralizing it. In this design, several behaviors of a client are base-rated, and the behaviors are treated in sequence. Every time a behavior is treated, the remaining untreated behaviors are base-rated to make sure that only the treated behaviors changed while the untreated behaviors did not. This strategy has been used extensively in clinical treatment research.

An experimentally active discipline is constantly seeking new ways of observing, measuring, and controlling the phenomena of interest. Efforts to extend the control techniques to a new range of phenomena are also made continuously. The amount of research done to solve practical problems and bring new range of phenomena under experimental control is often an indication of a discipline's degree of scientific progress.

Demonstrate Certain Effects

Finally, research may be done to demonstrate the effects of newly discovered variables. Research of this kind often results in the observation of new phenomena. Generally speaking, scientists start with a certain effect and then proceed to find out what caused it. The experimental search for the cause of an event involves the active manipulation of selected variables. If the event changes following such manipulation, then the manipulated variable may be the cause; if it does not, then some other factor may be the cause. In this manner, and with appropriate control procedures, the scientist determines what caused an event. It must be noted that in all such cases, the scientist has a clear understanding of the event but is not sure of the cause.

In contrast, the research study designed to demonstrate the effects of a certain variable starts with a causal variable. What is not clear in this case is the effect of that variable. This kind of research situation arises frequently, although it takes a keen observer to notice new variables whose effects are yet undetermined.

A new variable that may produce new effects is often discovered accidentally. In the field of stuttering, for example, Lee (1950, 1951) accidentally found that a speaker's speech becomes disturbed when a delay is introduced in the auditory feedback of one's own speech. Lee, an engineer, was working on some audio taping systems that accidentally introduced a delay in feedback and found himself "stuttering" under this condition. He and other researchers then began to investigate the effects of delayed auditory feedback more thoroughly to determine the full range of its effects on speech. It must be noted that in the beginning, Lee was not at all studying the effects of delayed auditory feedback on speech. The variable emerged accidentally, and its effects were then evaluated.

The literature on behavioral research contains many such examples of accidental discovery of certain variables whose effects were later investigated. Skinner (1956) documented several of these examples in his own research; the now well-documented effects of intermittent reinforcement on behavior was discovered entirely accidentally. At a time when Skinner was reinforcing rats with custom-made food pellets, he had to manufacture his own supply of pellets with a hand-operated machine that he had constructed. He was also reinforcing every lever press response (continuous reinforcement). As Skinner told the story:

> One pleasant Saturday afternoon I surveyed my supply of dry pellets and [found] that unless I spent the rest of the afternoon and evening at the pill machine, the supply would be exhausted by ten-thirty Monday morning. . . . [This] led me to . . . ask myself why every press of the lever had to be reinforced. . . . I decided to reinforce a response once every minute and allow all other responses to go unreinforced. There were two results: (a) my supply of pellets lasted almost indefinitely; and (b) each rat stabilized at a fairly constant rate of responding. (p. 111)

The above story points out several interesting aspects of the research process. Skinner did not hypothesize that intermittent reinforcement causes a more constant response rate than continuous reinforcement. Initially, he did not design a study to evaluate the effects of not reinforcing every response. Of course, he knew well what he had done that Saturday afternoon: He had changed the way the rats were reinforced. But he had no clear idea of what it would do to the response rate; he probably thought that it would make no big difference. But the data he saw on Monday morning were different. This led him to start a series of studies on the many different ways in which a response could be reinforced. These studies by Skinner and others (Ferster & Skinner, 1957) showed that different reinforcement schedules have characteristic effects on response rates and patterns. This area of research contains some of the most well-controlled and replicated evidence in behavioral research. More important, it showed how a variable discovered accidentally can suggest a new line of investigation to assess its effects more fully.

Physical and biological sciences also are full of examples of accidental discoveries of certain variables whose effects were studied subsequently. It is well known that penicillin was discovered accidentally (Batten, 1968; D. Wilson, 1976). In the process of culturing bacteria for other research purposes, Sir Alexander Fleming repeatedly found that a green mold that developed in the dish routinely killed his colony of bacteria. Some other scientist might have ignored the green mold, considered the death of the bacteria an accident, and perhaps proceeded to develop a fresh colony of bacteria. Although Fleming did this to a certain extent, the repeated deaths of bacteria forced him to take a closer look at the effects of the green mold. Eventually, the presence of the unexpected green mold led to the discovery of penicillin, whose effects were studied extensively in later experiments.

When the effects of a newly discovered variable are experimentally analyzed, the existence of new phenomena are simultaneously documented. When Lee analyzed the effects of delayed auditory feedback on speech, several interrelated phenomena concerning speech production and its continuous monitoring through auditory mechanism were documented. Skinner's discovery of the effects of reinforcement schedules led to demonstrations of new phenomena of response patterns under different arrangements of consequences. Fleming's discovery of penicillin led to the documentation of a host of biological phenomena relative to the treatment of various diseases.

The four kinds of reasons for doing research described in previous sections are not exhaustive, but they include the major factors that typically lead scientists to research and experimentation. Also, the reasons are by no means mutually exclusive; in fact, they are interrelated. Research done to satisfy one's curiosity may explain an event. Often, curiosity compels one to ask why a certain event is happening, and an answer to that question also may isolate the cause of the event. Curiosity can initially draw a scientist to a field of investigation. But soon, the scientist may be doing research to explain events (develop theories), solve practical problems, or demonstrate certain effects. It should also be clear that research done for any other reason will also satisfy the scientist's curiosity.

Research done to explain events can lead to additional research that may help solve practical problems. For example, an experimentally based explanation of language disorders should also suggest ways of treating or preventing them. Because an explanation always points to at least one cause of an event, additional research on the methods of manipulating that cause should provide a means of controlling that effect. Controlling a cause to produce an effect is a treatment procedure.

In a similar manner, research done to solve practical problems can eventually lead to an explanation of certain phenomena. For example, successful treatment of language disorders through certain environmental manipulations may suggest that certain variables facilitate language acquisition. The absence of those variables may contribute to language disorders. Unfortunately, a widely held assumption is that applied research cannot explain phenomena but can only manipulate them with the knowledge derived from basic research. However, well-controlled experimental treatment research can offer excellent suggestions on the controlling variables of successfully treated phenomena. This is because in solving practical problems, often the independent variables (causes) of the phenomenon of interest must be found. Obviously, the same causal variables can explain the phenomenon.

HOW IS RESEARCH DONE?

In this section, I shall not address the actual mechanics of doing research, for that is the running theme of this book, and the final part of the book contains more specific suggestions on how to do research. In this section, I shall present two approaches to describing research activity. Different ways of conceptualizing and describing research activity may impede or facilitate a more complete understanding of it.

It was noted earlier that the traditional view of research is that it is an extremely well-organized, formal activity; it was further noted that this view may be largely mistaken. A more accurate view of research is that it is always a formative, not necessarily formalized, activity. We shall take a closer look at the research process and contrast these views to emphasize that research is what some *people* do. In other words, research is a human activity that includes inital groping (in spite of methodological planning and subsequent methodological refinement) and, with some luck, leaps of the imagination.

The Formal View

It is not proposed here that there are two ways of doing research, one more formal and organized than the other. What is proposed is that research is *described* in two ways, and that all research is less formal and organized than published articles and textbook descriptions suggest.

The popular view of research is that it is a formal process with clear-cut steps and linear progression. According to the formal view, research involves an invariable, systematic, and step-by-step progression from the literature review to the problem, methods, results, and conclusions. However, this view of research is probably due to the format of published research. Those who write textbooks on research tend to support that view by omitting the process of research while describing the mechanics of organizing research already done.

A student of research methods who reads a published journal article to understand the process of research may gain the impression that the researcher knew everything from the beginning. It might appear that all that the researcher had to do was simply take the predetermined and incredibly clear steps of conducting the research. The student is apt to think that the experimenter had read everything about the past research well before the research problem was given its final form. Existing research being clear, the imagined brilliant researcher suddenly and inevitably generated the question that needed to be researched. The question as originally conceived must have been clear-cut and well formulated, for there is no indication in the article that the question was modified, was rewritten, or was not at all the original question considered for investigation. There is certainly no hint that the question investigated was one of several considered, or that it was initially quite fuzzy.

The student might then think that as soon as the problem was posed, the researcher knew what kind of results would be obtained, so a hypothesis was formulated. However, to avoid giving the impression that the investigator had a personal stake in supporting his or her guesses, a null hypothesis, which is essentially a prediction that the events investigated are not related, was proposed (see Chapter 3 for more on null hypothesis). The investigator then knew exactly what to do to test the hypothesis. It might appear to the student that there was no question as to what kind of design to use in the study. The design used must have been the only one available. If alternatives were available, the choice must have been easy and clear. The procedure of participant selection must also have been clear from the very beginning, because there is no indication of troubled decisions on this matter. All participants must have been readily available, and all the experimenter had to do was ask them to participate in the study. Furthermore, it may appear that the investigator was sure of the best method of measuring and manipulating the variables. In this manner, the student is likely to imagine that the scientist simply moved through a series of well-defined steps, which resulted in the conclusion of the study.

The student may further assume that once the data were collected, the predetermined method of analysis was applied to the results. Apparently, the meaning of the results was also unambiguously clear to the scientist; after all, the article talked about a definite number of implications that seem to have emerged full-blown in the order in which they were presented. With great ease, the scientist must have seen the relation between the study's findings and those of other investigations.

In essence, a typical journal article gives the student the impression that research is possible only when everything is brilliantly clear to the scientist.

Because the student has not heretofore seen anything so complex and yet so clearly and beautifully organized, research seems to be both a unique and formidable task.

That a student gains such an impression of the research process is not a fault either of the student who reads research reports or of the scientist who writes them; doing research and organizing it for publication are simply two separate activities. In writing a research article, the scientist describes the research question, the methods of investigation, the results, and the implications of those results. In this description, it is most efficient to omit the details of the research process. The process of doing research is full of various personal, practical, ideational, emotional, and organizational details that may not be entirely relevant to an understanding of what was done and what results were obtained. Furthermore, these factors, if chronicled in an article, may confuse readers. Besides, no journal will have space to print the story of research in addition to the research itself, no matter how interesting the story might be. Therefore, the preceding characterization of the research process that can be gleaned from journal articles is not meant to suggest that research reporting should reflect the complexity of the research process.

One would expect, however, that when research scientists talk about how they did their research or when authors write books on how to do research, the research process would be reflected. Unfortunately, many authors who talk or write about research paint an unreal picture of how they do it. The textbooks on research procedures, especially those based on statistics, are particularly vulnerable to this criticism. Textbooks typically reinforce the questionable notion of the clear-cut, step-by-step research process that the students gain from reading journal articles.

The Formative View

A research report documents (a) several decisions made by the investigator, (b) how those decisions were implemented, (c) what results followed that implementation, and (d) what the author thinks of those results. Decisions are made concerning the problem of investigation, what the previous research suggests, how the problem will be investigated, and how the results will be interpreted. However, these decisions should not be confused with the actual process of arriving at those decisions. Students who wish to know how to do research should gain an understanding of how such decisions are made. When this process is considered, a different view of how research is done emerges. Scientists who describe the process by which they made their own discoveries tend to create a synthetic vision of formality, clarity, logical precision, and inevitable movement through specific steps. In an article titled "A Plea for Freeing the History of Scientific Discoveries from Myth," Grmek (1981) expressed skepticism about the validity of many famous scientists' autobiographical accounts of the process of scientific discovery. Grmek believes that in describing their own past discoveries, many scientists resort to "rationalizing readjustment, whereby the actual sequence of events is transmuted in favor of logical rigor and coherence" (1981, p. 15).

Many authors who consider themselves competent researchers may be somewhat reluctant to talk about the typically uncertain, sometimes confusing, and generally groping nature of doing research. There may be an implicit assumption that "science" cannot be anything but utter clarity, beautiful organization, and superb efficiency. Scientific research may be thought of as entirely official, proper, prim, and uncompromising. However, when science is viewed as something people do, the emerging picture of the research process may be less magnificent, but it will be more real.

Research is more formative than formal. The formative view suggests that research is an evolving process. It is a process in which concepts, ideas, procedures, and skills emerge and develop gradually, sometimes slowly. A formative research process changes and improves. The formative view of research implies that even with much planning, research is an evolving process, not a process whose sequence and progression are fixed at the beginning. The movement from problem to discussion is not as certain, neat, and linear as a published article might imply. There is a beginning and an end to a particular study, but the boundaries are not always clear. More important, everything in between may involve many back-and-forth movements. Grmek (1981) stated that the typical textbook depiction of the linear ascent toward truth is a myth. He also stated that "neither the meanderings of individual thought, nor the advances of scientific knowledge within a community, proceed by successive approximations, always in the right direction, towards truth. The path to discovery is a winding one" (p. 20).

Research activity has patterns, but they are broad, general, and flexible. There are broad conceptual and methodological patterns. There are patterns pertaining to theory and practice. Unfortunately, most textbooks turn those broad and flexible patterns into specific and rigid steps of doing research.

The formal and clearly stated research question as it finally appears in a published article may barely resemble the early troubling but uncertain, vague yet haunting sensations that often are a coalescence of thoughts, images, and feelings about the phenomenon of interest. If questioned as to what he or she is doing at this stage, the scientist's answer might be more confusing than illuminating. The scientist's thoughts may appear not well organized at all. In all likelihood, at this stage some phenomenon is bothering the scientist, but there is no fully articulated research problem that can be investigated. At such a time, the scientist's speech, if he or she is willing to talk about the problem at all, will certainly not resemble the convention lecture given on the completed research a year later.

There may be a few exceptional scientists who, without much effort and time, can formulate significant research questions that, when investigated, yield meaningful data. In most cases, however, the emergence of research questions is a slow and formative process. Generally speaking, the beginnings of a research question may be felt after much reading on the issue. Some researchers may think of questions while talking about an issue or a topic. Others may sense potential questions while engaged in some practical work, such as working with a client.

Research itself is probably the most productive locus of additional research questions. Tentative research questions may emerge when the scientist observes something or while investigating a related problem. The results of an experiment might suggest additional questions for future investigation. The researcher may have found out that the method selected was not effective and that a different tactic might prove more useful. Thus, both effective and ineffective research can suggest valid questions to be investigated. Descriptive research might suggest questions for experimental research. Similarly, basic analysis of a phenomenon might suggest applied research questions.

A clinician who is a keen observer may think of many questions during treatment sessions or simply while watching client behaviors. An inefficient treatment should be an excellent source for treatment-related research questions. The clinician who has carefully broken down the treatment into separately manipulated components may be able to observe differential effects of certain components. The clinician may pursue such differential effects in a research study.

In most cases, extensive or intensive reading, keen observation, critical analysis of research literature, some experience in research, an understanding of logic and the philosophy of science, and critical thinking are all necessary to formulate significant research questions.

As noted before, most research questions are not very clear in the early stages. Furthermore, upon further thinking and reading, those that were clear to begin with may be judged the wrong kind of questions. The refinement of the question takes much thinking, and most questions undergo several revisions before they are ready for investigation. The relative emphasis on the variables within a question may be changed when the investigator thinks of a strategy to implement the experiment.

Once the question becomes reasonably clear, the scientist begins to think about the ways of answering it. Different methods can be used to answer the same research question. For example, the effects of a new stuttering treatment program can be tested within a single-subject design or a group design. In the former, all participants receive the experimental treatment. In the latter strategy, participants in one group receive treatment and the members of the other group do not, thereby serving as a control group. The investigator selects what he or she considers the best strategy to answer the particular research question, but the scientist's own investigative history probably plays a key role in that selection. Here too, the investigator is likely to go through a period of vacillation. Finally, a design may be selected for certain practical reasons. A group design, for example, may be selected simply because a certain number of participants happen to be available.

Various other aspects of the procedures of a study are decided one way or the other, often without any clear-cut guidelines or requirements. When there are no stringent guidelines, the investigator judges whether the selected procedure can be justified on some grounds. Also, a given course of action may be taken because no other option is available. For example, how many participants should be selected for the study? A group design would require more participants than a single-subject design, but in many cases, the answer depends simply on the availability of participants, especially in clinical fields. If 10 people who stutter are available for a study, the investigator decides to go with that number. It may happen that only 6 people who stutter are willing to participate, and the study has to be completed with them. When the report is written, however, it may seem to indicate that the planned and well-considered number of participants was 6. Indeed, planning may have nothing to do with the number of participants used.

Answers to many other questions may be similarly determined. What kinds of equipment will be used? In what facility will the experiment be conducted? Investigators construct new mechanical devices and buy new instruments when funds are available; ideally, the best available instrumentation must be used for the study, but in practice, most investigators use what is available. Sometimes, a problem already defined may have to be redefined or modified to accommodate the only available instrument. For example, an investigator who wanted to monitor different physiologic variables such as heart rate, muscle potential, cortical electrical potential, blood volume, and breathing patterns in people who stutter during treatment sessions might drop one or more of those variables simply because a multichannel polygraph that measured all of them was not available. Once again, practical exigencies, not planning, would have determined the variables selected for the study, but the written report is not likely to reflect this.

Many times, research problems sit on shelves collecting dust because the investigator does not have the time, participants, money, or all of these to complete the studies. Other problems may not be investigated because of methodological difficulties; an investigator may not see how a problem can be researched. In other situations, a problem that has been forgotten or neglected may suddenly be revived because a certain number of clients or type of client becomes available. The investigator will somehow make time and will convince himself or herself that the existing equipment, although not ideal, will do. During an incidental and entirely informal conversation with a colleague, a method to study a perplexing problem may emerge. Or, a recently published article may suggest an innovative method. Not infrequently, the investigator may think of a procedure while taking a walk or while just sitting and thinking about the problem. Suddenly, the problem sitting on the shelf is picked up and dusted off, and the investigator drops everything else and becomes immersed in the new study. Meanwhile, other research ideas maybe neglected.

In any discipline, there are probably countless studies that remain half-finished, or that were abandoned soon after they were begun. But the number cannot be too small. Many investigators are likely to have a few studies that were implemented to varying degrees and discontinued for any of a number of reasons. Maybe the investigator found out that it was not a great study (meaning it was bad) after all. Maybe the researcher came across a more interesting study or obtained some grant monies that forced attention into some other area of investigation. Perhaps the investigator got sick during the course of the study and never again had time to finish it. Furthermore, subjects may drop out, equipment may break down, or the investigator may move to another position. All of these not-so-formal reasons for discontinuing research are real and more common than the books on research methods lead us to believe.

A certain number of research studies that are completed may never be published. Again, objective data on the number of such studies are lacking, but editors of journals can testify to the number of rejected articles. An article rejected by one journal may be published in another journal; but still, many articles prepared for publication may never be published. Or, a completed research study may never be written up for publication. A study may have been completed without its flaws having been realized, but one look at the data may convince the investigator that the study is not worth publishing.

The sequence of research found in published articles gives an impression of an orderly progression through an invariable sequence. Most empirical research articles have a rigid sequence because scientific journals require it. An article starts with an untitled Introduction or the Review of Literature, proceeds to the Method, then to the Results, and finally to the Discussion or Conclusion. The article ends with References, Appendixes, or both. But this rigid sequence is rarely a reflection of how the research itself was conducted. In some cases, investigators have sufficient reason to do a study with only a minimal survey of literature. This is especially true when an investigator knows that no study of the kind being considered has been made. After the study has been made, a more thorough search of the literature may be conducted to determine if the new findings can be related to any of the old findings. Often, methodological considerations precede a more thorough analysis of the research problem itself. One may have a general idea of the research problem, such as an evaluation of two language treatment programs, but the more critical factor to be assessed at the very beginning may be the number of participants that are available for the study. This may then determine the design of the study. A researcher may not wish to use statistical methods of analysis, in which case considerations of data analysis may determine the design to be used. In this manner, the investigator considers factors sometimes in the sequence in which the paper is written but many times in a sequence dictated by the practical contingencies that affect the researcher.

It must be recognized, though, that some research practices are more rigid than others. The statistically based group research designs are relatively more rigid in their strategies than are the single-subject designs. Typically, in the group research designs, the study is completed the way it was planned even if it becomes evident that something is wrong with the study. The design itself is rarely, if ever, modified in the middle of an investigation. To the contrary, a study with a single-subject design may be modified when the data warrant a change. For example, if found ineffective, a treatment procedure in clinical research may be changed in a single-subject strategy, but usually not in the group strategy. The number of days for which the experimental treatment is applied may be predetermined in the group approach, but not in the single-subject approach. For instance, people who stutter may be treated for a fixed duration in a group design study. In a single-subject study, the same treatment may be continued until stuttering is reduced markedly or until it becomes evident to the researcher that it is no use to continue the experimental treatment. Such judgments, made during the course of the study, are considered undesirable in the group research strategy. However, the same judgment or similar judgments made prior to the implementation of the study are considered a part of good planning.

SERENDIPITY IN RESEARCH

We noted earlier that accidental events have often helped scientists discover new phenomena. That accidents lead to significant scientific findings also suggests that all research is not totally planned. By definition, accidental discoveries are unplanned, but they are scientific discoveries nonetheless. Some accidental discoveries have proved more valuable than the planned research during which such accidents happened.

Walpole's story *The Three Princes of Serendip* has given rise to the term *serendipity* in research (Cannon, 1945). The story goes that three princes, while looking for something that they never found, nevertheless found many interesting things that they had not thought of finding. Often, when looking for something, scientists may find something else. Such accidental discoveries may help scientists begin new lines of productive investigations. It was noted earlier that Fleming's discovery of penicillin was accidental, as was Skinner's discovery of the effects of intermittent reinforcement on response patterns.

A particularly fascinating story of accidental discovery in medical sciences is that of Ignaz Semmelweis, a Hungarian physician who worked in a maternity ward of the Vienna General Hospital from 1844 to 1848 (Sinclair, 1901). The hospital had two maternity wards, and Semmelweis worked in the first ward. An anguishing puzzle he faced was that in his ward, the death rate due to childbed (puerperal) fever among women after delivery was as high as 11%; but in the other, identical ward, the death rate was around only 2%.

Like most investigators, Semmelweis began to test various logical possibilities and opinions about the causation of the unusually high mortality rate. Unfortunately, none of the logical possibilities proved to be the cause of the death rate. He found that such variables as overcrowding, unexplained "epidemic influences," rough examination by medical students, the posture women assumed during delivery, and a variety of psychological factors all proved to be inconsistent with facts or specific manipulations. For instance, overcrowding was common to both the wards and hence could not explain a differential death rate. Reducing the number of examinations by medical students did not reduce the death rate. Semmelweis reasoned that unexplained epidemic factors must be common to both the wards.

The puzzle was eventually solved in 1847, but the solution did not come from any of Semmelweis's rigorous hypothesis testing. It came from an unfortunate accident. While performing an autopsy, a student's scalpel punctured a wound in the finger of his instructor, Kolletschka. Soon Kolletschka became violently ill with the same symptoms of childbed fever. He died, just like many women with childbed fever. This led Semmelweis to think that perhaps the "cadaveric matter" the student's scalpel had introduced into Kolletschka's bloodstream must be the cause of the disease. The medical students were not trained in the other ward that had the low death rate. In that ward, midwives who did not dissect cadavers delivered babies. It then dawned on Semmelweis that he, his colleagues, and the medical students regularly came to examine the women in labor soon after completing dissections. Possibly because they did not wash their hands thoroughly, the physicians and medical students themselves were the carriers of the deadly microorganisms that were introduced into the bloodstream of women in labor.

Semmelweis solved the problem when he ordered that before examining the women in the ward, all physicians and medical students wash their hands thoroughly with a solution of chlorinated lime. Consequently, the death rate in Semmelweis's ward declined to the level found in the other ward. As the Semmelweis story suggests, a problem is not always solved by a planned test of a formal hypothesis. An accident that reveals an unsuspected relation between events can solve a problem that had proved frustrating.

A source of accidental discovery that is not widely recognized is apparatus failure. All scientists know that instruments break down and that in most such cases they create problems for the scientist. Most scientists dread apparatus failure in the course of an experiment. Nevertheless, important discoveries have been made when apparatuses broke down in the middle of experiments. Two examples from behavioral research illustrate this. First, the discovery of operant extinction was aided immensely by a breakdown in the equipment Skinner was using to reinforce responses. In fact, one of Skinner's (1956) unformalized principles of scientific practice is that "apparatuses sometimes break down" (p. 109). As it happened, one day the food magazine, which was a part of the mechanical device used to automatically reinforce the bar press responses in rats, became jammed. Therefore, the rat's responses went unreinforced against the plan of the experiment in progress. The result was an extinction curve, which led to a series of experiments on the properties of extinction and on the functional relations between the prior reinforcement contingencies and later patterns of extinction.

The second example also comes from experimental research on conditioning and is provided by Sidman (1960):

> An experiment on avoidance behavior was in progress in which an animal was scheduled to receive only 20 percent of all the shocks that became due when it failed to make the avoidance response in time. A relay failure in the automatic programming circuit altered the procedure one day in such a way that every *fifth* shock was delivered *regardless* of whether or not the animal had made an avoidance response. The apparatus failure was discovered when the animal's usually stable rate of lever pressing began to accelerate, and continued to increase throughout the experimental period. The increased rate of avoidance responding in the face of unavoidable shock was so unexpected that a new research program was immediately launched, a program which has been productive for three years and is still continuing. (p. 9)

The phenomenon Sidman discovered because of an accidental failure of apparatus has come to be known as the Sidman avoidance, in which an organism has no prior signal of an impending aversive stimulus, and there is no escape, but each response postpones the aversive stimulus for a fixed period of time. It is known that the Sidman procedure produces a high and consistent rate of response, which is unusually resistant to extinction. Sidman's original finding has been replicated widely, and its human behavioral and clinical implications are extensive. But, the point to be made here is that the discovery of this important phenomenon of aversive conditioning was entirely due to a breakdown in instrumentation.

When experimental apparatuses break down, many scientists may be tempted to discard the data collected up to that point because of the "contamination caused by equipment failure." Usually, after having cried on the shoulder of a friendly colleague, the scientist will rebuild the apparatus and start all over again. In many cases, equipment failure can be a cause of worry, especially when all the data are lost and there is nothing to discover. However, the results produced by failures are always worth a serious examination. The investigator may find new problems for exciting research in those unexpected results.

Serendipity in research not only shows that not all research is thoroughly planned, but also that research need not necessarily test hypotheses. If research is done only to test hypotheses, then the chances for accidental discoveries are eliminated. In hypothesis testing, the scientist asks a question and then formulates a tentative answer, which is then put to experimental test. The results of such research studies are always evaluated in terms of their relation to the hypothesis. Anything not relevant to the hypothesis is not of interest. Because "accidental confirmation of a hypothesis" is a contradiction of terms, accidental discoveries must be necessarily useless. But this is not the case.

PLANNING IS STILL IMPORTANT

The view that research is more formative than formal does not imply that research is casual or that there is no need for planning or preparation. It must be noted that most accidental discoveries happen in the process of well-planned investigation. The scientist needs to be an intellectually prepared person. A thorough knowledge of existing research is usually necessary, if only to avoid the same conceptual or methodologic mistakes committed by other scientists. In the research process, evidence accumulates slowly and is built by the continuous, collective efforts of scientists. The building blocks of scientific knowledge are the little pieces of research done by a variety of researchers past and present. Therefore, researchers must be able to see interrelations among research findings, and this takes painstakingly achieved scholarship.

Good research also requires a working knowledge of the methods of manipulating and measuring variables. Some skill and experience in looking at data and thinking about their importance are also necessary. Undoubtedly, many questionable investigations are due to poor scholarship, inadequate technical skills, and lack of sufficient planning on the part of researchers.

The formative view of research does suggest, however, that research is a more flexible, open, human, sensitive, and practical activity than it is often depicted to be. At the conceptual and methodological levels, research is formative in the sense that different contingencies continuously affect the process. A good research scientist is always willing to go back and forth and to change ideas or the plan of an experiment. A scientist is not necessarily bound by rigid sequences that may not promote creativity. Such a scientist is sensitive to unplanned events that happen during the course of research and does not have the great investment in his or her own guesses (hypotheses) that seems to create a scientist's affliction called *hypothesis myopia* (Bachrach, 1969). Though he or she is knowledgeable regarding previous research findings, the scientist's thinking is not limited by those findings. The scientist knows that nature is likely to display events not suggested by previous research and not predicted by hypotheses and theories. Such a scientist is fully prepared to seize an unplanned and unexpected moment of creativity.

SUMMARY

- *Science* is a certain philosophy, a set of methods, and a certain behavioral disposition. *Research* is science in action.

- Scientists do research to
  — satisfy their curiosity about natural phenomena
  — explain events
  — solve practical problems
  — demonstrate certain effects

- There are two ways of describing how research is done: formal and formative. The formal view holds that researchers follow rigid, clear, and linearly sequenced steps from thinking about a problem to completing the study. The formative view holds that research is an evolving, changing, and improving process in which back-and-forth movements are common.

- Science is full of accidental discoveries of great importance. Even apparatus failure during research can generate significant findings. Such discoveries show that research is not always planned and that it need not always test hypothesis. The term *serendipity* captures the essence of the importance of accidental scientific discoveries.

- Good planning for research is still needed because accidental discoveries often are a part of well-planned research. Good findings rarely come from unplanned, unprepared, and haphazard research.

STUDY GUIDE

1. Distinguish between research and science.

2. Define research.

3. What are the bureaucratic reasons for doing research?

4. Describe the various reasons for doing research.

5. Explain why research done to satisfy one's own curiosity may not involve hypothesis testing.

6. What is the difference between private curiosity and scientific curiosity?

7. What is a scientific explanation?

8. Write a hypothetical statement of explanation of a selected communicative disorder.

9. What are the two kinds of practical problems scientists try to solve?

10. What is the name of the by-product of research that is successful in solving some practical problems?

11. Give two examples of scientists' in-house problems.

12. What kind of research results in the observation of new phenomena?

13. What are the two approaches to describing research activity? Compare and contrast the two approaches.

14. Why do students tend to have a formal view of research?

15. What is meant by the statement that "research is more formative than formal"?

16. Give an example of accidental discovery in scientific research. Find an example not given in this text.

Chapter 3

◆◆◆◆◆◆◆◆◆◆◆◆◆◆◆◆◆◆◆◆◆◆◆◆◆◆◆◆◆◆◆◆◆◆◆◆

Science and Its Basic Concepts

- Popular Misconceptions About Science
- What Is Science?
- Outcome of Scientific Activity
- Variables and Their Types
- Causality and Functional Analysis
- Experiment and Experimental Control
- Hypotheses in Scientific Research
- Theories and Scientific Reasoning
- Theories and Scientific Laws
- Data and Evidence
- Summary
- Study Guide

W e all seem to know what science is, but the formal question, "What is science?" is not always easy to answer. Experts have given different answers, each describing some aspect of science. However, there are many popular misconceptions about science and it is instructive to know what science is not. Some of these misconceptions may be entertained by persons who are otherwise educated but have not formally studied the philosophy and methods of science.

POPULAR MISCONCEPTIONS ABOUT SCIENCE

Probably the first and the most common misconception about science is that it is a certain subject matter. Many people think that science is physics, chemistry, or biology. Traditionally, certain subject matters have come to be regarded as sciences. Therefore, the popular opinion has equated science with those subject matters. Certain other subject matters, such as sociology or speech–language pathology, may not be regarded as sciences.

The misconception is understandable because scientists themselves have often defined science in terms of a "body of knowledge" that is systematic and verified. Some disciplines have a more systematic and verified body of knowledge and therefore are more likely to be equated with science. Other bodies of knowledge that are not as systematic, or that are still being verified, may not qualify for the title of science. The metaphoric notion of the "body of knowledge" is misleading if it is equated with science but appropriate if it is thought of as a product of science. A group of persons who engage in scientific activity over an extended period of time may produce knowledge that is consistent with the philosophy and methods of science.

Science is not the same as particular subject matters such as physics or biology, though it may be appropriate to say that some subject matters are more scientifically oriented than others. A subject matter is more or less scientific depending on the extent to which it applies the methods of science in investigating its subject matter.

A second misconception equates science with activities carried on in certain physical settings such as laboratories involving complex instruments. Laboratories and instruments that several scientific disciplines use are not always necessary or sufficient to make a piece of investigation scientific. For instance, scientific experiments can be conducted outside laboratories; they can be conducted on playgrounds or in shopping centers or living rooms. Experiments can be done in classrooms, industrial assembly lines, outer space, or underwater. Many experiments can be conducted with no complicated instruments.

A third misconception about science is evident in a confusion between science and technology. Designing and building computers, spacecrafts, bridges, and buildings are technological tasks. Technology often is the application of science in solving problems, but it is not necessarily the science itself. The confusion is understandable because technology provides highly visible examples of the application of science.

WHAT IS SCIENCE?

Science may be defined from three basic views that stress its different aspects. The three views are that **science** is (a) a philosophy, (b) a certain kind of behavior, and (c) a set of methods. I shall briefly describe each of these views. All three are necessary to obtain a comprehensive view of science.

Science as a Philosophy

Science is a certain philosophical position regarding nature and the nature of events. The philosophic foundations of science include *determinism* and *empiricism*. **Determinism** states that events are caused by other events. Events do not happen haphazardly; they are determined by their causes. Without this basic philosophy, scientific activity would not be meaningful; scientific activity is essentially a search for the causes of events.

The early history of science shows that laity and learned people had difficulty accepting the philosophy of determinism. People in most societies believed that events happened because of a divine design beyond the scope of human observation and investigation. Science, on the other hand, insists that events are caused by other events and that the causes can be observed, studied, and in many cases, controlled. Before the advent of science, theology and a closely affiliated branch of philosophy called *scholasticism* ruled the world of knowledge, understanding, and explanation. Both scholasticism and religion had their explanations of the physical, chemical, biological, and human world. Often, science found itself in conflict with traditional religious wisdom. Both science and scientists have suffered because of this.

It is well known that physical, chemical, and biological phenomena were among the very first to come under the scope of the philosophy and methods of science. Science replaced the notion that the earth is flat and that it is the center of universe. Science challenged the notion that human beings suddenly emerged because of divine creation. It showed that physical, chemical, and biological phenomena are lawful and that those laws can be discovered. The progress in such basic scientific analyses eventually led to technology, which helped solve many problems of living. Technology began to make life a little easier and thus reduced some of the resistance to science. Nevertheless, new inventions and discoveries provoke social resistance (Johnston & Pennypacker, 1993).

Generally speaking, resistance to the philosophy of science is less marked in the case of physical and chemical phenomena. As applied to biological phenomena, however, scientific philosophy still provokes considerable resistance. The continuous controversies over teaching science versus creationism in U.S. public schools testify to this persistent resistance to the philosophy of science.

The resistance to the concept that human behavior is predetermined is even more vocal. Human behavior has been the last stronghold of anti-scientific philosophy. Traditional religious philosophies that assert that human beings are created also tend to discredit the possibility that human behavior is determined. Human actions are supposed to be due to inner forces such as free will. Many people who readily accept the philosophy that natural events are caused by other events vehemently oppose the notion that human behavior has its causes that can be studied and controlled by the methods of science. In recent years, the science of human behavior has been one of the most attacked of sciences.

Within the domain of human behavior, higher human activities such as language and thinking have been a particular stronghold for the traditional, nonscientific philosophies of rationalism, mentalism, and scholasticism. For example, when the evidence that most forms of human behaviors can be analyzed by the methods of science became overwhelming, traditional thinkers insisted upon exceptions. Language and creativity seemed like an urgently needed exception if traditional concepts of human behavior were to be maintained. The nativists' strong rejection of the behavioral analysis of language is but one indication of this tendency.

The history of science shows that it has been somewhat easy to look at physical and chemical phenomena and analyze them objectively. Because scientists also are behaving organisms, a science of behavior requires that we analyze our own behaviors objectively. Unfortunately, looking at ourselves and analyzing our own actions has been a difficult scientific activity. The historical resistance to the concept of determinism as applied to human behavior may be part of this difficulty.

Another philosophical cornerstone of science, **empiricism** is a philosophical position that sensory experience is the basis of knowledge. Traditional (nonscientific) thinking would suggest that knowledge may be derived from rational thinking and intuition, or by mystical, religious, and divine revelations. To the contrary, science insists that valid knowledge is based on sensory experience. This experience must be socially and objectively verifiable; after all, even divine revelation can be an "experience." The methods of empiricism make experience acceptable to science.

The philosophy of empiricism requires **observation** and **measurement** of events scientists study. For the most part, observation is a sensory process. Observation requires that scientists come into sensory contact with the phenomenon under study. If different scientists establish contacts with the phenomenon and arrive at the same or similar values of measurement, then the probability is high that the phenomenon exists and does so in the manner measured. Once the existence of a phenomenon is confirmed through observation and measurement, the scientist is ready for the next step in which the phenomenon is manipulated. Such manipulations are called scientific experiments. Later chapters will take a closer look at both observation and experimentation.

Science as Behavior

The term *science* includes the actions and behaviors of scientists. Obviously, science is the result of what people called scientists do. The view that science is a certain kind of behavior is not well known because of the emphasis on objective methods, procedures, and philosophies in descriptions of science. While such an emphasis is entirely valid, people need to understand the behavior of scientists to appreciate the full meaning of science. Viewing science as the product of scientists' behaviors may have the best pedagogical value. Young people may understand science better when told how accomplished scientists tend to behave.

The view that science is a certain kind of behavior is relatively new. Behavioral scientists such as Skinner (1953, 1974) have insisted that the behavior of scientists is a subject of the science of behavior. Systematic analysis of the behavior of scientists has barely begun, partly because of the belief that scientific as well as literary creativity is mysterious and unique and thus beyond the scope of scientific analysis. There is some fear that an objective analysis of the process of writing a poem, painting a picture, or discovering some lawful relations in nature will adversely affect such valuable (but poorly understood) activities. Possibly, the resistance to a scientific analysis of the behavior of scientists and artists may simply be a part of the historical skepticism regarding determinism of human behavior.

Consistent with some of the misconceptions of science, there also are several misconceptions about scientists as people. Scientists are popularly depicted as impractical, fanciful, and unsociable. They may be considered maniacs who wish to control the world and all humanity. Scientists are often thought to be absentminded and slovenly. They may be described as cold, mechanical, and lacking in feelings and warmth.

As Bachrach (1969) put it, such a stereotypical notion of scientists is "arrant nonsense" (p. 111). More sensibly, scientists are described as curious people who often are dissatisfied with the existing explanations of events they wish to study. Skinner (1953) stated that scientists are disposed to "deal with facts rather than what someone has said about them" (p. 12). Curiosity, dissatisfaction with existing explanations, and a tendency to deal with facts all lead to a disposition to reject authority. The history of science shows that science "rejects its own authorities when they interfere with the observation of nature" (Skinner, 1953, p. 12).

A scientist is more willing than other people to set aside his or her wishes and expectations and let the facts and results of experiments speak for themselves. The scientist is interested in replacing subjective opinions and convictions with objective, demonstrated relations. As pointed out by Skinner (1953), intellectual honesty—the opposite of wishful thinking—is an important characteristic of scientists. A scientist may find that the results of an experiment are not as expected and predicted or that they contradict his or her own well-known theory. In such cases, an honest scientist would report the findings as they were observed, because "the facts must stand and the expectations fall. The subject matter, not the scientist, knows best" (Skinner, 1953, p. 13).

Another characteristic of scientists, according to Skinner (1953), is that they are willing to remain "without an answer until a satisfactory one can be found" (p. 13). Beginning students in many fields often are surprised when told that there is no satisfactory answer to certain questions. When students are told that scientists do not know precisely how language is acquired or how stuttering is caused, they find it hard to believe that "all those experts do not have any idea" and that the experts can live with such uncertainties. Scientists can tolerate such uncertainties because they are trained to reject premature explanations and theories. That something cannot be explained at a given time is generally less bothersome to scientists than it is to nonscientists. Instead of accepting whatever explanations that may be available, scientists tend to investigate.

Sometimes people think that when there is no good explanation, the knowledge that is available can be, or even must be, accepted. Such acceptance would be dangerous, however. Unfortunately, this practice often is encouraged by investigators who, after having advanced their own explanations, challenge others to either accept those explanations or offer better ones. Good scientists do not pay much attention to such challenges. A scientist need not propose a better explanation to reject a bad one. Explanations stand on their evidence, and if there is no acceptable evidence, they just do not stand. A scientist can examine alternative explanations and reject one in favor of the other. But an explanation also can be rejected in favor of none (Hegde, 1980a).

The debate over the Chomskyan innate hypotheses in the explanation of language acquisition illustrates this issue. During the 1960s, many linguists and psycholinguists who had proposed a variety of innate hypotheses to explain language acquisition had also repeatedly challenged nonnativists to either accept those hypotheses or offer better explanations. Addressing this kind of challenge, and referring to Chomsky's nativist theory, Goodman (1967), a philosopher of science, stated that although one may not have an alternative explanation for a phenomenon, "that alone does not dictate acceptance of whatever theory may be offered; for the theory may be worse than none. Inability to explain a fact does not condemn me to accept an intrinsically repugnant and incomprehensible theory" (p. 27). This again underscores the view that scientists are people who can go without an explanation.

Science as a Set of Methods

In addition to certain philosophies and behavioral dispositions, science is a set of methods. The definition of science as methods is generally better

understood than either the philosophy of science or the behavioral dispositions of scientists. This is understandable because in the teaching of science
and research, tangible methods receive greater attention than philosophies
and dispositions.

Science can be defined as a certain way of studying events and solving
problems. Science is a set of methods designed to investigate research questions in a manner acceptable to scientists. The methods of science can also
be described as rules that dictate scientists' conduct in carrying out a piece
of research. Violation of these rules produces questionable results. Therefore, scientists are trained in those methods so that they can engage in activities that produce valid knowledge.

The most important aspect of the methods of science is that they help
answer research questions. The methods are structural and conceptual means
of investigating research problems. The selection, formulation, and definition of research problems; selection of participants; specification of variables
or factors to be analyzed; the manner in which the variables are measured
and manipulated; and the techniques of data analysis are all a part of the scientific method.

Probably the most basic characteristic of the methods of science is that
they are objective. **Objectivity** is achieved when the methods and the results
are publicly verifiable. Public verification simply means that other scientists
can reproduce both the procedures and the results. Similar scientific procedures should produce similar results.

Of all the aspects of scientific methods, the most fundamental are observation, measurement, and experimentation. **Observation,** the systematic
study of a phenomena to note its characteristics, is a basic tool necessary for
all scientific operations. **Measurement,** which refers to assigning numbers
to properties of events, is another basic tool of science. Objective and precise
measurement is necessary to make a scientific analysis of a phenomenon. In
Chapter 5, observation and measurement are described in greater detail.

Once a phenomenon comes under systematic observation and measurement, **experimentation** becomes possible. Through experimentation,
scientists establish cause–effect relationships between events. The concept
of experiment is described later in this chapter.

To summarize, a comprehensive view of science includes the philosophical, behavioral, and methodological considerations just described.
Throughout the book, these aspects of science are addressed in different
practical and theoretical contexts.

OUTCOME OF SCIENTIFIC ACTIVITY

Science is said to have certain goals. However, when people talk about the
goals of science, they are actually talking about the eventual outcome of scientific activity. The term *goal* suggests that something that might happen in
the future affects scientists' behavior. Neither scientists nor others are affected

by future events. The question of the goals of science is the question of why scientists do what they do. Scientists do what they do because of their past and because of present contingencies, not because of some future events called goals. Why scientists do research cannot be answered by listing the goals of science. Therefore, consideration of the typical outcome of scientific activity is more meaningful. Only in a nontechnical sense are scientists after such outcomes.

A basic outcome of scientific activity is **description** of natural events (phenomena). After having observed an event, scientists describe its characteristics. Therefore, describing a phenomenon is usually the first step in scientific analysis. An adequate description of the characteristics of an event often is useful in taking additional steps such as experimentation and prediction. At this stage, mostly the observable properties of the event under study are described. A researcher observing the language behaviors of a 2-year-old child may note the conditions under which specified language behaviors are produced. The observation might answer questions about the number and types of language behaviors a 2-year-old child is able to produce under specified conditions of stimulation.

Some disciplines rely heavily on naturalistic observations. Ethology, for example, is a study of the behavior of animals in their natural habitat. Ethologists typically do not manipulate the animal's natural environment to see what effects follow. Rather, the goal is to understand the relation between animal behavior and its habitat, including the animal's social milieu. Similarly, astronomy is mostly observational, not because of choice but because of necessity. Nonexperimental, observational sciences do not seek to effect changes in the phenomena they study. However, in many branches of science, mere description of a phenomenon is not sufficient for a complete scientific analysis. This is because in the case of many complex events, descriptions tell us what is happening, but not necessarily why. Therefore, a description often leads to experimentation designed to find out why the event is taking place.

In the field of communicative disorders, descriptive studies and models are emphasized. This is partly understandable because other kinds of studies, especially those designed to develop theories or find the instigating causes of speech–language disorders, have been few, mostly inadequate, and therefore frustrating. This does not mean, however, that one should stop at the level of descriptive analysis. As discussed in later chapters, experimental analysis of the causal variables of speech–language behaviors is much needed. Such an analysis makes it possible to effect changes in disordered communication.

Another significant outcome of science is typically described as **understanding** natural phenomena. One does not understand an event when one does not know what causes it. No amount of description, therefore, is sufficient to achieve an understanding of a given event. Therefore, discovery of cause–effect relations is one of the most desirable outcomes of scientific activity. Cause–effect relations are discovered through experimentation in which some presumed cause is systematically varied to see the effects.

An outcome closely related to understanding an event is **explanation.** It often is said that science seeks to explain events. In a technical sense, an explanation is the specification of a cause–effect relation. Scientists explain events by pointing to their causes. Therefore, the two outcomes—understanding and explanation—are realized simultaneously.

A thorough understanding and a valid explanation often lead to the next outcome of scientific activity: **prediction.** In most cases, a demonstrated cause of an event will help predict the occurrence of that event. Scientific predictions are reliable to the extent the explanations are valid.

A final outcome that depends on the other outcomes is **control** of natural phenomena. In most sciences, scientists can control an event when they understand its cause and predict its occurrence. Events are controlled when they are changed in some manner. An extreme change is achieved when an event's occurrence is totally prevented. Other kinds of changes are obtained when some properties of the event are altered. The event may still take place but at a reduced magnitude, duration, or intensity.

Control may be an optional outcome of science. One might understand, explain, and predict an event but be unwilling to change it. To a certain extent, an option to control an event may be a matter of social policy. For example, experimental genetics might show that it is possible to create new forms of life, but society may not wish to exert that control. On the other hand, some sciences cannot exert significant control on most of the phenomena they study even though the scientists understand them and reliably predict their occurrence. Astronomy is a significant example. The movements of planets and resulting events such as eclipses are well understood and reliably predicted, but no control is exerted on these events.

Most of the outcomes of science depend upon one thing: the specification of cause–effect relations. Much of the methodological activity in advanced sciences seeks to isolate cause–effect relations among natural phenomena. Disciplines that do not focus upon this kind of activity usually cannot achieve other outcomes such as explanation or prediction. They also are less likely to be regarded as sciences.

VARIABLES AND THEIR TYPES

The basic method of scientific investigation is empirical analysis. This means that in many cases, the phenomenon to be studied is broken down into smaller components that can be observed more easily, measured more precisely, and manipulated more successfully. Very broadly defined phenomena often are not suitable for scientific investigation, especially during the early stages of investigation. In the analysis of a phenomenon, scientists first identify some specific aspect that can be defined in a narrow and precise manner. **Variables** are narrowly defined aspects of an event that can be measured and manipulated. In this sense, a phenomenon refers to a broad event, and variables are certain aspects of it.

Variables are specific aspects of events that change. Everything that exists varies across time and conditions. In fact, much of the methodology of science has been designed to isolate and (when appropriate) to control the sources of variability in naturally occurring events. Science seeks to analyze variables; they are what the scientist observes, measures, changes, and manipulates in some way.

All natural events are a bundle of variables—physical, chemical, biological, behavioral, and other kinds of variables. Articulation, language, fluency, and voice are the four large classes of phenomena with which the field of communicative disorders is most concerned. The "normal" as well as the "deviant" aspects of these phenomena create a host of specific variables that must be measured and manipulated. The phenomenon of language is a collection of such specific variables as the production of plural *s* or two-word phrases. The phenomenon of articulation contains specific variables relating to the production of various phonemes at different levels of response topography. Similar specific variables can be identified for other aspects of communicative behaviors.

A discussion of different types of variables can be helpful in gaining a better understanding of this important concept in scientific research and theories. The most important variables include the following: dependent, independent, active, assigned, and intervening.

Dependent Variables

The technical term for an effect is **dependent variable.** In many cases, scientific analyses start with some dependent variables that are the effects of unknown causes. Confronting an effect, the scientist may try to find its cause. In other words, the dependent variable is an event or an aspect of some event that needs to be studied and explained.

Many research questions contain a dependent variable. How do children acquire *language?* What are the causes of *aphasia* or *stuttering?* Why do some children fail to learn the correct production of *speech sounds?* What is the best way of teaching *manual signs* to people who are deaf? What causes high-frequency *hearing loss?* These are some of the many questions the communicative disorders specialist typically asks and tries to answer. Thus, language, aphasia, stuttering, speech sounds, manual signs, and hearing loss are all examples of dependent variables.

As the term suggests, the existence of dependent variables is contingent on some other variables. Dependent variables are said to be a function of causal variables. In other words, effects depend on causes; therefore, no causes, no effects.

Dependent variables are typically measured and monitored by the scientist, but they are not directly manipulated. They can be manipulated only indirectly and only when their causes are known. For instance, scientists cannot directly change stuttering. They can change it only when they have access to a treatment method that reduces it. They treat disorders and teach communicative skills only by manipulating teaching or treatment methods. This is what is meant by "indirect manipulation of dependent variables." Throughout a scientific study, scientists measure the dependent variables while they manipulate other variables expected to change the dependent variables. Such measures tell the scientists whether the manipulations are affecting the dependent variables. An educator, for example, may continuously measure language skills in children who are exposed to a teaching method.

To be useful in research, dependent variables must be defined in precise terms. They must be defined **operationally,** which means that the definition must specify how the variable will be measured. Language, for example, is too broad a dependent variable to be of use in particular research studies. Typically, some specific aspect of language, such as the production of certain morphemes, phrases, or sentences, is the defined dependent variable in research studies.

Independent Variables

While the dependent variables are the effects, the **independent variables** are the causes. Independent variables often are unknown, many times presumed, and sometimes accidentally stumbled upon. When a research question aimed at discovering a cause–effect relation is effectively answered, an independent variable will have been identified. For example, when data show that language disorders are due to some form of environmental deprivation, there is both a dependent variable (language disorder) and an independent variable (environmental deprivation). Similarly, when audiological research shows that prolonged exposure to high-frequency noise (cause) produces a type of hearing loss (effect), there is an independent variable and a dependent variable. Therefore, the specification of independent variables is crucial in any type of causal analysis. In many cases, the effect (i.e., the goal or objective) of successful scientific research is the description of an independent variable. Independent variables explain dependent variables because an explanation of an event is nothing but a specification of its cause.

Independent variables are measured and directly manipulated by scientists. When manipulated, an independent variable can induce systematic changes in a dependent variable. When there is no access to the independent variable of an event, the scientist cannot induce changes in that event. In the field of communicative disorders, all teaching and treatment methods are independent variables. One can effect changes in communicative behaviors only by manipulating those methods.

There are three important kinds of independent variables in communicative disorders. The first kind of independent variable explains normal communicative behaviors in general. The potential causal variables of oral and sign language, speech, voice, and fluency fall into this category. For example, one can ask what causes fluency or what causes language or phonological acquisition. Answers to such questions explain communicative behaviors in general.

The second kind of independent variable explains disorders of communication. Why do children fail to acquire language, phonological responses, or fluency? The same questions can be rephrased in terms of the causes of language, articulation, or fluency disorders. Such questions address the causes of disorders and diseases in a clinical science. The first and second kinds of independent variables can be counterparts of each other. For example, if language acquisition is made possible by parental stimulation (whatever that means), then a disorder of language may be due to deficiencies in such stimulation.

The third kind of independent variable is treatment techniques. Treatment variables are the causes of positive change in the disorder being treated. They can help change undesirable effects (diseases or disorders). As noted before, a scientist or a clinician cannot directly affect an event. The clinician must gain access to a treatment (independent) variable to effect changes in a disorder. The treatment variable is systematically manipulated so that the effects are eliminated or modified.

Most variables can be either dependent or independent. The status of a variable depends on the frame of reference of particular studies. A given variable may be independent in one study and dependent in another. For example, in one study, a clinician may try to show that speech-related anxiety causes stuttering. In this case, anxiety is the independent variable and stuttering is the dependent variable. The investigator may hope to show that systematic increases or decreases in experimentally manipulated anxiety produce corresponding changes in the frequency of stuttering. In another study, the investigator might try to show that when stuttering is reduced, speech-related anxiety also is reduced and that when stuttering increases, anxiety also increases. In this case, stuttering is the independent variable and anxiety is the dependent variable. Similarly, hearing loss is a dependent variable when its cause is investigated, but it is an independent variable when its effect on communication or academic performance is assessed.

Active and Assigned Variables

Typically, research studies involve many variables, only some of which the researcher controls. In experimental research, the investigator controls at least one independent variable. But the investigator might suspect the existence of other potential independent variables, some of which are not manipulable or simply not manipulated. An **active variable** is a manipulated independent variable.

Other suspected independent variables that may influence the dependent variable under study may be considered assigned variables. An **assigned**

variable is a presumed or potential independent variable the investigator does not or cannot manipulate. Assigned variables that cannot be manipulated include the characteristics of participants used in research.

In research involving biological organisms (including human participants), assigned variables are thought to play an important role. The typical assigned variables include such factors as age, gender, intelligence, socioeconomic status, occupation, education, ethnic and cultural background, physical and mental health, personality characteristics, and genetic predispositions. The actual effect of an active (manipulated) independent variable may be influenced to a certain extent by one or several of these assigned variables. For example, an investigator may try to determine the effects of a parent stimulation program on the rate of normal language acquisition. In this case, the parent stimulation program is the active, manipulated, independent variable. At the same time, the rate of language acquisition may be partly determined by assigned variables such as the child's intelligence, gender, age, and undetermined genetic predispositions. Obviously, the investigator cannot control such participant characteristics. They are treated as assigned independent variables whose contribution often is inferred.

In experimental research, it is possible to rule out the influence of most assigned variables. For example, an investigator can show that the parent stimulation program works regardless of children's intelligence, gender, and socioeconomic status.

Assigned variables are most troublesome in nonexperimental research, where investigators do not manipulate independent variables and do not control the potential variables. In certain kinds of research, participants are grouped on the basis of assigned variables. Subsequently, the groups may be shown to be different on some dependent variable. Then the investigator may conclude that the differences in the dependent variable are due to the difference in the assigned variables. For instance, a sample of children may be grouped according to the children's social class while their language performance is measured. Any difference in the performance of the groups may then be attributed to the participants' social classes. In this type of research, there is no control of potential independent variables, and therefore there is no assurance that the conclusions are valid. In Chapter 4, different types of research are described and compared in greater detail.

Intervening Variables

Of all the kinds of variables researched by social, behavioral, and biological scientists, the intervening variables are the most controversial. **Intervening variables** are events or processes that are supposed to be active inside a person's body. They are informally described as "in-the-head" variables. Mind, nervous system, and cognition are among the major sources of intervening variables. These variables are thought to provide a link between observed dependent and independent variables. Such a link is considered missing when only the observed cause–effect relations are described.

The study of human behavior and particularly that of language is replete with intervening variables. The emphasis on such presumed variables as language processing, linguistic competence, internalized rules of grammar, the theory of mind, knowledge of phonologic rules, and phonological awareness that is found in the current linguistic analyses demonstrates the use of intervening variables. Cognition, for example, is an enormous collection of a variety of intervening variables. The observable, productive language behavior is thought to be impossible without cognitive inputs and information processing strategies.

The historical roots of intervening variables lie in the philosophy of mentalism. **Mentalism** asserts that observable behaviors are a product of internal, mental (psychological) processes that are not observable; according to mentalism, the unobservable mind is the source of observable actions. In due course, the nervous system, especially the brain, became more attractive as a source of action. Various kinds of processes are supposed to underlie observable actions. A popular source of action in general, and language in particular, is cognition.

Intervening variables are attractive to theorists who believe that an explanation of observable behaviors lies in unobservable events taking place in presumed entities or processes. The main problem with intervening variables is that they are simply inferred from observable behaviors, often in the absence of any kind of experimental manipulations. The most questionable practice relative to intervening variables is that processes inferred from observable behaviors are immediately offered as explanations of those behaviors. For instance, the presence of cognitive processes is inferred from certain language behaviors; in turn, cognitive processes are offered as explanations of those language behaviors. Because they are not directly measured, observed, or experimentally manipulated, the explanatory status of cognitive processes is highly questionable. What is inferred from an action cannot explain that action.

CAUSALITY AND FUNCTIONAL ANALYSIS

As noted earlier, science is essentially a search for cause–effect relations in natural events. Basic and applied scientists as well as clinicians need to gain access to causes of effects that need to be modified, controlled, or eliminated. Diseases and disorders can be treated more effectively when their causes are known. Also, as noted before, when causes are specified, events are explained.

A problem in scientific analysis of causality is that dynamic sets of complex events cause other events. Because this has been demonstrated repeatedly, a basic assumption of science is that events typically have multiple causes. Multiple causation generates methodological and analytical consequences.

Multiple Causation and Levels of Causality

A basic assumption of science is that events typically have multiple causes. Because of their complexity, most events cannot be analyzed in total or all at once. Therefore, scientists analyze them at different levels of observation. At each level of observation, a cause may be found. This results in different causes at different levels of analysis. In many cases, it also is possible to identify multiple causes at the same level of analysis. This means that causes and effects are nothing but a string of events. Depending on the temporospatial locus of analysis, an event is a cause of the succeeding effect, which is in turn a cause of the next event in the string. For instance, in a given individual, a stroke is an immediate cause of aphasia, a ruptured blood vessel in the brain may have caused the stroke, high blood pressure may have caused the rupture, and poor eating habits and genetic predisposition may have caused the high blood pressure. However, at a given level of analysis, only one causal variable may be found (e.g., stroke as the cause of aphasia).

Although experimental demonstrations are rare, it often is thought that most communicative disorders are caused by a combination of genetic, neurophysiological, and environmental factors. Therefore, speech and language disorders can be analyzed at the levels of genetic, neurophysiological, and environmental events. At each of these levels, there may be multiple causes. Theoretically, many genetic conditions, some of which may be active simultaneously, can be causally related to a given disorder. Cleft palate, for example, can be a result of several genetic, teratogenic, and toxic factors. Neurophysiological variables may be genetically determined to a certain extent, but some of them may not have a clear-cut pattern of inheritance, thus making it difficult to identify potential genetic factors in given cases. Nevertheless, at the level of neurophysiologic functioning, multiple factors may cause a given disorder. The neurophysiologic mechanism may show an inherited weakness, an injury-based (environmentally induced) deficiency, or a disease-based problem. Similarly, an environmental analysis may show deficiencies in stimulation, reinforcing contingencies, or educational practices.

When different causes of a disorder are identified at different levels of observation, the causal analysis may be shifted to a more complex level. The investigator may now analyze potential interactions between different types of causes. For instance, an initial analysis at the genetic level may show that stuttering is partly determined by a genetic predisposition. Next, an analysis at the neurophysiological level might reveal neural and muscular aberrations in persons who stutter. A further analysis at the learning and conditioning level might show that certain types of conditioning or environmental variables are also important in the etiology of stuttering. Eventually, the investigator might analyze how these three types of causal variables interact to produce the final effect (stuttering).

It must be understood that a tentative determination of a cause at a given level may not necessarily negate the importance of causes at other levels of analysis. For example, the strong possibility that there are some genetic factors in the etiology of stuttering does not rule out the presence of environmental factors. Similarly, experimental demonstration of environmental factors does not negate the importance of genetic influence. It often is believed that genetic and neurophysiological explanations of behavioral phenomena will automatically discredit explanations based on environmental or conditioning variables. However, the philosophy of multiple causation does not support this belief. For example, the evidence that stuttering is associated with a genetic predisposition does not negate the experimentally demonstrated effects of a conditioning contingency. In the future, neurological investigations may be better able to describe what happens in the brain when someone stutters, but they would not minimize the importance of experimentally demonstrated effects of reinforcement or punishment contingencies. Similarly, future neurology may be better able to describe what happens in the nervous system when a child learns the alphabet or produces the very first word. Such a description, however, could not suggest that no environmental variables are involved in that learning process. The parents and teachers would still provide certain stimulus conditions and arrange certain response consequences.

Instigating Causes Versus Maintaining Causes

Some causes create an effect and other causes maintain it. **Instigating causes** create an effect, and **maintaining causes** sustain it over time. Many disorders, including those of communication, may have been caused by one set of causes and maintained by an entirely different set of causes. Possibly, an event may be caused and maintained by the same multiple causes. However, in many cases, instigating and maintaining causes may be different. Also, instigating causes might still be working while new maintaining causes may have been added. Alternatively, regardless of how it was started, an event may be maintained by different causes at different times.

In physical and medical sciences, the maintaining causes may not always be radically different from the original or instigating causes. Theoretically, the same infection, tumor, or injury can be the original cause and the maintaining cause of a given disease. This is not to say that either the cause or the effect is static. Both are in fact dynamic. They change and produce additional effects, which become new causes of new effects. Nevertheless, physical, chemical, or topographical similarities between the instigating and maintaining causes can often be identified. In disorders of human performance or behavior, however, the instigating and the maintaining causes could be entirely different.

Several hypotheses in communicative disorders illustrate this point. For example, it may be hypothesized that parental punishment of dysfluencies causes stuttering in young children. Thus, the instigating cause of stuttering may be parental punishment. However, if stuttering continues into adult life in the absence of parental punishment, the maintaining causes are clearly different from the instigating cause. One might hypothesize that the maintaining causes are negatively reinforcing events stemming from avoidance of difficult speaking situations. In this case, the maintaining causes may be diametrically opposed to the original causes (punishment vs. reinforcement). To take another example, the speech and voice disorders of a child with cleft palate might persist even after adequate surgical repair of the cleft. This persisting disorder cannot be attributed to the nonexistent cleft. In such cases, the disorder has a different set of maintaining causes.

It is well known that searches for the causes of communicative disorders have often been frustrating. At best, such searches have led only to speculative reasoning. When parents ask such questions as, "What caused my child's stuttering?" or "What is the cause of my child's language delay?" clinicians often go into a discussion of possibilities and conjectures that have only a general relevance—relevance only to groups of persons with the disorder. But such discussions are dissatisfying to the parents, who expect an answer relevant to their specific child. It also is equally well known that in the "diagnostics" of communicative disorders, clinicians do not diagnose anything, because within the medical model, diagnosis means finding a cause or causes of a given disease. Often, this failure to find causes of communicative disorders has led to a belief that clinicians should simply be descriptive and not worry about causes.

Description is only the beginning stage of scientific analysis. There is no substitute for a causal analysis in basic or applied sciences. The frustrating searches in the field have been concerned mostly with original causes of communicative disorders, be they organic or environmental. Such causes of communicative disorders have not been understood, perhaps for several reasons. One possibility is that the original causes may be physical or chemical conditions that are unavailable for examination as long as the disorder persists. Another possibility is that even if physical or chemical conditions do cause communicative disorders, such conditions may not be enduring. Therefore, those conditions may not be present at the time of examination, which is typically done some time after the manifestation of the disorder. Still another possibility is that the causal, physical, or chemical conditions are as yet unobservable because of technical limitations. Furthermore, there may be temporary environmental causes, which also are not detected upon later examination.

More is known about the maintaining causes of communicative disorders than the instigating causes. The search for environmental maintaining causes has generally been more productive and less speculative than searches for original causes. It is known that in treating many disorders of communication, clinicians alter possible maintaining causes and teach behaviors that are incompatible with the existing faulty behaviors. For example, a clinician who ignores misarticulations while reinforcing correct productions tries to alter the factors that may have been maintaining those misarticulations. Similarly, a language clinician who withholds all attention to gestures and grunts while reinforcing meaningful vocal productions is eliminating potential maintaining factors of inappropriate behaviors. Though the instigating causes of many communicative disorders are unknown, clinicians can still treat several disorders successfully. This suggests that clinicians generally manipulate maintaining causes of appropriate and inappropriate behaviors in their clients.

It is desirable to find the original causes of diseases and disorders. A knowledge of the original causes can be useful in preventing a disorder. To reap the applied advantages of original causes, they must be experimentally demonstrated, not just inferred from the effects. However, most presumed original causes are difficult to manipulate experimentally. Johnson's hypothesis that stuttering is a result of parental negative reaction to the child's normal "nonfluency" is a case in point (Johnson & Associates, 1959). For ethical reasons, negative parental reactions are not experimentally manipulable. For example, one cannot ask parents to react negatively to the occasional dysfluencies of fluently speaking children to see if stuttering develops.

EXPERIMENT AND EXPERIMENTAL CONTROL

As noted earlier, establishing cause–effect relations is the key to understanding, explaining, predicting, and controlling natural phenomena. To establish cause–effect relations, scientists engage in various activities including observation, measurement, and data analysis. However, the most important of these activities is an experiment because it is the most powerful of the strategies available to scientists to establish cause–effect relations.

The term *experiment* often is used loosely to indicate any type of research study. The term, however, has a technical meaning in science. Not every kind of research is an experiment. An **experiment** can be technically defined as the manipulation of an independent variable or variables under controlled conditions to produce systematic changes in a dependent variable or variables. There is no experiment unless the researcher has clearly identified at least one causal factor whose influence on a dependent variable is assessed while other potential causes are controlled for.

Manipulation of an independent variable is the most important feature of an experiment. It means that the effects of a causal factor are studied by introducing or altering that factor. The typical question that prompts an experiment is, "What happens when I do this?" and in this sense, the researcher is already clear about the potential independent variable. In clinical treatment research, an independent variable is **manipulated** whenever a treatment technique is introduced, withdrawn, reversed, or varied in some systematic manner.

A treatment is *introduced* when it is first applied, *withdrawn* when it is simply discontinued, *reversed* when it is applied to some other behavior or disorder, and *varied* when its frequency or intensity is altered. When the number of treatment sessions is increased or decreased, the strength of the independent variable is altered. Within given sessions, the frequency of applications of an independent variable may be changed. The frequency of reinforcer delivery, for example, can be changed within or across treatment sessions. Manipulations of an independent variable include these and other alterations introduced by the researcher.

Another important feature of an experiment is that the independent variable is manipulated under controlled conditions. **Controlled conditions** exist when extraneous independent variables are systematically ruled out. In other words, when establishing a cause–effect relation, the researcher must ensure that other potential causes were not also involved in the experiment. When several potential causes are present, it becomes impossible to determine the cause or the causes of the effect being analyzed. Thus, the essence of an experiment is manipulation of a single independent variable which produces an effect on the dependent variable under controlled conditions.

In clinical research, experiments are the means to demonstrate that certain treatment variables were indeed effective. Through experimental manipulations, clinicians can demonstrate that changes in disorders were brought about by particular treatment variables and that those changes were unrelated to other potential treatment variables. This type of research is discussed in Chapter 4.

The cause–effect relation isolated by an experiment is known also as a **controlling relation.** Well-designed experiments help isolate a controlling relation between two variables: The cause controls the effects. Controlled conditions, however, should not be confused with controlling relations. The term **controlled conditions** refers to various procedures designed to rule out the potential causes other than the one in which the researcher is interested. In essence, controlled conditions are structures of experiments, whereas controlling relations are abstract ways in which events are related to one another.

HYPOTHESES IN SCIENTIFIC RESEARCH

Hypotheses are predicted relations between two or more variables selected for an investigation. A good hypothesis specifies a dependent variable and at least one independent variable. Therefore, all hypotheses are statements of cause–effect relations between certain variables. Because hypotheses are typically formulated prior to the actual experimentation, they are predictive statements. A hypothesis predicts that when a certain event is present, a certain other event will follow as a consequence.

Scientific hypotheses contrast with everyday guesses, predictions, and assumptions about cause–effect relations. For the most part, hypotheses of everyday life are informal, sometimes vague, and rarely expressed in measurable terms. As a result, popular hypotheses are difficult to verify. Scientific hypotheses, on the other hand, are more formal, specific, and expressed in operational (i.e., measurable) terms. Because they are stated in measurable terms, scientific hypotheses are testable. Furthermore, unlike everyday guesses, good scientific hypotheses are based on systematic observations. Ideally, scientific hypotheses tend to be verified, whereas everyday hypotheses may lead to untested beliefs.

Although hypotheses bearing no particular relation to a theory are sometimes formulated and tested, most hypotheses are derived from a theory. In fact, hypotheses are the means by which theories are tested. A complex theory may give rise to a number of hypotheses, each of which is tested independently. If most of the hypotheses are verified with positive results, then the theory is said to have received experimental support.

Need for Hypotheses: Two Views

Whether hypotheses are essential in the conduct of meaningful empirical research depends upon the investigator's research style and philosophy. Traditionally, research is equated with hypothesis testing. It often is said that scientific research starts with a hypothesis. The statistical approach to research asserts that hypotheses are essential in empirical research (Kerlinger, 1986). It is argued that hypotheses give direction to research because they suggest what to look for. It is believed that without a hypothesis, there may be nothing to investigate. It also is believed that hypothesis testing is the most important—if not the only—means of verifying scientific theories. Moreover, the hypothesis is described as "the most powerful tool man has invented to achieve dependable knowledge" (Kerlinger, 1986, p. 25).

Advocates of the usefulness of hypotheses suggest that scientists should first formulate a hypothesis and then design an experiment to test that hypothesis. Depending on the results of the experiment, the hypothesis is either retained or rejected. When a substantial number of hypotheses derived from a theory are verified and accepted, the theory is validated.

An alternative view on the usefulness of hypotheses has been suggested by the experimental analysis of behavior (Bachrach, 1969; Sidman, 1960; Skinner, 1974). This view questions the need for, and the importance of, formal hypotheses in the conduct of research. Proponents of this view suggest that it is possible to investigate important research problems without the directive of formal hypotheses (Sidman, 1960; Skinner, 1956). Newton's famous statement concerning the research process is *Hypotheses non fingo*, which means "I do not make hypotheses." Skinner has also stated that he has "never attacked a problem by constructing a Hypothesis" (1972, p. 112).

Hypotheses, as noted earlier, are proposed after a research question has been formulated. In this sense, a hypothesis is nothing but the prediction of results of a planned experiment. Skinner (1972) said that one can ask a question and immediately proceed to answer it through an experiment. He saw the intermediate step of hypothesis formulation as an unnecessary exercise. Whether predicted or not, a well-designed experiment may produce results that throw light on the relation between the variables investigated. Because the experimental results are the final test of a relation between variables, the need to predict those results beforehand is not clear. Because it is the evidence that stands, not necessarily the hypothesis, it is best to ask a question and produce results through experimentation. The results then help shape a valid statement of cause–effect relation.

There are other problems with the formulation of hypotheses prior to experimentation. If one insists that all meaningful research should start out with a well-formulated hypothesis, it is hard to imagine how unsuspected relations between variables could ever come to light. Hypothesis testing minimizes the importance of accidental discoveries. And yet, as I noted in Chapter 1, many important scientific discoveries were made accidentally. By nature, accidental discoveries are unsuspected and hence unformulated in terms of an a priori hypothesis. Often, accidental findings are noted during the course of research designed to test formal hypotheses. The history of natural sciences is replete with examples of accidental discoveries that proved to be more important than the planned research during which such accidents occurred (Bachrach, 1969).

Another problem with formal hypotheses is that they can bias the investigator. A researcher who hypothesizes that *A* is the cause of *B* fully expects to support that hypothesis by the results of his or her experiment. If not, there would be no point in proposing that hypothesis. Theoretically, negative results should lead to a prompt rejection of the hypothesis. In practice, however, some investigators may show a tendency to explain away negative results in an effort to breathe life into their dying hypotheses. There is always the possibility that the hypothesis was true but that the results did not support it because of methodological problems, but in the absence of convincing evidence of such problems, the hypothesis must be at least temporarily rejected. This may not happen because of the researcher's belief and investment in the hypothesis.

The biasing effects of formal hypotheses are recognized by those who support their use. Because the need for hypotheses is taken for granted, statisticians have offered a unique solution to the problem of bias: the null hypothesis (Fisher, 1956). The term *null* means zero, and a **null hypothesis** is a statement of no relation between two variables. It also is known as a statistical hypothesis. If using a null hypothesis, an investigator who believes that *A* is the cause of *B* would actually propose that *A* and *B* are unrelated. For example, an investigator who thinks that the parental punishment of dysfluencies in speech causes stuttering would actually state that parental punishment and stuttering are unrelated. The investigator then hopes to show that this null hypothesis is not true and that parental punishment and stuttering are indeed causally related. When a hypothesis is stated in positive terms, the investigator expects to support it, and when it is stated in the null form, the investigator expects to reject it. Nonetheless, it is presumed that an investigator who proposes a null hypothesis instead of a positive one would not be biased in the interpretation of results.

It is highly questionable whether the null is an answer to the biasing effects of hypotheses. The null is no more than a surrogate for a positive hypothesis the investigator believes in. All knowledgeable readers of research papers know that a null hypothesis really means the opposite of what is stated. An investigator's efforts are directed toward rejecting a null hypothesis just as much as supporting a positive one. Therefore, when the results fail to reject a null, the investigator may try to explain the results away—the null was not what was really believed. The null is a facade and a transparent one at that. It is hard to imagine how it can help remove or reduce the investigator's bias. For these reasons, those who do not believe in the value of formal hypotheses do not take the null seriously. Skinner stated that in his research, "the null hypothesis finds itself in the null class" (1969, p. 81).

The biases of an investigator are a fundamental problem that cannot be eliminated by statistical devices and null hypotheses. Investigators who do not state a hypothesis may still exert biases in interpreting their results. Therefore, not stating a hypothesis is not effective as a means of overcoming one's own biases regarding the outcome of research. On the other hand, an explicit statement of a hypothesis commits an investigator to a public position. It can thus create an additional pressure on the investigator to support the stated position. Typically, hypotheses are derived from already published theories for which the investigator may be well known. In such contexts, formation of hypotheses can have an especially biasing effect on the interpretation of results.

Objective interpretation of experimental results requires rigorous intellectual discipline. This discipline is a part of the scientist's disposition to value evidence more highly than his or her opinions and expectations. Artificial devices such as the null hypothesis do not solve the difficult problem of investigator bias. The solution is to train scientists who are objective and who continue to be so because of their personal history, shaped mostly by education and experience.

THEORIES AND SCIENTIFIC REASONING

It is common knowledge that scientists build theories. Probably it is no exaggeration to say that most people equate theory building with scientific research. Many philosophers of science believe that the aim of scientific research is to develop theories. Theories help individuals understand events around them. Theories are valued products of scientific investigations.

A **theory** can be defined as a set of statements concerning a functional relation between a class of independent variables and a class of dependent variables. Therefore, a theory *explains* an event. In the technical sense, a clearly specified functional relation between variables is the heart of a theory.

In a more general sense, a theory can be described as a systematic body of information concerning a phenomenon. A theory begins with a thorough description of the event or the effect to be explained. It states the conditions under which the occurrence of that event is probable. The properties of the event, such as the topography (form), frequency, magnitude, intensity, and levels of complexity also are specified. Variations in the properties and the conditions associated with specified variations are described.

After having described the event, the theory explains the event by specifying why it occurs. In other words, the causal variable or variables are specified. In essence, a theory states that Y exists because of X. Furthermore, the theory may describe limitations of the discovered causal relation. It might specify any exceptions noted during the systematic, experimental observations. Finally, a good theory clearly specifies how it can be verified; in other words, a theory specifies conditions under which the proposed cause–effect relations can be verified by other investigators.

A hypothesis can be contrasted with a theory. A theory is a more comprehensive description and explanation of a total phenomenon. A hypothesis, on the other hand, is concerned with a more specific prediction stemming from a theory. Hypotheses are testable propositions derived from a theory. It is possible, however, to propose hypotheses that are not a part of theories. In either case, the scope of a hypothesis is more limited than that of a theory. For example, a theory of language disorders might explain all kinds of language disorders found in all age groups, whereas a hypothesis might be concerned with the specific language problems of a particular group such as people with mental retardation.

Inductive and Deductive Reasoning

Logic and reasoning play an important role in designing and conducting research studies and in the formulation of theories. As a part of philosophy, logic describes formal rules of correct reasoning. Because incorrect reasoning may lead to faulty experiments as well as faulty interpretation of results, it is necessary to understand the logical basis of science and scientific experiments. The early development of the scientific method was due to philosophers' interest in logic and reasoning. In fact, many early scientists were also the philosophers, logicians, physicists, and psychologists of their times.

The philosophers recognized two important modes of logical reasoning: deductive and inductive. Deduction and induction are a part of everyday reasoning as well, but they are used in a more formal manner in scientific thinking. These modes of reasoning are especially involved in the process of constructing scientific theories. Therefore, theories themselves often are described as either inductive or deductive.

Induction is reasoning from the particular to the general. Inductive reasoning starts from an observation of particular instances of an event and eventually arrives at some general conclusions regarding the nature and causation of that event. Every time an event is observed, such factors as the precipitating conditions, intensity, magnitude, and so on are carefully recorded. Observations of this kind are made until several individual instances of the event have been observed and described.

The observed individual instances are categorized to see if some common patterns emerge. It may be determined that whenever the event occurred, certain common conditions were also present, and whenever the event failed to occur, the common conditions were absent. For example, an audiologist might observe that whenever some patients took a certain prescription drug, their hearing thresholds were temporarily elevated and whenever they were free from the drug, their thresholds were lower. It also may be observed that when certain conditions systematically vary across instances, the magnitude of the event also varies. In the audiology example, whenever the dosage increased, the hearing thresholds were higher and vice versa. Such observations could result in a collection of reliable facts about the event.

The facts gathered through observation lead to certain conclusions regarding the nature and causation of the observed event. The scientist may conclude that the events that reliably precede an effect are the cause of the effect. A simple logical rule scientists follow is that causes precede effects.

In the inductive reasoning used in modern science, observation is not limited to describing the observed event or effect. Observation also includes experimentation, without which a valid theory cannot be built. Instead of waiting for the event to occur, a scientist may create it by manipulating what is believed to be the causal factor and then withdrawing the factor to see if the event disappears. The cause–effect relations receive their maximum support when such experimental manipulations are successfully carried out. When such experiments are repeated with comparable outcome, a theory may emerge out of the data.

Inductive reasoning is the method by which people draw conclusions based on their personal experiences. We know that it is not prudent to draw conclusions based on isolated experiences regarding an event or an individual. When similar experiences accumulate, certain conclusions may be considered more appropriate. For example, a person who knows nothing about the education of speech–language pathologists might come in contact with one of them and find out that the pathologist is a college graduate. The same person may later come in contact with another clinician who also is a college graduate. In this manner, the person may meet many clinicians, each with a college degree. That person may then conclude that all speech–language pathologists are college graduates. Inductive reasoning used in theory building is a more systematic use of this process with the added feature of controlled experimentation.

Deduction is reasoning from a general rule or set of rules to particular instances. Deductive reasoning starts with what are known as logical premises that are assumed to be valid. Premises are general statements, which suggest that given their validity, certain specific statements also are true. In other words, conclusions are deduced from valid propositions. A set of assumed and deduced statements is known as a **syllogism,** which is a logical device described by the ancient philosopher Aristotle. A syllogism starts with two general statements whose validity is assumed. For example, one may state that "All speech–language pathologists have a college degree" and "Jane is a speech–language pathologist." These two statements will then serve as the basis for the deduction, or conclusion, that "Jane has a college degree." Syllogisms, as described by Aristotle, are used in modern deductive logic with very little modification. Thus, deductive reasoning begins with generalities and ends with relevant specific instances.

In building a deductive theory, a scientist first makes a series of proposals. Of course, these proposals are based on observations that suggest the existence of certain cause–effect relations. In essence, a theory may be proposed on the basis of observations. From this theory, specific predictions may be derived. Predictions suggest that if the theory is valid, certain specific results must be observed. For example, an audiologist might make a theoretical statement that noise exposure is a cause of a certain type of hearing loss. If this theory is valid, a prediction that the frequency of that kind of hearing loss in people living in quiet, remote mountain communities is lower than that in people living in noisy environments should be true. Predictions of this kind are then put to experimental test. If the results of the experiment confirm the prediction, the theory is supported. If repeated experiments confirm various predictions of the theory, then that theory is accepted as valid.

Deductive theories are more commonly proposed in physical sciences than in behavioral sciences. In behavioral sciences, many have tried to develop such theories, but few have succeeded. This is because a large body of well-established facts is needed to attempt the formulation of even a rudimentary deductive theory. Compared to behavioral sciences, physical sciences have an impressive body of accepted facts and methods of observation; that is, physical sciences have a long tradition of experimentation which has produced a more solid data base. Because of this, better deductive theories can be proposed in physical sciences than in behavioral sciences.

An investigator who uses the deductive method proposes a theory without having conducted certain crucial experiments. Therefore, the investigator takes some risk in proposing a deductive theory. The ensuing experiments may support all, some, or none of the predictions made by the theory. The investigator is then expected to revise the theory in light of the evidence gathered or abandon it altogether. Further predictions of the revised theory are then tested experimentally. Thus, continued experimentation may appropriately modify and eventually validate a deductive theory.

It is useful to compare inductive and deductive theories. Both types of theories start with certain systematic observations of a given phenomenon. Questions are then raised regarding such aspects as the nature, frequency, and magnitude of the phenomenon under investigation. The two approaches immediately diverge, however. The investigator using the deductive approach will propose a theory, whereas the one using the inductive method will proceed to experiment. In other words, within the deductive framework, questions lead to answers that need to be verified, whereas within the inductive method, questions lead to experiments, which may supply the answers. The deductive method is quick in providing an explanation but slow in verifying it. The inductive method is slow in offering an explanation, but the offered explanation tends to be based on better evidence. Much experimental work lies *ahead* of a deductive theory but *behind* an inductive theory. The inductive theorist must resist the temptation to offer a theory without evidence, and a deductive theorist must resist the tendency to avoid the difficult course of experimentation after having proposed an explanation.

Most, if not all, of the differences between the two approaches lie in the process of theory construction, not necessarily in the final product, which is a validated theory in either case. Validated deductive theories are no different from validated inductive theories. Whether one builds a deductive or an inductive theory depends upon the state of the art of the scientist's subject matter and his or her personal dispositions shaped by the history of training, education, and experience.

Generally, the inductive method is somewhat safe in disciplines that do not have widely accepted dependent variables, methods of observations and measurements, or a relatively long tradition of experimentation that has produced data of some generality. Communicative disorders is still such a discipline. Therefore, the inductive approach may be the more desirable of the two strategies. Deductive theories in communicative disorders tend to be based on meager evidence and hence more speculative than they ought to be. Besides, it takes a substantial amount of time to verify a deductive theory, and in the meantime many persons may prematurely accept it as valid.

Other dangers of deductive theories are personal. Some of those who propose deductive theories may find it harder to face negative evidence that refutes their well-known position. In such cases, instead of revising or rejecting the theory, some investigators may be more inclined to find faults with the data. A much worse situation arises when investigators propose deductive theories but fail to launch a program of research to verify their theories. This type of mistake is quite common in many fields, including communicative disorders. Some deductive theorists seem to imply that their theories are already validated, because some evidence suggested them. Such a tendency betrays a misunderstanding of the deductive process. Initial observations help develop a deductive theory, but they do not validate it. The theory is validated only when experimental tests of specific propositions deduced from that theory produce positive results. When this difficult validation process is neglected, the deductive approach becomes an excellent refuge for armchair theorists whose easy victims are colleagues who lack a sophisticated understanding of logic and science.

THEORIES AND SCIENTIFIC LAWS

Validated theories allow scientists to move on to the next stage of scientific activity: formulation of scientific laws. **Scientific laws** are relatively brief statements of replicated or repeatedly confirmed relations between events; they are mostly predictive in nature. Compared with scientific laws, which apply to a narrowly defined set of events, theories are broader in scope. Theories may still have portions that need to be verified or evidence that needs to be replicated. Scientific laws, on the other hand, are statements that have received maximum experimental support. Scientific laws are tersely written summaries of replicated evidence. Therefore, scientists are more confident in scientific laws than they are in theories.

It takes a long tradition of experimental research for a discipline to state its laws. Laws cannot be based on controversial evidence. Therefore, what is needed is agreement among scientists that similar observations lead to the same or similar results. Therefore, whether a set of statements (theories or laws) is accepted as valid depends largely on the opinion of scientists in the field. Scientific evidence is always relative because no scientist can claim that all possible observations of the phenomenon under investigation have been exhausted. Though several scientists may have repeatedly observed the same cause for a given event, there is no assurance that some other cause of the same event will not emerge in a later observation.

The relativity of scientific evidence also means that evidence suggests probabilities and not certainties. Observed cause–effect relations may be more or less probable. When different investigators repeatedly observe the same empirical relationships between certain events, the probability that the relationships are valid is increased. In essence, continued accumulation of positive evidence increases the probability that a cause of the event investigated has been isolated. The continued efforts to gather more evidence may also help identify exceptions to the commonly observed relations. Special conditions under which the generally valid cause–effect relations do not hold may become evident. This will also help the scientist refine his or her statement of the cause–effect relations. When the evidence reaches a certain point of accumulation, scientists begin to think that a theory has been validated or that a more specific statement of a scientific law can be made.

DATA AND EVIDENCE

It is clear from previous discussions in this text that theories are validated by scientific evidence. At this point, it is necessary to consider the process of developing scientific evidence. The process typically starts with the observation and collection of data. **Data** can be defined as the results of systematic observation. When a scientist observes an event and records some measured value of that event, data begin to accumulate. Scientific data are empirical in the sense that they are based upon actual happenings that resulted in some form of sensory contact. This then may lead to a more systematic measurement of the phenomenon. Such measured values constitute empirical data.

As noted earlier, a phenomenon may be observed at different levels. As a result, the data generated by observations may vary in validity and power to support theories. At the first and the lowest level of observation, an event is witnessed and described. This results in **descriptive data,** which are data in the minimal sense of the term. Descriptive data are useful in identifying the properties of an event but not in supporting a theory. Generally, descriptive data pertain to dependent variables. Although they might suggest potential independent variables, descriptive data cannot isolate such variables.

At the second level of observation, an event may be witnessed and thoroughly described, and some aspect of that event may be systematically measured. For example, one might describe *and* measure the frequency of stutterings, misarticulations, and so on. This level of observation provides the investigator with more than mere descriptive data. It generates **quantitative data.** This is an improvement over the first level of observation, but these data still cannot explain the event or support a theory.

At the third level of observation, the event is not only described and measured but also systematically manipulated. At this level, the event is brought under experimental control. To manipulate the event, the experimenter may select and apply a potential independent variable. This level of observation is comparable to clinical treatment in applied settings. A disorder, for example, is described, measured, and treated to modify it. However, such treatment or the manipulation of an independent variable may have been done with no controls; that is, the experimenter may not have taken steps to rule out other potential causes. This level of uncontrolled experimentation yields **uncontrolled data.** In such cases, the resulting data may be suggestive of a cause–effect relation, but they still cannot support a theory.

The fourth level of observation includes everything specified under the third level, plus adequate controls to rule out the influence of extraneous independent variables. For example, the investigator may show that a clinical group that received treatment improved while a second comparable group, untreated, showed no improvement. This level of controlled experimentation produces **controlled data,** which are essential for supporting a theory. Controlled data can explain an event because the cause of the event will have been isolated through controlled experimentation. For the scientific community to accept the theory, however, an additional set of observations is necessary.

The fifth and the last level of observation is probably the most time-consuming and complex because it seeks to establish the generality of controlled experimental data. Experimental data established in one setting (laboratory or clinic), with one set of participants, by a given investigator, may or may not have generality. In other words, whether the same data can be obtained by other investigators in other settings with different participants is not known. **Generality** is the wider applicability of data and methods. A theory begins to gain a wider recognition only when its generality across settings, participants, and investigators is established. **Replication** is the method of establishing generality of experimental findings; it is the repetition of an experiment in different settings, by different investigators, and with different participants. Replication yields **controlled replicated data.** Replicated data are obtained at different stages. Therefore, at any one time, there may be a greater or lesser degree of replicated data supporting a theory. Replication will be considered in greater detail in Chapter 9.

Scientific data obtained at any level of observation are objective in the sense that they are publicly verifiable. To establish the reliability of some data, different observers observing the same event must report similar values of measurement. Verified and replicated data also are known as **scientific evidence.** In essence, evidence, not mere observation, supports a theory.

SUMMARY

- Science is a certain philosophy, behavioral dispositions, and a set of methods.

- As a philosophy, science believes in determinism and empiricism. Determinism means that all events have causes. Empiricism insists that all forms of knowledge are derived through sensory experience.

- As behavioral dispositions, science is what scientists do. Scientists tend to be objective, curious, nonauthoritarian, and skeptical of explanations not supported by data.

- Science is a set of objective methods used in investigating research questions.

- The outcome of scientific activity includes description, understanding, explanation, prediction, and control of natural phenomena.

- Scientists study variables that are narrowly defined aspects of events. The types of variables include dependent, independent, active, assigned, and intervening.

  — Dependent variables are the effects under study.

  — Independent variables are the causes.

  — Active variables are manipulated independent variables.

  — Assigned variables are presumed but not manipulated independent variables.

  — Intervening variables are presumed, unobservable, "in-the-head" independent variables.

- Science believes that events have multiple causes and that different levels of analysis reveal different causes. Instigating causes start an event and maintaining causes keep it going.

- Experiment, a central concept of science, is the manipulation of independent variables under controlled conditions to produce some effects or change some independent variables.

- Hypotheses are statements about yet-to-be-verified cause–effect relations. Some researchers believe that they are essential to research and others believe that they are unnecessary.

- A theory also is a statement of cause–effect relations, but it has a larger scope than a hypothesis. Many hypotheses may be derived from a single theory.

- Theories are built either through deductive or inductive reasoning. Using deductive reasoning, a scientist first proposes a theory and then verifies it. Using inductive reasoning, the scientist first experiments, and then proposes a theory based on the results.

- Scientific laws are based on replicated evidence; hence, they are more credible than hypotheses or theories.

- Data are the results of systematic observation. Data may be descriptive, quantitative, uncontrolled, controlled, and replicated. Controlled and replicated data are evidence that support a theory.

STUDY GUIDE

1. What are some of the popular misconceptions of science?
2. What are the three terms that describe science?
3. Define determinism. Illustrate your definition with an example from communicative disorders.
4. Distinguish science from technology.
5. What subject matters have witnessed the greatest resistance to the philosophy of science?
6. What is empiricism? What is its importance to science?
7. How do you describe a scientist as a person?
8. Define objectivity.
9. What are the outcomes of scientific activity? What is an optional outcome of science?
10. What are the two disciplines mentioned in the text that do not experiment much with their subject matter? Why?

11. Give an example for each kind of variable: dependent, independent, active, assigned, and intervening.

12. Name the variables in the following statement: Five-year-old children belonging to the upper middle class are more likely to produce grammatic morphemes at 90% accuracy than are children coming from lower socioeconomic strata. Mothers of the upper middle class read more to their children, and this may be the reason why the children are advanced in their language production.

13. What are the limitations of intervening variables?

14. Select a communicative disorder and illustrate the concept of multiple causation and levels of causality.

15. Does the discovery of a genetic factor in the causation of a disorder necessarily negate the importance of environmental factors? Why or why not?

16. Give an example of an instigating cause and a maintaining cause of a particular disorder.

17. Describe the elements of an experiment. Illustrate your description with a hypothetical experiment.

18. Discuss the need for hypotheses in scientific research.

19. What is a null hypothesis? Why was it suggested?

20. Describe a theory. Find a theory in your reading of the scientific literature. Identify the elements of that theory.

21. Give your own examples of inductive and deductive reasoning in everyday life.

22. What is a syllogism? Give an example of your own.

23. How are inductive and deductive theories built?

24. Distinguish between theories and scientific laws.

25. Distinguish between data and evidence. Describe the different levels of observation that produce different kinds of data.

Chapter 4

◆◆◆◆◆◆◆◆◆◆◆◆◆◆◆◆◆◆◆◆◆◆◆◆◆◆◆◆◆◆◆◆◆◆◆

Treatment Research

- What Is Treatment Research?
- Conceptual Issues: Consequences of Treatment
- Treatment Research: Logical and Empirical Constraints
- Group Treatment Research: Randomized Clinical Trials
- Single-Subject Treatment Research: Multiple Control Conditions
- Randomized Clinical Trials Versus Single-Subject Treatment Research
- Classification of Treatment Research
- Summary
- Study Guide

reatment research, a variety of clinical research, holds special relevance for clinicians and clinical researchers. Chapter 5 describes and contrasts several types of research. But because of its importance in speech–language pathology and all clinical disciplines, treatment research is discussed separately in this chapter.

Treatment research affects professional practice more than any other form of research. The clinician accountability, evidence-based practice, treatment selection, and consumer satisfaction with services received may all depend on reliable and valid treatment research. In private practice and hospital settings, third-party payment for services also may depend on available evidence to support treatment techniques offered to clients. To receive reimbursement, clinicians may have to justify the treatment procedures offered to clients. Such justifications may be acceptable only when they are based on treatment research evidence. Finally, it is an ethical responsibility of clinical researchers to experimentally evaluate treatment procedures before recommending them to professionals. Similarly, it is the ethical responsibility of professionals to use only those techniques that have received experimental support. Therefore, it is important to understand both the conceptual and methodological issues involved in conducting and evaluating treatment research.

WHAT IS TREATMENT RESEARCH?

Treatment research is a variety of clinical research designed and carried out to establish the consequences of treatment applications. Treatment research may be uncontrolled or controlled. Each variety may be original or a replication. Replications, in turn, may be direct or systematic.

Uncontrolled treatment research is designed to document improvement in clients who receive it. Case studies that report improvement in clients who receive a given treatment illustrate this type of treatment research. Because uncontrolled treatment research does not use the experimental method, it cannot claim effectiveness for the technique (Hegde, 1998a). All clinicians, too, can document improvement without claiming effectiveness for the procedure used.

Controlled treatment research is designed to establish a cause–effect relation between a treatment procedure (independent variable) and positive changes (dependent variables) in clients who receive it. Controlled treatment research is designed to claim effectiveness for a procedure. It is carried out under controlled conditions that help rule out the influence of other (extraneous) variables that could also produce positive changes. Controlled treatment research needs an experimental design of the group or single-subject variety.

Directly replicated treatment research is designed to find out if improvement or effects documented in an uncontrolled or controlled study can be reproduced by the same investigators in their original setting with different clients. There will be no change in the treatment method, setting, or the clinicians; only new clients will define direct replications. Successful direct replications establish the reliability of previously documented improvement or effectiveness.

Systematically replicated treatment research is designed to find out if other clinicians, in other settings, using other clients, will get results comparable to those documented in uncontrolled, controlled, or directly replicated studies published by the original investigators. Systematic replications may also involve the original investigators if they change some aspect of the treatment procedure to increase its effectiveness. Others who conduct systematic replications also may modify the treatment or apply the treatment to clients who differ on some characteristics (e.g., age or gender) from the original set of clients. Successful systematic replications document both reliability and generality of improvement or effectiveness reported in earlier studies for a treatment. **Generality,** also known as external validity, refers to the extent to which a researched treatment may be recommended for general use. Issues and procedures related to generality and replication of treatment research studies are addressed further in Chapter 10.

CONCEPTUAL ISSUES: CONSEQUENCES OF TREATMENT

A treatment is offered with the expectation that it will produce certain measurable and favorable changes in clients. An ineffective treatment will produce no consequences. These changes are the consequences of treatment and may be described as *improvement, effects, effectiveness, efficacy, efficiency,* or *outcomes.* Distinction among some of these concepts is appropriate, but distinction among others may be questionable. Conceptual clarity helps scientists design treatment studies and evaluate evidence stemming from such studies. In making valid conceptual distinctions, the conditions under which a treatment was offered and the purpose for which the changes were measured must be considered (Hegde, 1998b, 2001).

Improvement

A common consequence of treatment offered in routine clinical settings is improvement in clinical conditions or skills targeted for enhancement. Improvement contrasts with effectiveness. **Improvement** is documented positive changes in client behaviors while the clients receive treatment in routine professional settings. Improvement in clinical conditions that follows routine treatment does not mean that the treatment was effective, necessary, or that the client would not have improved without the treatment. Treatment that was offered and improvement that followed are correlated events with no assurance of causation. Therefore, improvement should never be misinterpreted as effectiveness.

Under routine clinical conditions, professionals are expected to document improvement that follows treatment, not treatment effectiveness. Positive changes that document improvement will justify treatment from a clinical and social standpoint; it will enhance clinician accountability. Improvement data will convince other clinicians that the clients who receive a treatment benefited from it.

Improvement is a direct consequence of treatment offered under uncontrolled clinical conditions. Direct consequences are immediate and are contrasted with certain indirect or delayed consequences which include generalization and maintenance. Direct consequences are positive changes in the skills to which the treatment has been applied. Frequency of target skills are the most common direct measures, but the measures may be of intensity, amplitude, duration, intertrial interval, and so forth.

Treatment Effects

Treatment effects are documented positive changes in the health status, behaviors, or skills of individuals who receive intervention under controlled experimental conditions designed to demonstrate that the documented positive changes are due to the treatment itself. Controlled experimental conditions help assert that variables that could produce the same effect but were not manipulated in the experiment did not contribute to the observed effects. For instance, to show that a certain treatment is effective in teaching language skills to children, the researcher needs to demonstrate that neither the child's teachers nor parents could take credit for the positive changes in the child's language skills. In essence, then, to claim effects for a treatment, one should show a cause–effect relation between the treatment and the changes that follow.

To demonstrate a cause–effect relation between a treatment and the changes that follow, one should show that there would be no such change when the treatment is absent and that changes do appear when the treatment is present. Several experimental methods are available to demonstrate the effects of treatment and their absence. These methods are classified as group designs or single-subject designs, described respectively in Chapters 8 and 9.

Treatment effects are immediate and direct consequences of applying a treatment procedure. Direct effects should be first demonstrated before measuring such indirect consequences as generalization or maintenance. In single-subject designs, direct effects are measured continuously (see Chapter 9). In group designs, such effects are measured in pretests and posttests (see Chapter 8). In either case, direct effects of treatments are typically measured objectively. Quantitative increases in the skills taught are more easily documented than indirect changes that follow in natural environments as in the case of generalized responses. Direct effects are temporally close to the treatment offered under controlled conditions. Therefore, such effects help establish a cause–effect relation between treatment and the changes in skill levels.

Generalized Consequences

Generalized consequences of treatment are additional and indirect changes in the target behaviors or related skills (Hegde, 1998a). Clinicians hope that a client who learns certain limited skills under treatment will topographically expand them within and outside the clinic with no additional treatment. For instance, a child might expand a phrase learned in clinic into sentences and produce them at home. A client who learns to respond reliably to certain stimuli in the clinic may then give the same responses to new stimuli in natural settings. Speech learned in formal clinical situations may be produced in more natural communicative situations.

Measurement of generalized consequences is more difficult than measurement of direct consequences observed in the clinic. Limited expansions observed in the clinic are more readily measured than complex changes that take place in natural communicative situations. Such complex changes are not always obtained without additional clinical effort. For instance, the parents of a child with language disorders may have to be trained in evoking and reinforcing the clinically established skills and their expanded versions at home.

Generalized consequences, though highly desirable from a clinical standpoint, are not necessary to claim that a treatment was effective. Direct consequences observed under controlled conditions are sufficient to claim treatment effectiveness. However, generalized consequences enhance the meaningfulness of clinical services or treatment research results. Because they are more natural, more useful, more socially recognizable, generalized consequences of treatment help establish clinical validity of treatments.

It is generally difficult to claim that generalized consequences were indeed produced by an experimental treatment because of the time that typically separates them and the possibility of extraneous variables generating generalized consequences. Such consequences are at best correlated with treatment with no assurance of a cause–effect relation between the two sets of events. In essence, generalized consequences are neither necessary nor sufficient to claim treatment effectiveness.

Maintained Consequences

Maintained treatment consequences are clinically established skills that continue to be produced over time. Only the direct consequences of treatment (treatment effects or improved skills), generalized indirect consequences, or both may be maintained across time and situations. When only the direct consequences are maintained, the client will have derived somewhat limited benefit from treatment. When both the direct and generalized consequences are maintained, the treatment will have produced more meaningful, long-term, and presumably more satisfying results for the clients. Maintained consequences imply that the treatment offered was socially and personally meaningful; thus they establish the clinical validity of treatments offered.

Although important and highly desirable, durability of direct effects of treatment does not mean that the treatment was indeed effective. Maintained skills are no basis to claim a cause–effect relation between treatment and the skills maintained. Whether the treatment was offered under controlled conditions or in routine clinical situations is of no consequence. At best, maintained consequences, along with generalized consequences, may be correlated with treatment with no assurance of causation. One will have to assume that if treatment consequences were maintained, some lasting independent variables in the natural environment have gained control over the dependent variables (skills and behaviors). In other words, the time that lapses between treatment and maintained consequences will offer plenty of opportunities for other variables to come into play. Only additional experimental analysis, if successful, can help establish that maintained consequences are due to treatment. Unfortunately, it is impractical to sustain an extended experimental analysis in the natural environment. In essence, then, maintained consequences, like generalized consequences, are neither necessary nor sufficient to claim effects for a treatment procedure.

Treatment Outcomes

In recent years, treatment outcomes have gained much professional attention in education and health care. Currently popular and often market-driven outcomes research in health-care professions raises important issues of both scientific and professional value. Treatment outcomes are currently of great concern to service providers and those who financially support those services. Unfortunately, there is a danger that outcomes will be confused with effects of treatments. Should there be such a confusion, outcomes research will replace or diminish the treatment efficacy research. Several sources do not make a distinction between the methods of efficacy research and those of outcomes research (Kendall, Flannnery-Schroeder, & Norton-Ford, 1999; Smith & Sechrest, 1998; Yates, 1998). A clear distinction between treatment effects and treatment outcomes is necessary to maintain the integrity of both kinds of research.

Treatment outcomes are generalized, maintained, indirect, and clinically valid consequences of treatment with no assurance that treatment caused them. Outcomes are essentially an extended notion of improvement because they are not established through controlled experiments. Careful documentation of outcomes will help justify treatment and its cost to society. Professionals gain credibility when outcomes of their services are socially acceptable. The goals of outcomes research are often described as (a) finding out what works and what does not; (b) documenting functional status of clients; (c) forming general health perceptions; (d) documenting overall quality of life; (e) assessing service quality with a view to improve it; (f) assessing consumer satisfaction with services, and so forth (Frattali, 1998; Hicks, 1998; Robertson & Colburn, 1997). Most of these goals are addressed through clinical measurement of dependent variables, not through experimentation.

Unfortunately, outcomes research rarely finds out what works and what does not. Outcomes research is not treatment effects research. That there might be a confusion between experimentally established treatment effects and nonexperimentally (clinically) measured outcomes is evident in certain definitions and descriptions of outcomes. For instance, Donabedian (1980) defined outcome as "a *change* in the current and future health status *that can be attributed* to antecedent health care" [italics added] (p. 82). The phrase *attributed to antecedent health care* suggests that outcomes are the effects of treatment. Outcomes, however, are not the same as effects for two reasons. First, only an experimentally demonstrated effect can be attributed to its manipulated cause. Second, outcomes are clinical measures of extended improvement with no experimental manipulations. So far, outcomes research has not used experimental methods, and it is unlikely that it will to any great extent. Like generalized and maintained consequences, outcomes may at best be correlated with treatment. Therefore, outcomes and effects should be defined differently.

Systematic documentation of socially and personally meaningful changes in a client's health status, functional communication or other skills, satisfaction with services, general well-being, and so forth are highly desirable. Nonetheless, outcomes research rarely has asked: What techniques produce acceptable outcomes under controlled conditions? It typically asks: Are acceptable outcomes of routine clinical services documented? Outcomes research data are meaningful only if it is first established that the treatments used are effective. Outcomes in the absence of such controlled efficacy data are ambiguous and may be unrelated to treatment.

An important aspect of good treatment outcomes is that to obtain them, one should select personally and socially meaningful targets for intervention. A child with a language disorder, for example, may be taught either language skills unrelated to academic success or those that are closely related. Carefully selecting language skills that increase the child's chances of academic success is likely to produce functional outcomes of treatment for that child. Similarly, a patient with aphasia who experiences naming problems may be taught the names of family members, pets, and medications, or some names of objects not relevant to his or her living environment. The two sets of target behaviors will produce different outcomes for the patient.

In essence, then, outcomes are a composite notion of expanded improvement that includes meaningful target behaviors selected for intervention, generalized and expanded production of clinically established target behaviors, and maintenance of those behaviors over time. All aspects of outcomes are measured under uncontrolled conditions.

Validity and Generality of Treatment Research Data

For a treatment technique to be recommended for general practice, research data should exhibit internal validity, statistical (inferential) generality, clinical generality, and clinical validity. **Internal validity** is the degree of assurance that the treatment was the cause of positive changes observed in clients under controlled experimental conditions. The higher the internal validity of an experimental treatment study, the greater the level of confidence with which one can accept that the treatment (and no other factor) caused the noted changes. Internal validity is achieved by using an experimental design that helps rule out extraneous variables. See Chapter 7 for a further discussion of internal validity and the factors that negatively affect it.

Generality, also known as external validity, is the degree to which the results of a treatment research study may be extended to other people who need the same treatment but did not participate in the study. There are different types of generality subsumed under two major types: statistical and clinical. A related concept that has some consequences for generality is called clinical validity.

Statistical generality is the extension of a study's conclusions to all individuals in a population when an investigator draws a random sample from that population and then randomly assigns individuals to different groups of an experiment. It should be noted that statistical generality is treated here as a special case of external validity. As such, generality or external validity should not be equated with statistical generality because generality also includes nonstatistical types of generalities (e.g., logical generality).

Group experimental designs are claimed to have statistical generality. The claim is acceptable only if (a) a representative sample of participants was randomly selected from a population, (b) most, if not all, of the randomly selected participants agreed to participation, (c) the selected participants were then randomly assigned to the different groups of the study (e.g., experimental and control), and (d) randomly selected and assigned participants completed their study participation without significant drop-out. If these conditions are met, a group treatment researcher may conclude that all those people in the population who have not participated in the study also will benefit from the treatment. Unfortunately, no randomized treatment studies fulfill these conditions. Even in randomized clinical trials, the participants are self-selected, not randomly selected. Therefore, statistical validity of randomized treatment studies is a cherished, but rarely (if ever) attained goal.

Another problem with statistical generality is that under ideal conditions, the results of a study may be extended to the population as a whole, but not to any individual. Statistical generality allows a clinician to make general, quantitative statements about treatment effects on a large number of individuals. For instance, based on statistical generality, one might make the statement that a given treatment may be effective to a certain extent or may be effective in a certain percentage of clients who receive it. The same generality will not allow a clinician to say that a given client will or will not benefit from treatment. This is because statistical generality is a one-way street: it goes only from a large, randomly selected and assigned sample to still larger population. It does not go from the sample to one or more individuals. Practitioners, though, are typically pressed for an answer in relation to a given individual. While it is helpful to know that a majority of people who receive a given treatment will benefit, a particular client or the family may want to know whether the client will or will not benefit from the treatment. Statistical generality is of no help in answering that question. Clinicians who wish to respond to individuals who ask questions about treatment effects in their particular case will have to look for logical generality. See Chapter 7 for more on statistical generality.

Clinical generality, the other main type of generality, is especially relevant to treatment research. **Clinical generality** is the extent to which the conclusions of a study may be generalized to other clinical parameters. Several clinical parameters are important in clinical generality. These include different clients, settings, experimenters, and response classes. In essence, practitioners need to know if a researched treatment will yield the same or similar effects in different settings when applied by different clinicians to different clients or different kinds of clinical problems. See Chapter 7 for details on these different types of clinical generality.

In generalizing the conclusions of a treatment study to other clients, logical generality is important. **Logical generality** is the extent to which the conclusions of a treatment-effects study may be extended to individual clients. A type of clinical generality, logical generality is the strong suit of single-subject designs that give good descriptions of individuals who served in a treatment study. In other words, single-subject designs give profiles of participants. Practitioners can match the profile of a study participant to a given client. If the profile of a client matches the profile of the client who benefited from a treatment, then the practitioner can assume that the treatment may be effective with his or her client as well. If the profile of a client matches that of a participant in a study who did not improve, then the practitioner may refrain from extending the technique to that client. Such differential application of a treatment procedure is not possible with statistical generality. Logical generality, too, is a one-way street; it goes in the direction that is opposite to statistical generality. The conclusions can only be extended from a single-subject design to individual clients, not to the population of clients.

Clinical validity, a concept related to clinical generality, is the degree to which the consequences of a treatment are socially and personally meaningful. To be meaningful, the consequences of a treatment should enhance the quality of life, which may mean changes in different aspects of life, depending on the nature of treatment and the condition for which the treatment was offered. Clinically valid medical treatments should reduce the death rate, enhance the overall quality of life, improve the health status, instill a sense of well being, or increase the level of physical activity. Just a reduction in symptoms may not assure clinical validity of treatments. In communicative disorders, clinical validity is assured when the clients who receive treatment show significant gains in social interaction, personal and occupational communication, improved academic performance in the case of children, and so forth. Here too, just a reduction of symptoms—for instance, a reduction in stuttering in the clinical situation—may not assure clinical validity of a stuttering treatment. One might also insist that, for the treatment to have clinical validity, the treatment gains should be sustained over time and across situations. In other words, generalized and maintained consequences also may help justify clinical validity of treatment procedures.

Sometimes, broad and meaningful consequences of treatments are referred to as *clinically significant changes* (in contrast with *statistically significant changes*), but clinical validity is not always statistically based. Internal validity, statistical generality, and clinical generality do not automatically assure clinical validity. For instance, it is sufficient to show that a treatment effectively reduced stuttering under controlled experimental conditions to claim internal validity for the method. However, if the resulting fluency did not generalize to natural settings; was not maintained over time; and did not cause positive changes in the person's social, academic, personal, or occupational life, then the technique did not have clinical validity. When a treatment's effect is replicated with other clients in other settings, generalized to nonclinical settings, and maintained over time, external validity may be assured, but still clinical validity may be in doubt. For instance, a child with limited language skills may be taught to produce certain nonfunctional words that may then be produced in natural settings and maintained over time, but this newly acquired skill may not result in improved academic performance and social interaction, thus negating clinical validity. Therefore, to be totally successful, a treatment method should not only have internal validity, but also clinical validity.

All kinds of generality are achieved through replications of the original study to show that the results apply in different settings, to different people, and when the method is used by different clinicians. To achieve an acceptable degree of internal and external validity, researchers should rule out certain factors that negatively affect them. These factors are described in Chapter 7.

Treatment Efficacy Versus Effectiveness

There is a distinction sometimes made between treatment efficacy and effectiveness. Those who make this distinction define *efficacy* as the effect realized under ideal conditions of a treatment given in controlled experiments and *effectiveness* as the actual effect realized in the real-world experiments that are not as well controlled (Agency for Health Care Policy and Research, 1994; Hoagwood, Hibbs, Brent, & Jensen, 1995; Kendall & Norton-Ford, 1982). The distinction implies that when a treatment study's controls are good, the result is efficacy and when they are poor, the result is effectiveness. This is an artificial distinction that does not have conceptual or methodological consequences. If real-world experiments do not produce as good an effect as those observed in better controlled and perhaps laboratory-based treatments, then the difference obviously is due methodological deficiencies of the real-world experiments. It is better to analyze reasons for failure to obtain the same results as those found in better controlled results. Giving the results of poorly controlled studies a euphemistic name (such as effectiveness) will not help clarify the problems and will not encourage efforts to solve them. To compound the problem, the term *effectiveness* has always meant that a cause–effect relation is established with reasonable degree of certainty. Furthermore, experimental control is not categorical; it is a matter of degree. Few if any laboratory studies are so perfect as to deserve a different term for the effects they document. If the real-world clinical experiments are so poorly designed as to require a new name for their effects, then their effects probably are not trustworthy. Therefore, in this book, the terms *effectiveness* and *efficacy* are used synonymously.

TREATMENT RESEARCH: LOGICAL AND EMPIRICAL CONSTRAINTS

The goal of treatment research may be to (a) describe client improvement; (b) measure generalization of clinically established behaviors and their expansions; (c) record maintenance of clinically established behaviors and their expansions; (d) describe functional outcomes of treatment; (e) establish effects of specific treatment procedures; (f) document generality through direct replication of previous findings on treatment techniques; and (g) document generality through systematic replication of previous findings.

Of the various goals of treatment research, the one that seeks to establish the effects of a given treatment is perhaps the most important. All other goals, including improvement, generalization, maintenance, functional outcomes, and generality through replications can be more confidently pursued only after establishing the effect of a treatment. If a treatment's effects are unknown, then other goals, when realized, remain ambiguous. For instance, when a treatment whose effects have not been experimentally established is associated with improvement, generalization, maintenance, or functional outcomes, one would not know whether to attribute such consequences to treatment or to some other variable that could also produce those consequences. Therefore, while other goals are clinically important and socially valuable, treatment effects need to be established to meaningfully interpret other consequences that follow the treatment's routine application.

It is generally agreed that a treatment's effects may be established only through controlled experimentation. Technically, a controlled experiment establishes a cause–effect relation between two variables. Clinically, a controlled treatment experiment demonstrates that the clients actually needed the treatment and that without treatment, they would not have improved. This demonstration justifies treatment, its cost, and the effort involved in offering it and getting it.

There are two major approaches to conducting controlled experimentation in treatment research: the group design approach (described in Chapter 8) and the single-subject approach (described in Chapter 9). Both design strategies help establish that (a) treatment was the cause of changes in the clients, (b) no other variable was responsible for the changes, and (c) the clients would not have improved without it. In establishing treatment effects, researchers in both design approaches adhere to certain logical constraints and create certain empirical conditions.

Logical Constraints and Empirical Conditions Necessary To Claim Treatment Effects

While a researcher is busy showing that a treatment is the cause of changes in the clients who received it, many other factors may quietly contribute to the change. When this happens, the claim that treatment is the sole cause of the effects is invalid. To convince others that the treatment alone produced the changes, the researcher must arrange experimental conditions such that other potential factors cannot account for the changes documented in the clients. This action is typically referred to as *ruling out extraneous variables*. Extraneous variables are not ineffective variables; they are potent variables that could produce the same effect the treatment could or did produce. They are extraneous only to the purpose of the experiment, which was to show that a treatment alone produced the effect.

A researcher, for example, may use a new technique to teach language skills to children with autism. The researcher may establish initial baselines or pretest scores to show that the children did not produce the language skills targeted for intervention. The researcher may then teach the new language skills with the treatment. After a period of teaching, the researcher may measure the targeted language skills in probes or posttests. Observing that the probe or posttest scores are higher than the baselines or pretest scores of the children, the researcher concludes that the treatment was effective. A critic may point out that the study did not produce evidence for the treatment's effectiveness because the researcher did not rule out extraneous variables.

For example, the critic may point out that the study only showed that the children's language skills improved under the teaching method, but why they improved is not clear. The documented improvement may or may not be due to the treatment. The language skills of the children probably would have improved without treatment, because many children's language skills naturally improve as they grow older. (This is known as the maturation factor, discussed in Chapter 7.) The language skills probably improved because the parents began a home language stimulation program after the child was assessed and the parents were counseled. The language skills may have improved because of the special education teacher's efforts in the classroom. Perhaps the siblings, too, may have played some role in stimulating language skills in the children with autism. These are examples of extraneous variables; they could produce the same effect as the language treatment procedure. But the researcher's claim concerned only the language treatment, not these extraneous variables. Therefore, the critic will contend that the study did not produce evidence for the treatment's effectiveness. More technically, the critic may contend that the researcher's study did not have *internal validity;* in other words, the researcher did not rule out extraneous variables and hence did not convince others that the treatment alone produced the language changes. The critic will remind the researcher that the study was an uncontrolled case study and did not have the power to establish a cause–effect relationship between the treatment and the language changes in the children.

Ruling out extraneous variables is a logical, not exclusively a methodological, matter. Methodologically, the researcher cannot (a) prevent maturation in children, (b) convince parents not to stimulate language in their children, (c) ask teachers not to do anything with language skills, and (d) refrain siblings from engaging in social communication. Therefore, ruling out extraneous variables does not mean that the variables were removed or minimized. Instead, the researcher arranges some empirical conditions such that the extraneous variables play their usual role, but nonetheless the changes are demonstrated to be the effect of a treatment. Once the correct empirical conditions of an experiment are created, the conclusion that the treatment alone was effective is a logical exercise.

Empirical conditions of an experiment that are necessary to make a logical claim of causation may be illustrated with an example of experimental group research design. In a group design, for instance, the investigator may draw a random sample (a smaller number) of clients or students from a defined population (e.g., all children with autism living in a certain geographic area). The children may then be randomly assigned to either the experimental group or the control group. The treatment to be evaluated will then be offered to only the children in the experimental group. If positive changes occur only in the experimental group children, the researcher may claim that the treatment was effective because the extraneous variables were ruled out. Once again, this is done on a logical basis, by pointing out that (a) if maturation were to be responsible, the language skills of children in the control group would also have improved, but they did not; (b) if the parents' language stimulation were to be responsible, randomly selected parents in the two groups would have stimulated language equally in their children, but again, children in the control group did not gain in their language skills; (c) if teachers' work were to be responsible for improved language skills in the experimental group, skills in the control-group children should have also improved because the children in the two groups attended similar or similarly diverse schools; and finally, (d) if improvement in language skills of the experimental group was due to the siblings' language interactions, then the skills in the control group should have improved, because they had similar sibling interactions. A single-subject design study may rule out extraneous variables just as effectively, albeit with different experimental conditions (see Chapter 9). Note again that these are logically based conclusions that the treatment was the cause of the effect (improved language skills) even though the extraneous variables were not methodologically removed or diminished.

Although there are many complications, the basic logic of causation is simple. Logically to claim a cause–effect relationship, certain conditions must be met. For instance, (a) causes precede effects, and effects follow causes; (b) causes and effects cannot be the same events, so they have to be different; (c) causes and effects are temporally separated, so they cannot co-occur in such a way as to be confused; (d) causes are typically multiple, which means that most events are caused by several factors; (e) among multiple causes, some may be sufficient to produce an effect, which means that when they are present, effects are present and no other factor needs to render a helping hand; and (f) causes may be necessary but not sufficient, which means that without them the effects will not appear, but unless some other factors also are present, their presence will not automatically result in the effect (Clatterbaugh, 1999; Heise, 1975; Rothman & Greenland, 1998a; Ruben, 1990; F. Wilson, 1985).

In scientific experiments, a cause is called an independent variable and the effect a dependent variable. An experiment is a means to show that an independent variable (e.g., treatment) is the cause of a dependent variable (e.g., changes in the skill level, health status, symptom reduction). An independent variable is experimentally manipulated to show corresponding changes in the dependent variable. In clinical terms, a treatment is introduced, withheld, withdrawn, reintroduced, and so forth to show changes in the skill or health status. Depending on the results of such experimental manipulations, an investigator may conclude that an independent variable is indeed a cause if (a) the effect appears when the independent variable is introduced, and (b) the effect disappears when the independent variable is withdrawn or withheld (Clatterbaugh, 1999; Heise, 1975; Rothman & Greenland, 1998a; Ruben, 1990; F. Wilson, 1985). When systematic manipulations of treatment in a controlled experiment are followed by predictable changes in the dependent variable, extraneous variables will have been ruled out.

GROUP TREATMENT RESEARCH: RANDOMIZED CLINICAL TRIALS

Controlled experiments may include an experimental group that receives treatment and consequently changes, and a control group that does not receive treatment and does not change significantly; this is generally known as the group design approach to treatment evaluation.

This section gives an overview of some methodological aspects of treatment research involving groups of participants. Chapter 8 describes specific designs this approach offers.

Random Selection of Participants for Clinical Trials

The group design approach offers several specific designs to evaluate treatment effects (see Chapter 8 for details). Among these designs, the classic pretest–posttest control group design is the most frequently used experimental design to establish treatment effects. In clinical literature, especially in medicine, studies that purport to use the pretest–posttest control group design are typically called *randomized clinical trials* (RCTs). However, RCTs do not precisely adhere to the requirements of the pretest–posttest control group design; therefore, it is more appropriate to say that RCTs are loosely based on the pretest–posttest control group design.

Randomized clinical trials are experimental treatment efficacy studies in which selected individuals of similar characteristics are divided into two or more groups, one of which may receive no treatment or a placebo, or all of which may receive a different treatment. The purpose of RCTs is to establish the absolute effect of a treatment offered to one group compared with a control group (which receives a placebo or does not receive any treatment), or to determine the relative effects of multiple treatments when all groups receive a specific treatment. A clinical trial is the same as a controlled treatment experiment. The term *randomized* refers to the procedure an investigator uses to select participants and form different groups to evaluate one or more treatments.

It is generally believed that in 1948, Sir Austin Bradford Hill reported the first prototype of an RCT in *The British Medical Journal* (Randal, 1998; Silverman & Altman, 1996). Hill assessed the effects of streptomycin on pulmonary tuberculosis in patients randomly selected across several hospitals in England. This study was also the first in which the investigators (who read chest X-rays to evaluate the effects of treatment) were blinded; that is, they did not know who had the treatment and who did not. In subsequent decades, RCTs became the established method to experimentally assess medical treatment effects.

In RCTs, the concept and the technique of randomization are important and related to participant selection. There are two issues in participant selection. First, when a treatment is compared with a no-treatment control group (or placebo) or one treatment is compared against other treatments, the individuals in the two or more groups should be similar; if not, the conclusions will not be valid. Second, when a treatment study is completed, the group design researcher's aim is to claim statistical generality. To accomplish these two goals, the researchers must draw random samples that represent the larger population.

A **sample** is a smaller number of individuals who represent a larger population of individuals with defined characteristics relevant to a study. The results of a study can be extended to the larger population only when the sample represents the population. A **population** is a large number of individuals with defined characteristics from which a representative sample is drawn. For instance, a population may be defined as all children who stutter in Grades K–12 in California public schools. Another population may be defined as all those who have experienced a stroke in a given calendar year in the United States. Populations may be defined more or less narrowly. Researchers may define limited regional populations and large national populations (e.g., all voting-age persons in the United States). It should be noted that random selection is not haphazard. It is an unbiased method of selecting participants. The different methods of random selection that are available vary from the ideal to the most compromised. The ideal may be difficult to achieve, but the most compromised will not serve any purpose.

Probability Sampling

The ideal random method of participant selection is called **probability sampling,** which is a method in which the participant selection is unbiased, all members of the defined population are available and willing to participate in the study, and each member of the population has an equal chance of being included in the sample. There are several variations of probability sampling. The best of the probability sampling methods is **simple random sampling,** in which a required number of participants are selected by such unbiased methods as a lottery. Unfortunately, simple random sampling is rarely achieved in experimental research.

In clinical treatment research, simple random sampling is particularly impractical because entire populations of clients and patients are rarely identified. Even when practical, simple random sampling begins not with the defined population, but only with an accessible population. For instance, in an aphasia treatment study, not all patients with aphasia living in a state or even a city may be accessible. Only those who have sought clinical services may be accessible. This already represents a compromise in probability sampling because those who are not seeking services are excluded.

Nevertheless, once the accessible population is identified, the required number of participants may be drawn randomly by using published tables of random numbers or by the common lottery method.

Systematic sampling is another probability random selection procedure in which the selection is made with a specified sampling interval. In this method, 1 in K (K standing for a specific number) will be selected to achieve the total sample. For instance, in selecting 200 clients from a list of 2,000 in an accessible population, the researcher might select every 10th person on the list. Systematic sampling is more convenient than simple random sampling. It might serve the purpose of obtaining a representative sample well if the list of accessible persons in the population is complete, unbiased, and all selected individuals participate in the study.

Stratified random sampling, yet another practical method of probability sampling, is a method in which the population is first divided into groups according to unique characteristics, and the required number of participants is selected from each group. Groups that contain homogeneous individuals with common characteristics are called **strata.** Typical strata that are used in clinical research include patients from different socioeconomic classes, educational backgrounds, disorder or disease severity levels, and so forth. Essentially, any factor that might influence the treatment outcome may be a stratum. Populations typically contain several of these strata, and just as typically, the proportion of individuals within a given strata varies. For instance, people living in a given geographic area may include persons who are more rich than poor, more highly educated than undereducated, more single than married, or more belonging to one ethnic group than another. When this is the case, the researcher will draw a **proportional stratified sample,** in which the number of selected individuals from a given stratum will reflect the size of that stratum. The larger the stratum, the greater the number of participants selected. Within each stratum, participants are selected randomly.

Cluster sampling, a variation of probability sampling, is a method in which the required number of participants is sampled in stages, each stage being identified as a cluster and serving as a sampling unit. Cluster sampling is sometimes referred to as *multistage sampling* because the sampling units are drawn from successive stages. For example, an investigator may wish to draw a national random sample of children with language disorders in the elementary grades. The investigator might initially decide that she will draw a sample of students from 10 U.S. states that roughly represents children in all the states. In Stage 1 cluster sampling, the investigator will randomly draw 10 U.S. states from the list of 50 states. The randomly drawn states form the initial cluster. In Stage 2, she will randomly draw a certain number of school districts, say 10, to form the second cluster. In Stage 3, she will draw a random sample of five schools from each district, resulting in the third cluster. She will then select children with language disorders in each of the 5 schools. The children are the final sampling unit, and the investigator reached them by successive and progressively smaller clusters.

Cluster sampling is more manageable than simple probability sampling, especially when one is dealing with a large population with defined characteristics. Unfortunately, the more manageable the sample, the less accurate it might be in representing the total population.

Nonprobability Sampling

Even more practical than some of the variations of simple random (probability) sampling is nonprobability sampling. Strictly speaking, **nonprobability sampling** is a compromised nonrandom sampling with no assurance that the sample represents the population. By definition, nonrandom samples cannot fulfill the mathematical requirement of the probability theory on which random samples are based. In nonprobability sampling, all individuals of specified characteristics in the population are not identified and all do not have the same chance of being included in the sample. As with probability sampling, nonprobability sampling allows various techniques, some better than others.

Convenience sampling is a variety of nonprobability sampling in which participants are selected simply because they were available. Also known as *accidental sampling*, convenience sampling is often used in clinical treatment research. Patients who are seeking clinical services, students in regular or special education classes, and college students enrolled in courses are all groups of typical participants in many kinds of experiments. Such groups are selected because they are available, not because they represent a population.

Consecutive sampling, a variety of convenience sampling often used in clinical research, is the recruitment of participants as they become available over a period of time. For example, patients who seek treatment in a medical facility may be recruited to participate in a new drug treatment evaluation study. The required number of patients may be recruited over a period of time, not all at once as in probability sampling. This type of sampling is frequently used in medical treatment research. Researchers may continue to sample patients for a treatment study over a period of months or even years. Patients who seek clinical services during such extended times may be screened, and those who meet the selection criteria may be included in the study.

Note that participants selected because of convenience are self-selected, not randomly or objectively selected. **Self-selection** means that the participants are selected by themselves to a study, not by the investigator using some unbiased method such as the simple random selection. Until multiple systematic replications of the study are completed, the results of a study that involved self-selection cannot be extended to others who did not participate in the study. Self-selection, however, may be a factor in all samples, including simple random samples drawn for clinical treatment research. This is because drawing a simple random set of individuals for a treatment study is not the same as having them in the study until its completion. Many patients who are randomly selected refuse participation or drop out of a study. Eventually, those who accept the new treatment will all have been self-selected.

Quota sampling, a method similar to stratified sampling, requires the investigator to select a fixed number of people belonging to different categories in the population. For instance, an aphasia treatment researcher may select 5 persons in their 50s, 10 persons in their 60s, and 20 in their 70s to reflect the increasing number of older individuals who suffer strokes and other conditions that cause aphasia. This method is an improvement over purely convenient sampling in which selected individuals may not be as diverse and may be much less representative of the population; in the example of aphasia, a convenient sample may consist mostly of 70-year-old patients because of the possibility that relatively more from this age group seek treatment.

Snowball sampling—a nonprobability sampling common in clinical treatment research—is a practical method in which participants themselves find other participants in a chain referral manner. Each or most of a small number of persons initially selected may find other participants in a snowballing fashion until the required number of participants is found and recruited. Also known as *reputational sampling,* this method is useful when the researcher cannot find individuals with specified characteristics and depends on patients to spread the word among their friends, colleagues, and relatives and make referrals to the investigators. The investigator will screen the referred persons to see if they meet the study's selection criteria. This technique may not be productive in clinical research involving diseases or disorders of low frequency, but the method may be effective in recruiting individuals from some hidden populations (e.g., drug addicts, gay or lesbian people in certain communities). This method also may be used in some genetic research, where an initially selected client helps recruit a family member who has the same disorder who then starts a snowball effect to recruit others.

Purposive sampling is a nonprobability method of handpicking individuals because they have special characteristics that are necessary for the purpose of the study. Note that in all sampling techniques, including probability sampling (simple random sampling), participants meet certain criteria because the population itself is defined in terms of those criteria (e.g., all 70-year-old individuals who have had a stroke in the past 3 months). Still, the individuals are not handpicked, not even in the convenient sampling method (although convenient and purposive sampling techniques are similar). Purposive sampling, in some of its applications, may be similar to snowball sampling, too. But the hallmark of purposive sampling is an effort to find individuals with narrowly defined characteristics.

Purposive sampling is useful in general clinical and treatment research. For instance, a clinician may design a child language stimulation program that parents conduct at home. In this case, the clinician's goal is to find out if (a) the parents may be adequately trained to implement the program at home, and (b) when the program is implemented, whether the children's language skills increase. The clinician may reason that for the initial study, he needs mothers or fathers with college degrees who can devote the required amount of time to get trained and then implement the program at home. A convenient sample of parents whose children attend the clinic may not give the kinds of parents the researcher is looking for. A simple random sample, even if practical, may yield too many parents who do not qualify. Therefore, purposive sampling may be the best choice. To handpick parents for the study, the clinician may check the case histories of children with language disorders and interview available parents; obtain information on their education, occupation, and available free time; and judge their level of sophistication, motivation, commitment, and so forth.

Purposive sampling typically sacrifices generality while gaining specificity. A researcher who wishes to generalize results to others in the population will not use purposive sampling. Once a study shows an effect for a procedure with a purposive sample, subsequent studies can use more representative samples to establish the generality of findings.

Random Assignment of Participants

Within the group design approach, participants randomly selected from a population are randomly assigned to either the experimental group (or groups) or the control group. **Random assignment** is an unbiased method of forming the experimental and control groups and based on the mathematical assumption that each participant has the same probability of being included in any of the groups to be formed for a study. For instance, in a study that involves two groups—a control group and an experimental group—all randomly selected participants have the same chance of being selected to the control group or the experimental group. If two treatments are offered in a study, all participants have the same chance of getting either Treatment 1 or Treatment 2. If the participants were matched, one in each matched pair will be randomly assigned to the experimental group and the other will be assigned to the control group. Random assignment of participants eliminates any investigator bias that might influence who gets treatment, who gets which treatment, or who does not get any treatment.

Random assignment assures **sampling equivalency,** which is the similarity of participants across groups formed for a study. Sampling equivalency is important because the group design approach is based on the assumptions that (a) the people in the groups were similar to begin with; (b) the presence of treatment in the experimental group was the only difference the investigator created; and therefore, (c) any difference in the group performance observed at the end of the experiment must be due only to the treatment offered to one group. Random assignment helps validate these assumptions.

It is important to note that random selection and assignment serve different purposes. Random selection assures that the sample is representative of the population from which it was drawn. Therefore, the investigator can extend the conclusion of the study to the population. Random assignment, on the other hand, assures that the two or more groups of a study were equal to begin with. Therefore, the investigator can conclude that any changes observed in the experimental group should be due to the independent variable that was absent in the control group.

In most studies on medical, behavioral, or educational methods of treatment or teaching, random assignment is possible, although true random selection is not. Nonetheless, random assignment may not always eliminate bias, even when the investigator's bias has been eliminated. There are several other sources of bias that may negatively affect the results of a study. First, randomly assigned participants may or may not stay in their assigned groups until the end of the experiment. Different kinds of participants may differentially drop out of the experimental and control groups; that is, those who dropped out may be different kinds of participants than those who stayed in the study. For instance, participants with greater severity of the problem under investigation may drop out of the experimental group, creating the possibility that the treatment will look better than it actually is. Second, some participants assigned to a traditional treatment may refuse that treatment and demand that they receive the new treatment being offered to others. Consequently, those who remain in the traditional treatment group may not be comparable to the ad hoc group that evolves for the new treatment. Third, some participants who were assigned to the control group with no treatment may demand that they receive treatment. Again, as a consequence, the two groups that are eventually formed may be different from those originally formed. Fourth, when a new treatment whose effects are completely unknown is being evaluated or when a treatment that poses known risks is being evaluated, only very sick or terminally ill patients may volunteer for that study. Patients with better prognosis may necessarily be included in the traditional treatment or no-treatment control groups, creating group disparities. These and perhaps other factors may induce bias that will make results questionable even if the participants were initially randomly assigned to the groups.

Matching: An Alternative to Randomization

An alternative to randomization is called **matching,** a procedure in which selected characteristics of one participant are matched with the characteristics of another. When it is not possible to gain access to a large population of participants, all of whom are willing to participate, the investigator may recruit available participants and then match individuals to achieve sampling equivalency.

Matching pairs of participants is a method in which the investigator matches pairs of participants on known (relevant) variables and then randomly assigns one member of each pair to the experimental group and the other to the control group. For example, suppose that an investigator knows that in the treatment of articulation disorders, the severity of misarticulations is a significant variable influencing the treatment outcome. In this case, the investigator may find pairs of participants who are equal in severity of misarticulation. One member of each pair will be assigned to the control group and the other to the experimental group. Another pair of participants may have a different level of severity. Matched pairs can be created on multiple variables. For example, pairs of participants can be matched on age, gender, socioeconomic status, intelligence, occupational background, and so forth.

When matching pairs of participants is impractical, scientists can use **equivalent frequency distribution** in which two groups are matched not on individual characteristics but on group averages of relevant variables in the two groups. If age, severity, and intelligence of participants are considered relevant variables in a particular investigation, a comparable distribution of these variables in the two groups may be obtained. For example, the mean IQ of the experimental and control group participants may be 110 and 108, respectively, with a standard deviation of 4.5 and 5.2. The distribution of the variables is considered comparable when the mean and the standard deviation of the measured values of those variables for the two groups are comparable. This technique of matching is less precise than the paired-participants procedure, but it is more practical. Individuals are not matched one-to-one, but the groups are matched on a statistical basis.

Limitations of Matching

The most serious limitation of matching is that, under the best possible circumstances, it can create two groups that are comparable on known variables only. Investigators match participants on characteristics considered important because of available information. The groups may still differ on variables that have an effect but were unknown and hence were not considered in matching the participants. Using the example described previously, it is possible that a family history of misarticulation or the presence of other communicative problems may be important variables, but because of no prior research on them, they are not considered in matching the participants.

Matching participants in clinical research poses serious practical problems. It is difficult to find pairs of clients who are similar on one or more relevant variables. Many clients will have to be rejected because another client who shares the same characteristics selected for matching is not available. The clinical researcher often cannot afford this luxury of rejecting available and willing participants. Equivalent distribution of variables in the two groups may be more feasible, but it still requires a large pool of participants. Furthermore, individuals across two groups formed on the basis of equivalent frequency distribution may still be very different because comparable means may not assure comparable individuals.

Theoretically, random selection and assignment assure equivalence on all of the relevant variables, known and unknown. Therefore, randomization is preferred to matching. In most clinical trials, randomization, not matching, is used to form the two or more groups for experimentation.

Treatment Administration

Once the groups are formed and before the treatment is offered, all participants are assessed to establish the pretreatment measures that will be compared against the posttreatment measures. Such pretreatment assessments are called pretests in the group design approach. In medical research, diagnostic protocols and laboratory measurements of relevant aspects of health and disease (e.g., blood tests or radiological tests) constitute pretests. In behavioral and educational research, various skills and behaviors may be measured during pretests. Pretests may be standardized test scores (e.g., scores on a language performance scale or a test of articulation) or specific measures obtained on each participant (e.g., a speech or language sample from each child participant or the frequency of self-injurious behaviors in a child with autism).

Completion of pretests sets the stage for experimentation. One or more treatment groups receive their respective treatments and a no-treatment control group goes without any treatment. In such treatment studies, additional opportunities for biased observations arise. The clients or patients who receive treatments and the investigators who make systematic observations of people during the course of the study may all introduce bias into the results. Procedures have been designed to control for this bias.

Single or Double Blinding

Bias introduced by participants may be significant in certain studies. For instance, patients who receive a new drug for arthritis may feel better simply because they know that they have been receiving the new drug, not because the drug is doing any good. They may report reduced pain to the measurement team, but there may be no objective basis for this. Experts who measure the various effects of a new drug, depending on positive or negative—but always subjective—evaluation of the drug, may record greater or lesser effect of the drug, again with no objective basis.

To eliminate or reduce participant and researcher bias in reporting or recording the treatment effects, investigators in medicine use a technique known as *blinding*. **Blinding** is a method in which the information about who gets what treatment or no treatment is withheld from the participants, investigators who measure the effects, or from both the parties. In **single blinding,** only those investigators who measure the treatment effects are unaware of their patients' treatment or no-treatment status. In **double blinding,** both the measurement team and the participants are unaware of the participant status. In other words, neither the patient nor the medical personnel in charge of measuring the effect of the treatment under investigation, has the knowledge of the group membership.

In medicine, administering a placebo to the participants in the control group is a standard method of blinding the participants. Originally, a **placebo** (meaning *to please* in Latin) was a dummy treatment given to patients just to please them. Placebos were thought to be especially useful with intellectually unsophisticated or generally uninformed patients. In 1807, Thomas Jefferson, who found out that his physician friend had prescribed more fake medicines than real ones to his patients, is reported to have called it a "pious fraud" (Kaptchuk, 1998). In the past, physicians used them in routine practice. Currently, placebos are offered to control group subjects in medical treatment evaluation studies. The notion of placebo has been extended to many forms of treatment evaluation. The typical pharmacological placebo in drug evaluation studies is a lactose tablet. A typical physical placebo (such as those used in physical therapy research) may be some kind of a sham movement or exercise regimen, administered with the help of a mechanical device to enhance the placebo effect. In psychological research where different forms of psychotherapy and counseling are evaluated for their effects, the placebo may be a neutral discussion or conversation with a therapist (Hrobjartsson & Gotzsche, 2001).

In 1955, Beecher first claimed that dummy treatments (placebo) can produce an effect. Analyzing 15 medical treatment studies, Beecher asserted that 35% of 1,082 patients receiving a placebo experienced relief from symptoms. In subsequent years, the placebo effect was generally accepted, and a need to control for it in treatment research was widely recognized (Kienle & Kiene, 1997). When evaluating the effects of a treatment, investigators were expected to have a control group that received only a placebo to distinguish the true effects of medication given to the experimental group. To claim effects for a new treatment, the experimental group that receives the real treatment should show an improvement that is over and beyond any placebo effect observed in the control group. When a placebo is used, the treatments and patients are coded and those who administer the treatment and placebo, and those who measure the effects (and maybe patients as well) are unaware of the meaning of patient codes. The codes are broken only after the study is completed. The patients and their treatments are identified only after all data have been collected and before the data are analyzed.

The placebo is not a practical method of blinding the participants in some kind of treatments. It is most effective in drug evaluations where the control participants swallow a dummy pill on the same schedule as those in the experimental group who receive the medication. It is impractical to blind participants to surgical procedures, although some ethically questionable sham surgeries have been performed on control group participants (see Chapter 16 for details). Most behavioral treatment and educational teaching methods cannot be blinded, although in some cases, dummy activity that looks like treatment may be offered to the control group. However, it is hard to conceal teaching sign language to deaf children and offering positive reinforcement for fluency to persons who stutter.

Recently, medical researchers have questioned the very existence of the placebo effect (Hrobjartsson & Gotzsche, 2001; Kaptchuk, 1998; Kienle & Kiene, 1997). Making a reanalysis of the studies Beecher (1955) used to claim the placebo effect, Kienle and Kiene (1997) concluded that none of the studies showed any placebo effect. Their general conclusion is that placebo effects have not been documented in any of the studies, before or since Beecher's publication. Apparently, some placebo-group members will have received other treatments whose effects were ignored. In some studies, recipients of placebo may have deteriorated, a fact also typically ignored. Studies that have compared placebo with no treatment have generally failed to show a placebo effect, which is typically (and perhaps erroneously) claimed when a placebo is compared against a new or established treatment. It makes sense to say that placebo effect is possibly due to some other variables because the term *placebo effect* is an oxymoron that claims that nothing produces something (Kaptchuk, 1998).

On the other hand, Hrobjartsson and Gotzsche (2001) suggested that in RCTs in medicine, a small placebo effect may be seen only when the dependent variable measured is pain felt by patients. That is, the sensation of pain, more than any other symptom, may be subject to the placebo effect. The placebo effect is more likely to be documented when it is measured or reported subjectively. Again, pain is subjectively reported and evaluated, and hence the possibility of a placebo effect in pain management. Objective measures of treatment effects are less likely to be affected by the placebo. For instance, laboratory measurements of the dependent variable (e.g., blood analysis or radiological findings) are unlikely to be affected by placebo (Hrobjartsson & Gotzsche, 2001). Even subjective reports of improvement in pain may not be a placebo effect. The improvement may be due to several factors that Kienle and Kiene (1977) describe as the more valid reasons for reported improvements attributed to placebo: spontaneous recovery from symptoms, regression to the mean, natural fluctuation of symptoms, patients' tendency to please physicians, concurrent treatments the placebo group members may have received, and so forth (Kaptchuk, 1998).

The role of placebo effect in speech and language treatment is unclear, and perhaps highly questionable. Objectively measured production of grammatical morphemes or phonemes by children with language delay, rates of stuttering in adults who stutter, swallowing skills in patients with dysphagia, and communication skills in persons with aphasia, just to name a few, are unlikely to be affected by sham treatment.

Once the groups are formed and decisions are made about blinding, pretests are administered to members of both the groups to establish the pretreatment measures of the dependent variables. Ideally, the pretreatment measures of the dependent variable should be comparable across the two groups. If they are not, the groups are different. Investigators then may recruit additional participants and assign them to the groups to make them more equal.

Control and Experimental Groups

Treatment administration may begin after obtaining acceptable pretest measures. In most behavioral and educational research, blinding is relatively uncommon, and the new treatment or teaching method is applied to the experimental group and withheld from the control group. Although the classic notion of a control group is that it does not receive treatment, there are studies in which a control group may receive a treatment. As noted before, placebo control groups in medical research receive a dummy treatment. Offering dummy treatment is not typical of behavioral and educational research and is full of ethical complications in medical research.

In some medical, behavioral, and educational research, a control group may receive a standard treatment while the experimental group receives the new treatment being evaluated. For instance, a medical research team may administer an established medicine for patients with arthritis in the control group and a new drug for those in the experimental group. A special educator may use children who are hard of hearing who receive standard reading instruction as the control group while offering a new method of teaching reading to the experimental group. This strategy helps avoid the ethical dilemma of not offering treatment to individuals who need it. It also helps evaluate whether the new treatment produces better outcomes than a standard (common, established) treatment.

At the end of the treatment or teaching period, the investigator administers posttests to both the groups. Posttests may take a variety of forms, depending on what was initially measured on the pretests and what was treated. In medicine, symptoms may be subjectively evaluated, along with objective laboratory measures of various disease and health status of patients. In behavioral and educational settings, pretests may include measures of target skills that were initially pretested and later taught. The pretest–posttest scores are used to make a variety of statistical analyses of the treatment effects, mentioned briefly in the context of specific group designs described in Chapter 8.

SINGLE-SUBJECT TREATMENT RESEARCH: MULTIPLE CONTROL CONDITIONS

A second experimental approach to evaluating treatment effects is the single-subject approach. This approach, too, uses the same logic of experimental control and establishment of cause–effect relations. Its methods and certain conceptual bases, however, are different from those of the group design approach. While the group designs use a control group to demonstrate that a treatment is effective, single-subject designs use control conditions to do the same. Just like control groups, control conditions help rule out the influence of extraneous variables.

Single-subject designs use multiple control mechanisms within a single study. A description of these control mechanisms follows. The major single-subject designs themselves are described in Chapter 9.

Experimental Control Through Multiple Control Conditions

In most group designs, the control group that does not receive treatment provides the basic control mechanism to rule out the influence of other variables. Because the single-subject designs generally do not use control groups, they rule out extraneous variables in other ways.

Several control mechanisms within the single-subject strategy help rule out the influence of extraneous variables. Together, they provide a comprehensive tactic of isolating the effects of independent variables on dependent variables. The control mechanisms variously employed in the single-subject strategy include replication, withdrawal, reversal, reinstatement, criterion-referenced change, rapid alternations, baselines, and simultaneous multibaselines.

Replication

One of the important characteristics that distinguish the single-subject strategy from the group strategy is the replication of experimental conditions, and hence the treatment effects within individual participants. The group designs typically introduce the treatment once, and when it is discontinued, there is no reintroduction of treatment. Therefore, within the group design strategy, there is no recapturing of a state after the dependent variable has been changed. The experimental group that shows change remains changed, and the control group that does not show change remains unchanged. Therefore, there is no replication of conditions in the group strategy.

In the single-subject strategy, the treatment condition, the control condition, or both are changed from one state to the other. During the course of an experiment, one or more of the earlier states are recaptured. In other words, the effects of the independent variable are shown once by introducing it and thereby changing the dependent variable; the effects are shown a second time by removing the independent variable thereby changing the dependent variable a second time. A preexperimental state or an approximation of it is recaptured. The simplest of the single-subject designs, the *ABA* design—which involves a baseline *A*, treatment *B*, and withdrawal of treatment *A*—replicates the original steady state.

In the *ABAB* design, a baseline is first established *A*, a treatment is then introduced *B*, subsequently withdrawn *A*, and finally reintroduced *B*. This design replicates the pretreatment steady state or baseline once (the two *A* conditions). In addition, the design replicates the treatment effects as well (the two *B* conditions).

When the relative effects of two or more treatments are evaluated, the single-subject designs repeatedly present and withdraw treatment variables. A series of replications may thus be achieved to observe different patterns of responses under the two treatment procedures. When the interactive effects of two treatments are evaluated, one treatment is withdrawn and reintroduced against the background of a constant treatment variable. In this manner, target response rates under treatment and no-treatment are established repeatedly.

Repetition of treatment or no-treatment condition in the same participant is called the **intrasubject replication,** by itself, not the strongest of the control procedures. However, when an effect is repeatedly demonstrated and repeatedly neutralized, the experimental operations gain credibility. When intrasubject replication is combined with other control procedures, it can be effective in ruling out extraneous variables.

Intrasubject replication must be distinguished from **intersubject replication,** in which a treatment effect is replicated across individuals. Most single-subject designs involve both intrasubject and intersubject replication of treatment effects. When multiple participants are used in a single-subject study involving a design such as the *ABAB*, the same treatment effects are demonstrated repeatedly both within and across participants.

Withdrawal of Treatment

In using **withdrawal** as a control mechanism, the treatment that was in effect for a certain duration is discontinued. The measurement of the dependent variables is continued to document their gradual reduction in frequency. Such a withdrawal can also demonstrate control of the independent variable over the dependent variable.

In a clinical research study, for example, the clinician may wish to find out whether production of morphological features can be reinforced by verbal praise. After establishing the baseline production levels of selected morphologic features, verbal praise may be made contingent on the production of those features in phrases or sentences. When an increase in the production of these behaviors becomes evident, the clinician may withdraw verbal praise. The selected stimuli are presented continuously in an effort to evoke relevant verbal responses to see if the production of the morphemes decreases. If they do, the clinician may conclude that the treatment variable was responsible for the initial increase and the subsequent decrease in the morpheme productions. Figure 4.1 shows the visual effects of the withdrawal procedure in which a target behavior increases under treatment and decreases under withdrawal.

Withdrawal of treatment in single-subject designs is not the same as the termination of the treatment followed by the posttest in a group design. The withdrawal of treatment is a sensitive operation in that it is supposed to demonstrate the presence and the absence of the effects corresponding to the presence and the absence of the independent variable. In the group strategy, the treatment is not terminated to show that the effects are reduced or eliminated. Also, researchers in the group strategy do not need to have the treatment effect neutralized; they have the control group to show that when there was no treatment, there was no effect.

Withdrawal of treatment and the resulting decrease in the response rate help rule out the effects of history and maturation, the important extraneous variables (see Chapter 9 for details). If events in the life of the participants are responsible for the changes observed during treatment, then the withdrawal of treatment should have no effect on the response rate. If the behavior increases when the treatment is applied and decreases when it is

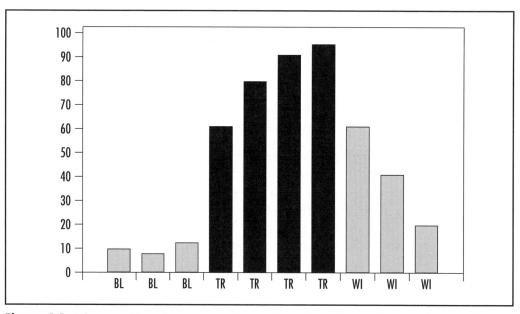

Figure 4.1. The controlling effects of the withdrawal procedure. A target behavior that is stable under baseline (BL) increases when treated (TR) and decreases when the treatment is withdrawn (WI).

withdrawn, then the probability that events in the life of the participants are responsible for the changes is reduced greatly. Similarly, if biological or other internal changes taking place in the participants are responsible for the increase in the behavior during the treatment condition, then such an increase should at least be maintained, if not continued, when the treatment is discontinued.

As a control procedure, withdrawal has its disadvantages. It can be clinically undesirable because the treatment effects are neutralized even if only temporarily. This poses no serious problem in basic laboratory research in which various independent variables are introduced and withdrawn to create and remove their effects. For example, in animal research, some response such as bar pressing can be increased by reinforcing it and decreased by withholding the reinforcer. This way, the experimenter can bring the bar-pressing response under experimental control and rule out the influence of other variables. In clinical situations, however, withdrawal of treatment and the resulting decrease in the target behavior is not appropriate. Withdrawal serves an experimental purpose, but it damages the clinical purpose of keeping and enhancing the behavioral change the treatment produces. Therefore, it is not a control method of choice in clinical research. However, withdrawal can be used in combination with other control procedures in which the treatment is reestablished.

The other problem associated with withdrawal is that the investigator needs to judge when to withdraw treatment. There are no objective rules to do this, but certain patterns of responses dictate the decision. The researcher must see a change that can be objectively judged when the treatment is introduced before it is withdrawn. Once the change reaches a convincing level, the treatment should not be continued. In other words, it should be withdrawn as early as possible so that the baseline or an approximation of it can be recaptured. However, when the response rate under treatment is highly variable, withdrawal may be delayed to find out if a continuation of treatment will stabilize it at a level higher than the baseline.

A more troublesome phenomenon could occur when the behavior initially increases under treatment but slowly or abruptly begins to decrease in later treatment sessions. While this is happening, withdrawal is inappropriate because it will only show a continuation of the trend already established during the treatment phase. The investigator once again may wish to continue treatment for awhile to determine if the declining rate of response can be checked or even reversed. A point may still come, however, when the treatment is withdrawn in spite of a persistently declining rate of response. Although the results cannot be interpreted clearly in this case, the suggestion is that the treatment perhaps has had only a temporary effect or actually no effect at all. The issue must be addressed in additional research.

Finally, if the response rate does not approximate the baseline rate when the treatment is withdrawn, the results cannot be interpreted. The possibility that some extraneous variable is responsible for the change observed during the treatment condition cannot be ruled out.

Reversal of Treatment

Reversal of treatment is an alternative to withdrawal. Sometimes, the terms *withdrawal* and *reversal* are used interchangeably. However, this practice is avoided here because of the procedural differences between them. In withdrawal, the treatment is simply discontinued. In **reversal,** the treatment is applied to an alternative, incompatible behavior. That is, the treatment is not withdrawn altogether; it is withdrawn from the particular behavior for which it was applied only to apply it on some other behavior.

Another way of looking at the distinction between withdrawal and reversal may be helpful. While withdrawal is a short- or long-term termination of treatment, reversal involves an intrasubject but interbehavior replication of treatment. Initially, the investigator hopes to show that the application of the treatment to behavior *A* resulted in an increase in that behavior. The treatment of behavior *A* is then discontinued. Next, the investigator demonstrates that an application of the same treatment to behavior *B* (reversal), increased behavior *B* while decreasing behavior *A*. This documents experimental control on both the behaviors, resulting in interbehavior–intrasubject replication. In essence, withdrawal is a singular procedure, but reversal is a dual procedure that includes withdrawal of treatment from the original behavior and its application to an incompatible behavior.

A hypothetical example will clarify this dual process. Suppose a clinician treats a client who stutters by reinforcing durations of fluency in conversational speech. A stable baseline of fluency and stuttering is established before the initiation of treatment. Reinforcement of fluent durations in speech results in a marked increase in fluency. At this time, the clinician cannot conclude that the reinforcement is responsible for the change because factors such as history and maturation have not been ruled out. At this point, the clinician stops reinforcing fluency and starts to reinforce stuttering, a response that is incompatible with fluency. As a result of the reversal of the treatment contingency, fluency decreases and stuttering increases. This then demonstrates that the reinforcing contingency is indeed responsible for the changes in fluency as well as stuttering.

Reversal has some of the same problems as withdrawal. Initially, the investigator must decide when to withdraw treatment from the first behavior according to the suggestions offered earlier. Then the investigator must select a behavior that is incompatible with the first behavior. Unless the behavior to be reinforced next is incompatible with the original behavior, a partial replication of the treatment effect may be all that can be achieved. The original behavior may or may not show a swift and concomitant change when the treatment is applied to a compatible behavior.

For example, in the treatment of a client with a language disorder, the clinician may first apply the treatment to the production of regular plural allomorph *s* in words. After having seen a substantial increase in the production of this allomorph, the clinician may decide to reverse the treatment. Now, the clinician must make sure that the behavior to be treated next is incompatible with the plural allomorph. The best strategy is to reinforce the production of the same words used in training the plural allomorph but in their singular form while showing the plural stimulus items. When the plural responses to plural stimulus items decrease, the singular responses to the same stimulus items increase. Should the clinician reinforce the present progressive -*ing* or some other behavior that is not incompatible with the plural allomorph, the production of the latter may not show a concomitant change under the reversal condition.

Reversal presents special problems in clinical research; therefore, other control procedures are preferred. The procedure requires that the clinician increase the frequency of an undesirable behavior after having increased its counterpart—a desirable behavior. Whenever it is used, the treatment for the original, desirable target behavior is reinstated in the next phase. This then shows that the undesirable behavior decreases, and its counterpart increases a second time. Thus, the treatment achieves its clinical goal.

When it takes several sessions to increase an incompatible, undesirable behavior, the experimental strategy is inefficient and perhaps totally unacceptable from the clinical standpoint. The parents or other members of the client family may react negatively to the clinician who first teaches a correct response and then spends a considerable amount of time and energy teaching the incorrect response. In institutional research, staff members who are asked to reverse the treatment may be reluctant to do so (Barlow & Hersen, 1984). For example, aides in an institution for persons with mental retardation who are asked to reinforce gestures instead of the word responses that had been reinforced may not be willing to follow this reversal procedure.

In a more conservative use of the reversal strategy, the clinician can make sure that both the reversal and reinstatement of treatment are achieved in a single session. If the clinician is not sure of this possibility, the reversal strategy may be avoided. In the example of language treatment research, if the clinician is not confident of increasing the production of the singular morpheme in relation to plural stimulus items (reversal) and then increasing the correct production of the plural allomorph in relation to plural items (reinstatement)—all in a single session—reversal may be avoided.

In many cases, it is possible to reverse and reinstate treatment in a single, perhaps a little extended, session. Also, the wrong responses need not be increased to the 100% level and stabilized there. Though there are not quantitative guidelines on this, an increase from a low, 10% to 15%, error rate to a moderately high, 40% to 50%, error rate may be considered adequate for the purposes of control. The clinician can then reinstate treatment for the correct response. The correct response rate under reinstatement can also be achieved quickly. When reversal and reinstatement are thus achieved in a single session, the client is not sent home with an increased or increasing rate of wrong responses.

Reinstatement of Treatment

Reinstatement of treatment is yet another strategy of control within single-subject designs. To use **reinstatement** as a control procedure, treatment is reintroduced when it has been either withdrawn or reversed. Thus, it is a contingent control condition that has a cumulative control effect within a design. It is contingent upon withdrawal or reversal that will already have demonstrated some control over the dependent variable. The reinstatement of treatment then adds additional control.

Reinstatement may be an optional control strategy in basic research. In nonclinical settings, a behavior shaped or taught can be eliminated by withdrawal. Along with this, another behavior may be increased with reversal. However, in clinical research reinstatement of effective treatment is almost mandatory when the control procedures of withdrawal or reinstatement are used.

The concepts and procedures of withdrawal, reversal, and reinstatement, though separate, are closely related. They also converge on the concept of replication. A single withdrawal replicates the baseline condition by showing an initial increase from, and then a decrease to, the baseline response rate. A single reversal replicates the treatment effect twice, first by showing that the initial target behavior increases and then by showing that the incompatible behavior increases under reversed contingencies.

When a treatment is withdrawn and then reinstated once, the effects of treatment are demonstrated three times: first when the treatment is initially applied, second when the treatment is withdrawn, and third when the treatment is reinstated. In the first and third cases, an increase in the frequency of the target behavior is demonstrated. In the second case, a decrease in the frequency is demonstrated. Together, the three demonstrations strengthen the possibility that the extraneous variables were controlled. Figure 4.2 shows the effects of a single withdrawal and reinstatement of a treatment.

When a treatment is reversed and then reinstated once, the treatment effects are demonstrated six times. The first demonstration occurs when the treatment is first applied to the target behavior which shows an increase; the second occurs when the treatment is withdrawn and the target behavior decreases; the third occurs when the treatment is reinstated for the target behavior which shows an increase again; the fourth occurs when the incompatible behavior decreases when the target behavior is treated; the fifth involves an increase in the incompatible behavior when the treatment is applied to it; and the sixth is evident when the incompatible behavior decreases under reinstatement of treatment for the target behavior. Figure 4.3 shows these demonstrations with the hypothetical target example of fluency (target, 1) and stuttering (incompatible behavior, 2).

A combination of reversal or withdrawal with the reinstatement procedure can provide a convincing demonstration of the treatment effect by making it difficult to explain the results on the basis of extraneous variables.

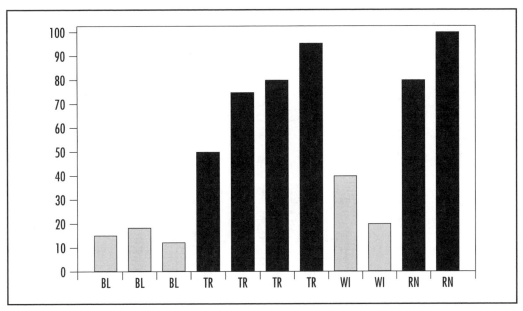

Figure 4.2. The controlling effects of a single withdrawal and reinstatement of treatment. A stable and low rate of a target behavior during the baseline (BL) increases during treatment (TR), decreases during withdrawal (WI), and increases again during reinstatement of treatment (RN).

When systematic changes are associated with the experimental manipulations of withdrawal or reversal on one hand and reinstatement on the other, the probability that the changes are due to those manipulations increases.

Criterion-Referenced Change

In one of the single-subject designs, some level of control of extraneous variables is achieved by showing that the dependent variable changes in relation to a criterion, and the criterion is changed several times in subsequent stages of the experiment. Thus, the criterion-referenced change is reliable, and multiple changes in target behaviors are consistent with changing treatment criteria.

The criterion-referenced change has not been used frequently in demonstrating the experimental control of independent variables (Barlow & Hersen, 1984). The basic idea of **criterion-referenced change** is that if changes in a dependent variable approximate a preset criterion, and if whenever the criterion is changed the dependent variable also changes in accordance with the new criterion in force, then the experimental control is demonstrated. In this case, the changes in the dependent variable follow a more predictable pattern that corresponds to the changing criteria.

A hypothetical example can illustrate the criterion-referenced change. An investigator may wish to find out if the amount of homework done by a

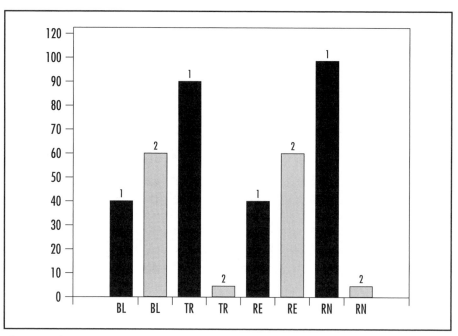

Figure 4.3. Six demonstrations of a treatment effect with a reversal and reinstatement. Fluency (1) and stuttering (2) are baserated (BL) and then fluency is treated (TR). The treatment is reversed (RE) and finally reinstated (RN) for fluency. Note the corresponding changes in the two incompatible behaviors.

child is a function of the reinforcement contingency. To rule out the influence of factors other than the reinforcement contingency, the investigator may devise a series of changing criteria that the dependent variables may track. For example, initially the child may be asked to complete five academic tasks in a given time. This is the initial criterion to which the dependent variable is held. The investigator will continue to measure the number of tasks completed. Reinforcement is provided for task completion. Suppose that in due course, the child stabilizes at the five completed tasks required by the criterion. After this, the investigator changes the criterion to eight tasks, and the child's behavior reaches and stabilizes at this level. In subsequent stages, the criterion is changed to 10, 14, 16, and 18 tasks. If the number of tasks completed by the child reaches and stabilizes at each new criterion in force, a certain degree of control over the dependent variable becomes evident.

If the dependent variable does not reach the criterion or stabilize at that level, then the control is not evident. Capricious changes unrelated to the criterion in force will also invalidate the data. To demonstrate an acceptable degree of control, the dependent variable should closely parallel the criterion in force.

Criterion-referenced change is probably the weakest of the control procedures available within the single-subject strategy. By itself, it does not provide for a no-treatment control condition, which is inherent to withdrawal and reversal. However, such control procedures can be incorporated into criterion-referenced change. Treatment may be withdrawn at some stage to determine if the behavior returns to at least one of the previous levels. Or, by periodically switching back and forth to a higher and a lower criterion, bidirectional control over behavior may be demonstrated. This also provides replication at the repeated criterion levels. The control function demonstrated by criterion-referenced change is illustrated in Figure 4.4. (Criterion-referenced change is involved in a design known as the *changing criterion design*. This design is described in a later section of this chapter.)

Rapid Alternations

Another form of control used in some of the single-subject designs is the rapid alternation of two or more conditions. The conditions may include treatment and no treatment, or two or more treatments. Of course, two or

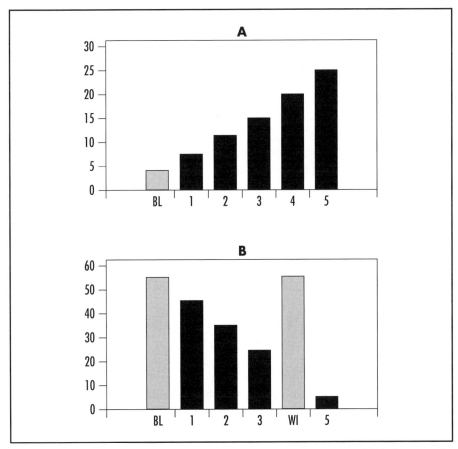

Figure 4.4. Criterion-referenced change showing control over a desirable behavior with an initial baseline and five changing criteria that increases the behavior (A). The lower portion (B) shows changing criteria decreasing an undesirable behavior with an added withdrawal (WI) feature that shows a temporary increase.

more treatments may be alternated along with no-treatment conditions as well. Quick changes in experimental conditions and corresponding changes in target behaviors define **rapid alternations** as a control mechanism.

Rapid alternation of conditions may be a control procedure because of the possibility of showing dependent variable changes that are equally rapid and consistent with the alternations of conditions. For example, when treatment and no-treatment conditions are alternated, the dependent variable may show appropriate increases and decreases. When the treatment is repeatedly introduced and withdrawn with results showing appropriate changes, the investigator increases the probability that the changes are due to the rapidly changing conditions of the experiment.

Rapid alternation of treatment and no-treatment conditions is not the same as treatment conditions interspersed with baseline conditions. In the latter strategy, one can initially baseline a behavior and introduce a treatment that will be continued for a certain length of time. After the behavior shows a convincing change, the treatment may be withdrawn until the client returns to the baseline. This second baseline may also be continued until the behavior shows a change toward the baseline. Then once again the same or even a different treatment may be introduced and maintained for an extended time. This strategy attempts to expose the participants to treatment and baseline conditions for a duration needed to produce changes that differentiate the conditions.

On the other hand, in rapid alternation of treatment and no-treatment conditions, there is no attempt to continue either the treatment or the no-treatment condition until some change is judged to have occurred. Each session involves a different condition, and the treatment and no-treatment conditions may be alternated even within sessions. In rapid alternations, the investigator expects to show a data trend over a time involving several alternations.

In the rapid alternation of two or more treatments, an initial baseline may be established, although it is not always required. The purpose of such a strategy is to determine the relative effects of two or more treatments, not the absolute effect of either of them. Therefore, baseline or any other form of control procedure is not necessary, though it is desirable. The control function of rapid alternations involving two treatments (X_1 and X_2) is illustrated in Figure 4.5. Note that Treatment 1 was more effective than Treatment 2 in increasing the target behavior from its baseline level.

A clinician, for example, may wish to evaluate the relative effects of two kinds of stimulus items in teaching vocabulary items to a child with mental retardation. The stimulus variables to be evaluated in the study may be actual objects and pictures that represent the words to be taught. During the training, objects and pictures may be rapidly alternated. However, through such alternations, training trials on a given word will have a constant type of stimulus. Each stimulus type may involve several target words. Over several rapid alternations, several words may be taught with each of

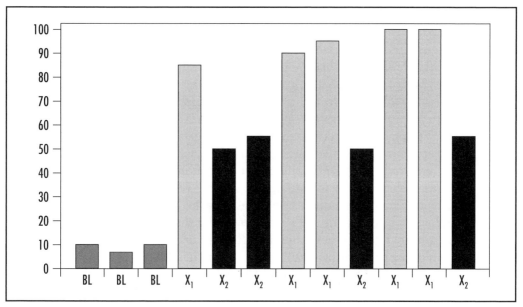

Figure 4.5. The demonstration of experimental control with rapid alternations of two treatments (X_1 and X_2). Note that in increasing the frequency of the target behavior, Treatment 1 was more effective than Treatment 2.

the two types of stimulus materials preceding specific targets. The data may be analyzed in terms of the number of training trials (or sessions, or both) needed to achieve an operationally defined training criterion for the set of words taught with objects versus pictures as stimulus antecedents. Or when the number of sessions is held constant, the number of words learned within the two procedures can also be analyzed. Such analyses can reveal the differential effects of the two stimulus variables.

Rapid alternation of two or more treatments, by itself, does not provide for strong controls within a design. That is why it is more suitable for evaluating relative, not absolute, effects of two or more treatment variables. When the alternations involve treatment and no-treatment conditions, appropriate controls exist to rule out extraneous variables. Lacking such a control condition, the multitreatment alternations can only identify which one had a greater effect on the dependent variable. However, control conditions such as a withdrawal of all treatments can be built into the alternating sequence. In that case, questions regarding whether treatments had any effect when compared to no treatment can also be answered.

Baselines

An important and almost invariably used control strategy within single-subject designs is the baselines or baserates of responses. **Baselines** are rates of responses in the absence of the independent variable whose effects are the subject of experimental analysis. They also are described as *natural rates* of responses and the *operant level* of responses. Baselines document the frequency of the dependent variable before the independent variable is introduced. The absence of treatment during baseline condition makes it the control condition within single-subject designs. The dependent variable measures obtained in the treatment and baseline conditions can be compared to assess the treatment effects.

It must be noted, however, that a mere baseline at the beginning of the experimental manipulation does not rule out extraneous variables. If a study includes only the baseline and treatment conditions, it has the same deficient control that is seen in one-group pretest–posttest design. In the single-subject terminology, this is an *AB* design which cannot rule out the influence of history or maturation. The improvement shown by the participants under a treatment condition within an *AB* study may be due to the events in the lives of the participants or to the intraparticipant biological changes. Therefore, what is needed in addition to a baseline is either withdrawal of treatment, reversal of treatment, rapid alternation, or criterion-referenced change. Baselines serve a control purpose only in conjunction with one of these procedures. Most frequently, baselines and either withdrawal or reversal are used to demonstrate the internal validity of experimental operations.

There is an exception to the rule that baselines must be combined with other control procedures to eliminate or minimize the influence of extraneous variables. The exception constitutes simultaneous multibaselines, which are described in a later section.

Baselines established before the introduction of treatment must fulfill certain standards of acceptability which are called **baseline criteria.** An overall consideration is whether the baselines are adequate to evaluate the treatment effects in conjunction with the treatment and other control conditions. There are three criteria that must be applied in evaluating the adequacy of baselines.

The first criterion to be applied is **reliability through multiple observations.** Unlike pretests in a group design, which normally involve a single observation of the dependent variable, baselines are held to an initial criterion of multiple observations. A single measurement of the dependent variable is inadequate because of its unknown reliability. By definition, reliability is consistency across measures, and therefore, multiple measures are needed to make sure that the frequency with which the dependent variable naturally occurs has been documented. It has been suggested that at least three separate observations are needed before the adequacy of a baseline can be evaluated (Barlow & Hersen, 1984). In fact, three observations may suggest that either additional measures are needed or the behavior has stabilized so that the treatment can be introduced.

The second criterion to be applied is that of **stability of the measures.** A highly variable baseline does not permit a valid comparison with the response rate under the treatment condition. If the rate of response is constantly fluctuating from observation to observation, then the treatment effects may be buried in this variability. However, variability itself can have some patterns, and it is important to note them.

If the response rate is variable in a predictable fashion, it has a pattern, which is better than variability with no pattern whatsoever. For example, the behavior may show a consistent increase in one session and decrease in the other session, and the overall data may show this duplicating pattern. Or the measures may show no pattern in the first few observations, and then a pattern either of stability or of alternating increases and decreases may emerge. Yet another possibility is that the variability may be too high in the beginning, but gradually its extent may be reduced though no pattern emerges. Baselines with no pattern and unpredictable variability are not acceptable.

A stable response rate is the one **without a trend** and without unpredictable variability. A trend is evident when the rate of responses either increases or decreases over time. A stable response without a trend is considered the ideal baseline. When the pretreatment baseline is stable, it is relatively easy to detect the effects of the independent variable.

A stable baseline is difficult to obtain in many cases, and fortunately it is not the only acceptable baseline. Baselines with certain trends are acceptable, as long as the trends themselves help establish a strong effect of the independent variable. Therefore, baselines with a clear trend in the direction that is opposite to the changes to be created by the experimental manipulations are acceptable. For example, in a study designed to evaluate the effects of time-out on stuttering, the clinician observes the rate of dysfluencies in conversational speech over several sessions. The measures of dysfluencies may show an increasing trend over the baseline sessions; this is sometimes referred to as a **deteriorating baseline** (Barlow & Hersen, 1984) because the problem to be treated is getting worse. Deteriorating baselines are acceptable from a scientific as well as ethical standpoint. Scientifically, treatment is expected to produce an opposite trend in the data. If time-out is effective, it will not only check the deterioration in stuttering but will also reverse the trend. Indeed, a treatment that reverses a deteriorating baseline can be considered a strong one. Ethically, deteriorating baselines require that the researcher intervene. If the participants' problem is getting worse by the day, the researcher will have to place client welfare ahead of any research demands.

A trend that is clearly not acceptable, both scientifically and ethically, is one in which the behavior to be increased shows consistent improvement over the baseline sessions; this is an **improving baseline.** For example, a clinician who baserates fluency and stuttering may find that there is a clear trend toward increased fluency and decreased stuttering across baserate sessions. In such cases, treatment cannot be instituted simply because the positive effects of the treatment, if any, will be confounded with the baseline trend of improvement in fluency. With such a trend, one will have to assume that fluency would have improved in the absence of treatment. Furthermore, it would be ethically unjustified to offer treatment for a problem from which people are recovering without professional help.

The best course of action to take when baselines are unstable without a pattern is to continue measurement until an acceptable pattern or trend emerges. Basic research has repeatedly shown that when the conditions are well controlled and observations are repeated, variability eventually dissipates. It is easier to take this course of action in basic research than in clinical research, however. In clinical settings, baselines cannot be extended indefinitely. The clients who serve as participants also are seeking treatment for their problem, and because one of the strengths of the single-subject designs is an integration of treatment and clinical service, the treatment must be introduced as soon as possible. At the same time, a highly variable baseline will not permit conclusions regarding the effects of treatment being evaluated. Therefore, one has to make a judgment regarding both the acceptability of the baselines and the duration for which they can be extended. The clinical researcher will have to weigh the advantages and disadvantages of continuing the baseline measures or introducing the treatment.

Another way of handling variability, which has proved successful in basic research, is to make variability itself the subject of experimental analysis. For instance, when dysfluency rates do not stabilize in spite of repeated observations, the clinician may begin to wonder why and think of strategies to find out. It is possible that the conditions of observation are not constant. The time of making observations, the method of evoking speech, or the topics discussed may have been variable. If the conditions have been constant, then perhaps factors in the life of the individual are affecting the dysfluency rates. Are there patterns of events that are related to the changes in the dysfluency rates? Such an inquiry also is relatively easily conducted in basic research, where the entire life and genetic history of an experimental animal is under the control of the investigator. However, a serious attempt to find out the sources of variability may be fruitful, though difficult, in applied settings. Possibly, it may be found that a woman's variability in stuttering is related to premenstrual and menstrual conditions. Another person's stuttering variability may be due to the frequency with which he or she has meetings with the boss before coming to the baseline sessions. Still another person's stuttering variability may be due to fluctuating marital problems at home.

Although tracking the variability of behaviors is worthwhile because it can lead to new information, it does involve taking a step back from the immediate clinical task at hand. The treatment will have to be postponed until the question of baseline variability is resolved. Obviously, this is not always desirable in clinical situations.

The third criterion to be applied in evaluating the baseline adequacy can be called a **potential for contrast;** baseline and treatment response rates should contrast with each other to convincingly show that a treatment was effective. A very high or very low baseline can be either acceptable or not acceptable, depending upon the direction in which the dependent variable is expected to be changed by the treatment variable. For example, a high rate of stuttering is acceptable, because the treatment is supposed to lower it. However, a high rate of fluency (with a negligible rate of stuttering) may be unacceptable because there is not much room to show the effects of treatment.

The best baseline provides a good contrast to the treatment condition. The behavior that is very low in the baseline condition may be shown to be very high in the treatment condition. When the reversal procedure is used in the later part of an experiment, the rates of manipulated behaviors may contrast with each other. An incompatible behavior the experimenter manipulates will be high, and the other will be low.

In some cases, the potential for contrast may make it possible to accept a highly variable response rate after all. Once again, a hypothetical example from stuttering may help. Assume that the stuttering is highly variable with no clear pattern. But the clinician may find out that although there is a wide range to the variability, the lowest level of stuttering, replicated a minimum of three times, is still considerably high. Let us say that over repeated observations, the least amount of dysfluency ever recorded is 15%, with a variability range of 15% to 37%. In this case, the clinician may decide to introduce treatment in spite of the variability, on the assumption that the treatment will bring stuttering to such a low frequency that there would still be a contrast. When a treatment is successful in virtually eliminating the disorder along with its variability, then the resulting contrast will have justified the introduction of treatment at a time when it would normally be considered undesirable.

Introduction of treatment on the basis of a potential for contrast in the face of high variability can be risky, of course, but taking risks is a part of all research activity. It is appropriate to introduce treatment when the variability gives the clinician a clear and solid floor so high that the treatment can be expected to lower it to a level that would provide a good contrast. In this case, one guideline that a clinician may use is the expected amount of change in the dependent variable. If a large effect that comes close to eliminating the behavior is expected (and supported from past research or experience), the clinician may introduce treatment in spite of a range of variability. However, if only a small degree of change is expected of the treatment, the clinician should continue baseline observations or seek an analysis of the reasons for variability. If either of these options is precluded, for whatever reason, the study may be abandoned and the client may be treated.

The basic strategy of analysis used in the single-subject designs requires contrasting levels of response rates in the adjacent conditions of most experiments. A contrastive shift in the rate of response must be evident in the treatment condition compared with the baseline condition. When the treatment is withdrawn, the declining (and decreased) response rate should provide a contrast with the increasing (and increased) response rate found in the treatment condition. Or, when the reversal follows treatment, the behaviors that changed in the opposite direction should contrast.

Although contrast helps demonstrate experimental control, a lack of contrast between certain conditions also is part of the analysis in single-subject designs. The baseline and the withdrawal conditions are expected to show a lack of contrast. In reversal designs, the behavior from which the treatment is withdrawn is expected to show the same lack of contrast, although its counterpart would provide increased contrast. The various baseline patterns that illustrate stability, pattern, and the presence and the absence of contrast are illustrated in Figure 4.6.

Ideal baselines are rarely achieved in clinical research unless one is willing to extend the observations to extents that often are impractical or unethical. Therefore, in the final interpretation of the data, a variety of factors, not just the stability of the baseline, must be taken into consideration. Such factors as the degree of variability, the existence of helpful patterns in variability, the presence of a high and stable floor, the expected magnitude of treatment effects, the degree of contrast in conditions that should be contrasted, and a similarity of patterns in conditions that need to be comparable help evaluate the internal validity (control) of given experiments.

Simultaneous Multibaselines

The final form of control used in the single-subject strategy involves simultaneous multibaselines. Normally, a single, stable baseline of a single target behavior is established before the treatment is started. This is the kind of baseline that was discussed in the previous section. In simultaneous multibaselines, several behaviors are observed before the introduction of treatment, and baselines are established on all of them. The baselines are repeated throughout the course of the experiment.

As noted earlier, single pretreatment baselines do not demonstrate control by themselves; they must be combined with one of the other control strategies. On the other hand, simultaneous multibaselines can demonstrate experimental control by themselves. For example, an investigator may obtain baselines of four grammatical features in an effort to establish the effectiveness of a language treatment program. Suppose that each of the behaviors is at the 0% baseline. The clinician then treats one of the grammatical features, increasing its production to 90% accuracy. Then, the other three morphemes are baserated again to show that their frequency did not change because they were not treated. The second morpheme is trained next, and the remaining two morphemes are baserated to document their unchanged status in the absence of treatment. In this manner, every time a behavior is brought under control, the baselines of unchanged behaviors help document the effects of treatment.

The visual effects of the control feature of the simultaneous multibaselines on four target behaviors are illustrated in Figure 4.7.

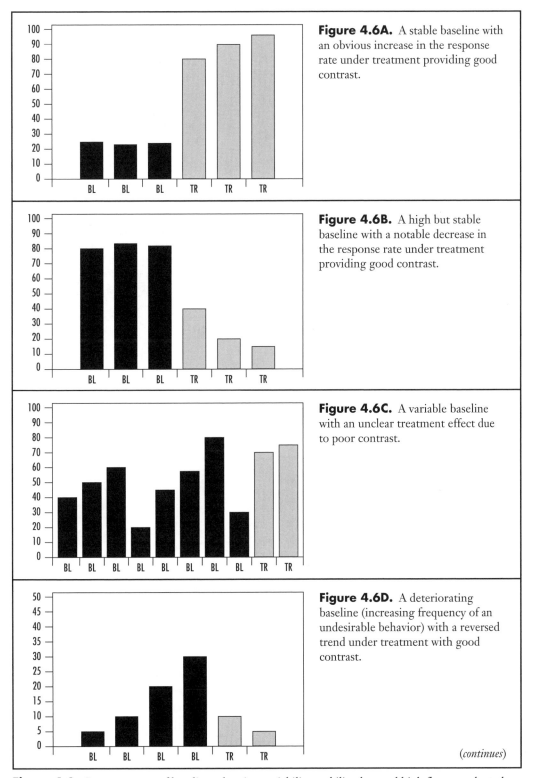

Figure 4.6A. A stable baseline with an obvious increase in the response rate under treatment providing good contrast.

Figure 4.6B. A high but stable baseline with a notable decrease in the response rate under treatment providing good contrast.

Figure 4.6C. A variable baseline with an unclear treatment effect due to poor contrast.

Figure 4.6D. A deteriorating baseline (increasing frequency of an undesirable behavior) with a reversed trend under treatment with good contrast.

(*continues*)

Figure 4.6. Seven patterns of baselines showing variability, stability, low and high floors, and good and poor contrast.

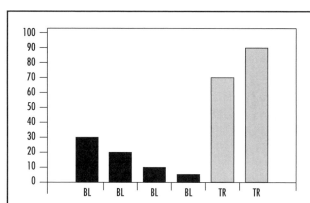

Figure 4.6E. A decreasing baseline (increasing frequency of a desirable behavior) with a reversed trend under treatment with good contrast.

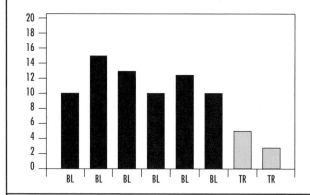

Figure 4.6F. A variable but acceptable baseline because of a high floor (10%) that provides good contrast with the treatment effect.

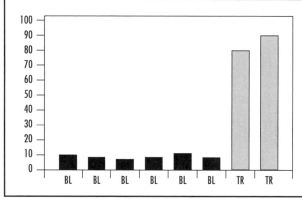

Figure 4.6G. A variable desirable behavior providing a low floor for a high contrast when the behavior increases significantly when treated.

Figure 4.6. *Continued.*

The multibaselines can be behaviors of the same or different participants. The baselines may also be situations where a particular behavior of a given individual is measured. When different participants constitute simultaneous multibaselines, participants are treated in sequence and baselines are repeatedly established on untreated participants. Unchanged behaviors of untreated participants help rule out the influence of extraneous variables. When different situations are the multibaselines, the same behavior is treated in sequence in different situations, and the rate of that behavior in

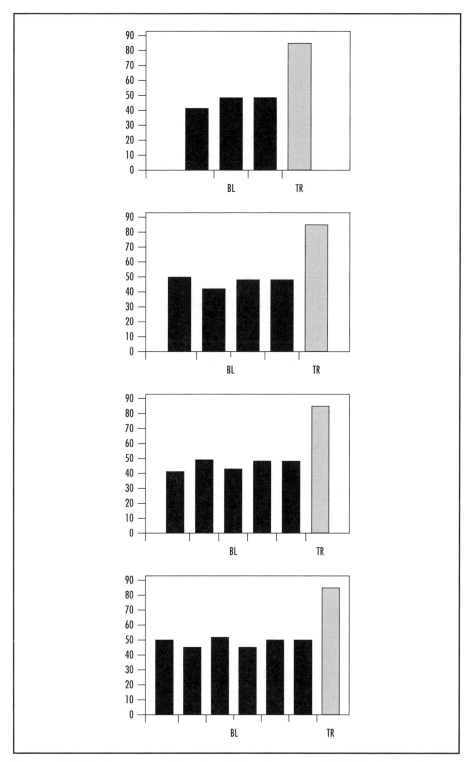

Figure 4.7. Simultaneous multibaselines (BL) and treatment (TR). Baselines are longer for behaviors that are treated later in the sequence. Each behavior increases only when treated.

untreated situations helps demonstrate the effects of the treatment. These three versions of the simultaneous multibaselines correspond to the three versions of the multiple baseline designs described in a later section of this chapter.

The logic of the simultaneous multibaselines comes close to that of the group design strategy. In group experimental designs, untreated participants serve the control function. In simultaneous multibaseline strategy, untreated behaviors, participants, or situations serve the same function. Unlike in the group design strategy, all participants receive treatment in designs that use simultaneous multibaselines as control procedures, however. The simultaneous multibaseline control procedure has been used extensively in clinical and educational research because it does not require clinically questionable strategies of withdrawal or reversal.

RANDOMIZED CLINICAL TRIALS VERSUS SINGLE-SUBJECT TREATMENT RESEARCH

Randomized group designs are well established in medical and surgical treatment research. Many medical researchers promote the RCTs as the "gold standard" of treatment research and conduct a large number of them. Annually and globally, several hundred RCTs are typically in progress. Many treatment researchers in communicative disorders, too, tend to favor RCTs of communication treatment procedures although such trials are few and far between.

Single-subject treatment approaches and RCTs are based on the same logic of causes and effects. They both use the experimental method to show that the treatment was the cause of improvement in people who receive it. Nonetheless, there are some important conceptual as well as methodological differences between the two approaches. Therefore, it is necessary to consider the following in understanding the differences between the two approaches: experimental control and internal validity; statistical and clinical generality; self-selection in randomized clinical trials; ethical issues with control groups; and treatment research in medicine versus communicative disorders.

Experimental Control and Internal Validity

The first concern of any treatment researcher is to establish good experimental control and achieve internal validity by ruling out extraneous variables. Under acceptable conditions, both RCTs and single-subject treatment research can achieve good experimental control and internal validity for the results. It should be noted that no experimental treatment evaluation is ideal or perfect. All treatment researchers are forced to make certain compromises because of practical exigencies. Too many and too serious compromises in methods of a study, however, will invalidate the results. For instance, a researcher using the randomized group design usually cannot select participants randomly from a defined clinical population. The researcher may recruit available people for participation. This may be an acceptable compromise assuming that the researcher will not claim external validity or statistical generality for the results. On the other hand, the researcher who fails to randomly assign participants to different groups will have made an unacceptable compromise. In that case, the researcher cannot claim internal validity for the results because there is no assurance that the two groups were equal to begin with.

Single-subject researchers, too, may make acceptable and unacceptable compromises. For instance, before introducing the treatment to be evaluated, single-subject treatment research requires stable baselines of target behaviors with little variation across baseline sessions. In some cases, such stability of target behaviors may be difficult to obtain. The investigator then may make an acceptable compromise and introduce treatment if the variability is within a certain range and the treatment produces large effects that override the variability. On the other hand, an investigator who introduces treatment when the target behaviors are highly unstable and the treatment effects are unclear against the background variability will have made an unacceptable compromise.

As noted in previous sections, RCTs use control groups to demonstrate internal validity and experimental control whereas single-subject designs use control conditions. Both are equally good in demonstrating the effectiveness of treatment procedures.

Statistical Generality Versus Clinical Validity

As defined previously, statistical generality refers to the degree to which the conclusions of a study based on a randomly selected and assigned sample may be extended to the population and logical generality is the extent to which the conclusions of a treatment study may be extended to individual clients who are similar to those who have served in a single-subject treatment study. Clinical validity, on the other hand, refers to the degree to which the treatment effects are personally and socially meaningful to those who experience it. Group and single-subject designs differ much on statistical generality, logical generality, clinical validity.

Historically, proponents of group experimental designs have claimed that the results of studies that use large numbers of participants may be extended to the population (D. T. Campbell & Stanley, 1966; Kerlinger, 1986). In other words, the assertion is that the results of group experimental designs have statistical generality whereas those of single-subject designs do not have it because of their small number of participants, constituting a nonrepresentative sample. It is true that one or a few single-subject design studies that show a treatment was effective cannot claim statistical generality. In other words, results of unreplicated single-subject studies cannot be extended to the population. Results of single-subject studies can be extended to the population only after demonstrating the same or similar effect in direct and systematic replications. The issue, however, is whether group design studies can demonstrate statistical generality without replications.

The claim of statistical generality for group designs is questionable on two major grounds. First, generality of treatment effects is always a matter of replications, not of experimental designs. The sample size is irrelevant to generality. In medical research, results of large clinical trials that included thousands of patients have later been questioned (e.g., studies on mamographic screening for breast cancer; see Gotzsche & Olsen, 2000). No clinician can assume that because a large number of patients have reacted to a treatment positively in a randomized clinical trial, all patients will react the same when different clinicians administer the same treatment to different patients in varied settings. Any kind of generality should be demonstrated, not assumed. To make sure that the treatment is effective with most patients treated in a variety of settings, studies should be replicated by different clinicians in varied settings. Randomization provides no shortcut to generality.

Second, statistical generality may be achieved in nonexperimental survey research, but not in treatment research in clinical disciplines, including medicine and speech–language pathology. In survey research, the concern is to predict behaviors of large groups of people. Behaviors of particular individuals do not matter. For instance, a national pollster (e.g., the Gallop Poll or the Harris Poll) is not interested in predicting the opinion or voting preferences of specific individuals. The pollster and the politician who pays for the poll results are both interested in the opinions and voting preferences of a majority in the population. Sample surveys (see Chapter 5 for details) can make a statistical prediction of a group's preference or behavior. This is because the pollster can and does draw a truly random sample of the population (e.g., voting-age persons). Such samples reflect the dispositions of the population. On the other hand, treatment researchers rarely, if ever, can draw a truly random sample of the population of clients or patients. The best the treatment researcher can do is to assign selected participants to two or more groups randomly. Random assignment does not assure any kind of generality, however. Random assignment can assure only that the groups were equal to begin with and that any difference at the end of the experiment must be due to treatment only. In other words, random assignment assures internal validity, not generality.

In essence, because the participants are not randomly selected from a population in RCTs, such trials cannot claim statistical generality. Any suggestion of random selection of participants is currently indefensible because of government regulations on human participant protection in all kinds of research. Essentially, no participant is randomly selected for RCTs. All participants select themselves, an issue addressed next.

Self-Selection in Randomized Clinical Trials

Before 1974, there were no laws in the United States to prevent abuse of human participants in experimental or nonexperimental research. Human participants were often not told about the purpose and methods of the experiment in which they were about to participate. In many cases, they were actively mislead by the scientists. While testing new and dangerous drugs, for instance, patients were led to believe that they were getting some safe and effective treatment. Such instances as not treating patients with syphilis to see what happens to them or injecting healthy patients with tumor cells have been documented (Beecher, 1966). When these and many other abusive practices in biomedical research came to light, the U.S. Congress passed the National Research Act of 1974 (P.L. 93-348) to prevent such abusive and dangerous research. See Chapter 16 for a short history and review of human participant protection measures.

Currently, in most countries where biomedical and behavioral research is conducted, potential human participants should give informed consent to participate. The research protocol and the human participant protection procedures should be reviewed and approved by an independent committee, formally known as *institutional review boards* and more popularly called *human subjects protection committees* (see Chapter 16 for details). Of all the procedures involved in protecting human participants, the informed consent has serious consequences for initial selection of participants and their eventual and complete participation until the end of a treatment study. These consequences negate randomization, and therefore, eliminate any possibility of statistical generality. Obviously, it is more important to protect human participants than it is to achieve statistical generality. Nonetheless, the inevitable consequences of informed consent on participant selection process must be clearly understood.

Aspects of informed consent that affect the participant selection process include the following. First, potential participants must be fully told about the purpose and methods of the study. Second, the potential participants must fully understand the potential risks and benefits of treatments they will receive. Third, after fully understanding the objectives, methods, benefits, and risks of a study, all individuals should give free and voluntary consent to participate. Fourth, all participants who initially give voluntary consent to participate are totally free to withdraw any time during the course of the study. Fifth, all participants retain a right to demand alternative treatments to which they are not assigned, demand or reject the experimental treatment, refuse to be a part of a control group that does not receive treatment, and simply drop out of a study without giving any reason. When these conditions are fulfilled—all researchers are legally required to fulfill them—there is no random selection or assignment of participants in so-called RCTs.

Treatment researchers initially identify potential participants who are available in clinics and hospitals. They rarely start with a population of patients all of whom have the same chance of being selected. Obviously, those with the same disease or disorder who are not seeking treatment are not in the potential participant pool. A researcher may randomly select patients among available patients; however, this is not random selection from a population of patients. It is now well established that a large number of potential participants who have been randomly selected for a study refuse to participate. In medical research, it has been documented that many primary care physicians do not refer their patients to experimental treatment evaluation because their patients who need urgent treatment may be assigned to a risky new treatment, to a no-treatment control group, or to a fake treatment placebo group (Taylor, 1985). Consequently, those who eventually agree to participate do not constitute a randomly selected sample. In fact, investigators no longer can select and keep patients in a study; it is the patients who select an investigator and then continue only if they want to.

The self-selection process continues to operate even after obtaining informed consent from individuals who do agree to participate, because the initial consent to participate does not require participants to finish the study. After obtaining informed consent, researchers randomly assign participants to experimental and control groups. An individual's assignment to new treatment, an established treatment, or a placebo control group may or may not be revealed, depending on the blinding procedure. The self-selection tendency begins to exert its greatest influence when patients find out or suspect their group assignment. Patients who are assigned to a risky new treatment (the treatment being evaluated in the study) may demand a well-established older treatment. To the contrary, when it is suspected that the new treatment involves fewer risks than the older treatment, patients may refuse to receive the older treatment. Many who are assigned to the placebo control group may demand treatment, the new or the old, depending on the situation. Some who are assigned to placebo group may simply drop out of the study to seek treatment outside the scope of the study. Those who find either treatment unattractive also may drop out of the study. Furthermore, those who have received one or the other treatment but are disappointed with its effects may drop out as well. Finally, some individuals who reluctantly accept an undesirable treatment may not comply with the treatment protocol, inducing data distortions. A consequence of all of these self-selection tendencies is that those who complete the new treatment regimen are even more self-selected than the initial, already self-selected volunteers. As a result, the new treatment will have been evaluated on a special group of individuals. Therefore, there is nothing random about their selection or assignment.

Bias introduced by self-selection of participants makes it difficult to extend the conclusions of a study to the population. This is because self-selected individuals may not represent the unselected individuals in the population. There is now plenty of evidence that volunteers and those who stay with a study until its completion have different characteristics than those who do not volunteer or who drop out after volunteering. Medical journals have shown that those who volunteer to participate in research on new treatment for a disease tend to be poorer, less educated, and more seriously ill than those who refuse participation. A majority of those who volunteer for new treatment study lack health insurance and will have had a poor health status. On the other hand, those who volunteer to participate in a study designed to enhance health status or prevent diseases are more affluent and better educated than those who refuse participation in such studies (Gorkin et al., 1996; McKee et al., 1999). In any case, those who initially volunteer to participate and those who eventually complete the study do not represent the population to which they presumably belong. Therefore, the typical claim that RCTs or group experimental designs that use large numbers of participants have statistical generality is an unacceptable claim.

Because of the human participant protection procedures, participants in single-subject research also are self-selected. Self-selection does not pose a serious problem when statistical generality based on a single study is not claimed. It poses a problem only when the mistaken claim of statistical generality is made based on a single RCT. Single-subject researchers typically avoid this mistake.

It is true that eventually researchers want to establish treatment procedures that work with a larger number of individuals with given diseases or disorders. That is, statistical generality is a worthy goal. Unfortunately, it cannot be achieved by a single study of any kind. It can be achieved only by systematically replicating a treatment study in different settings, by different investigators, and by recruiting a variety of patients or clients. Multiple replications that repeatedly sample small number of participants to study them intensively are more likely than RCTs to contribute more to statistical generality.

Ethical Issues with Control Groups

All participants in single-subject designs experience treatment even if the treatment offered initially is withdrawn for a short duration of time in certain of the designs. When a no-treatment control group is used in group designs, the treatment is denied to members of that group. When a placebo control group is used, a fake treatment is offered to members of that group. The placebo-control group is the same as the no-treatment control group except that the members of the former group are misled to believe that they may be getting the real treatment. Treatment denial and placebo controls raise much more serious ethical concerns than temporary withdrawal of treatment found in some single-subject designs (e.g., the *ABAB* design and its variations, see Chapter 9).

The ethical issues related to no-treatment or placebo controlled RCTs are addressed in greater detail in Chapter 16. In medicine, placebo control is more often used than no-treatment control. Note that treatment denial or sham treatment may be unethical and socially unacceptable, except in certain highly circumscribed situations (e.g., a total absence of a treatment for a disease except for the one being evaluated). Unfortunately, far too many medical treatment studies are still conducted with no-treatment or placebo controls.

Placebo procedures in surgical treatment research raise the most serious ethical questions In some studies, placebo control group patients in heart surgery research have had their chest cavity cut, opened, and then closed without taking any remedial steps to give the patient an impression that the intended surgical procedure had been carried out on them. In studies on Parkinson's disease, holes were drilled in the skulls of placebo control group patients' to simulate intracerebral transplantation of fetal mesencephalic tissue (Brody, 1998; Dekkers & Boer, 2001; Morris, Zaritsky, & LaFever, 2000; Verdu-Pascal & Castello-Ponce, 2001). Such invasive procedures performed on control group subjects who, instead of receiving some benefit or even no benefit, expose themselves to significant risk, pain, and suffering are hard to ethically justify.

Those who believe that RCTs are the only means of establishing treatment effects accept the ethical problems as inevitable. In most behavioral research, control conditions (e.g., baselines, treatment withdrawal, treatment reinstatement, multiple baselines) will satisfactorily establish treatment effects with no control groups. In most medical research, too, control conditions will work fine. The same patients' symptoms or health status may be measured under baseline, under administration of new medicine, and under temporary withdrawal of medicine which is reinstated as quickly as possible. All patients will be treated in this arrangement. Single-subject designs are quite effective in disease prevention studies. For instance multiple baseline designs will work well in studies on weight loss, smoking cessation, cholesterol reduction, exercise programs, and so forth. Other single-subject designs will work just as well. While all treatment studies raise some ethical issues, single-subject designs minimize the ethical dilemmas more satisfactorily than the RCTs.

Treatment Research in Medicine Versus Communicative Disorders

Although the basic logic of establishing cause–effect relationships is the same in all sciences, there are some important structural and practical differences between treatment research in medicine and speech–language pathology. In fact, all behavioral (nonmedical) treatment or teaching procedures, including those used in counseling, clinical psychology, social work, physical therapy, health science, occupational therapy, special and regular education, and so forth contrast with medical procedures in certain important respects. Therefore, it is necessary to understand the nature of treatment in these disciplines to objectively evaluate the different options available for treatment research.

In medicine, treatment research is typically conducted in three phases. In Phase I trials, new drugs are tested to evaluate their safety, not effectiveness. Whether a drug produces a toxic effect is the main concern in Phase I trials. A small number of individuals (typically 10 to 30), mostly healthy volunteers, are tested. There is no random selection or random assignment of participants in Phase I trials. There are no control groups either. Treatment that passes the Phase I trial is advanced to Phase II trials in which 50 to 100 patients with the target disease may be tested. A few Phase II trials may use randomization and a control group, but most do not (Finn, 1999; Meinert, 1986; Pocock, 1983). Phase II trials involve homogeneous participants selected with clearly specified criteria, as against RCTs that use heterogeneous participants.

Treatments that pass the first two phases are advanced to Phase III trials in which the new procedure is experimentally evaluated. Only Phase III trials are RCTs involving experimental and control groups. Large numbers of patients in multiple centers and multiple countries may be selected for participation. Trials involving multiple centers and countries also involve hundreds of medical personnel helping collect data.

Randomization in Phase III clinical trials is limited to an initial random assignment of available patients to the experimental and control groups. As noted before, there is no random selection from a defined population, and the random assignment is continuously subverted by ethically justified patient decisions; consequently, all participants in RCTs are self-selected. In any case, the effects of a new treatment are often evaluated in an experimental group compared against control groups that receive either a standard treatment, no treatment, or a placebo.

Important differences emerge when RCTs in medicine are compared with treatment research in speech–language pathology and many other allied health professions. Institutional, economic, and scientific distinctions need to be considered. Nationally and internationally, many medical hospitals are large institutions that house great numbers of patients who may at least initially consider participation in treatment research. Such a large participant pool is typically not available in speech–language pathology. Limited participant pool also characterizes clinical psychology and several other health-related professions. Within the medical discipline, such specialties as surgery and psychiatry also face a dearth of participant populations for treatment research. For instance, RCTs are fewer and use few participants in surgery and psychiatry. While in medicine, some large-scale studies have used a few thousand to 40,000 patients in multiple centers, psychotherapy research has used an average of 12 to 13 patients (Pocock, 1983; Shapiro & Shapiro, 1983). In speech–language pathology, large-scale studies are few, and the number of participants rarely exceeds a few dozen.

Economic factors that distinguish treatment research in medicine from that of speech–language pathology may be even more powerful than the institutional differences in service delivery. Most RCTs in medicine, simultaneously conducted in multiple centers in several countries, are fully supported by global pharmaceutical companies who are anxious to bring their product to market. Legally, drugs cannot be marketed without extensive experimental evaluations. Therefore, the pressure to conduct treatment research in medicine is much higher than that in such disciplines as communicative disorders, education, clinical psychology, counseling, and so forth. The legal requirement to evaluate new procedures and the enormous financial stakes involved in developing and marketing new treatment products in medicine force drug and other treatment product manufacturers to support global RCTs. Additionally, government and private agencies offer a significant amount of financial support for medical treatment research. Compared to this, the amount of financial support available for conducting large-scale treatment research in speech–language pathology is miniscule. Small-scale studies on behavioral techniques, such as those done with single-subject designs, are more practical, and hence, more often performed and reported.

Scientific distinctions include the nature of independent and dependent variables in speech–language pathology and medicine. Treatment (independent variables) in medicine is relatively easily administered by a large number of well-trained individuals in multiple centers. New drugs being evaluated have clear prescriptions on how much, when, and how to administer to selected patients. A large number of medical technicians in different countries can administer treatment with little variation in procedures.

For several reasons, treatment in speech–language pathology, compared to that in medicine, is difficult to administer to a large number of individuals. First, being behavioral in nature, treatment in speech–language pathology is not as standardized as drug administration. Even though many procedures are clearly described (e.g., the discrete trial procedure in language treatment, syllable prolongation in stuttering treatment, or cueing hierarchy in treating naming deficits in patients with aphasia), their administration may be as varied as the number of clinicians who use them. Speech–language pathologists do not follow strict treatment protocols, although it is possible to train them to do so. Such training will be necessary in any treatment research. If the treatment research is an RCT, multiple clinicians will have to be trained to follow a strict treatment protocol. The required training expense may be prohibitive to most treatment researchers.

Second, compared to medical treatment, treatment in speech–language pathology is more labor intensive. Stuttering treatment for a child or an adult might take 9 months of individual therapy, offered twice weekly, in sessions lasting 45 to 60 minutes. Similarly, treatment of language and phonological disorders takes months of regular therapy. Treatment of aphasia may last a year or more. RCTs on such speech and language treatments with a large enough number of participants to be meaningfully randomized will involve an incredible number of clinician–client contact hours. Such treatments cannot be administered by technicians or aides. On the other hand, the administration of most drugs in RCTs may require a few minutes of daily patient contact, is likely to be over in a few days or weeks, and is typically accomplished with the help of large numbers of readily available nurses, medical technicians, and other aides.

Third, training a large number of speech–language pathologists to administer treatment uniformly in a large RCT will pose significant practical and economic hurdles. The task of training medical personnel in following a drug administration protocol for a randomized study would involve much less effort, training time, and research funds than training a large number of speech–language pathologists to administer a treatment for stuttering, phonological disorder, or aphasia. Until funds for treatment research in speech–language pathology are increased geometrically, this kind of clinician training will be impractical. Without such training, data generated by RCTs in speech–language pathology and related disciplines will be uninterpretable.

Fourth, the nature of dependent variables or skills taught to clients with communicative disorders also poses problems for speech–language pathologists conducting RCTs. Similar to treatment administration in speech–language pathology, documenting changes in communication skills due to treatment is more labor-intensive, riddled with controversies, and takes more time than documenting changes due to medical treatment. This problem can get compounded beyond practicality in a large RCT that may require multiple measures of the dependent variable to achieve reliability. Although unreliable dependent variable measurement is a problem in medicine as well (e.g., questionable results of a single laboratory test for blood cholesterol), reliability can be more easily achieved with multiple measures that are less time consuming than in speech–language pathology (e.g., recording, transcribing, and analyzing multiple language samples for each of hundreds of children in a randomized language treatment study).

The differences between treatment research in medicine and communicative disorders suggest that small groups of participants, studied intensively, will produce more practical and valid treatment efficacy data. Relatively small number of homogeneous individuals may be studied either with group designs or single-subject designs. Participants may be randomly assigned to groups, but no statistical generality will then be claimed. Both the single-subject and group design studies will eventually claim generality only on the basis of successful direct and systematic replications.

CLASSIFICATION OF TREATMENT RESEARCH

Treatment research is done at various levels. At certain levels, treatment research does not establish that the treatment indeed caused the changes in clients who received it. As noted before, treatment research may document improvement, generalized consequences, and functional outcomes or may establish a cause–effect relationship between treatment and its effects. Therefore, the first criterion in classifying treatment research is **causality,** or the degree of experimental control used in studies that evaluate different treatment procedures (Hegde, 1998a, 1998b).

The second criterion to be used in classifying treatment research is **generality,** or the presence, absence, and degree of replication; generality is the extent to which the conclusions of a treatment study may be extended to all those who need or could benefit from the same or similar treatment. When the results of a treatment study are replicated, professionals may use the technique with greater degree of confidence.

The first criterion of causality produces treatment research at two major levels: uncontrolled and controlled. The second criterion of generality results in three major levels: unreplicated, directly replicated, and systematically replicated treatment studies. The two criteria interact with each other to produce six levels of treatment research: (a) uncontrolled unreplicated, (b) uncontrolled directly replicated, (c) uncontrolled systematically replicated, (d) controlled unreplicated, (e) controlled directly replicated, and (f) controlled and systematically replicated (Hegde, 1998b). I will now address these six levels of treatment research and the evidence they create.

Uncontrolled Unreplicated Treatment Research

Treatment research is uncontrolled when it does not use an experimental design and, therefore, lacks internal validity. A study is unreplicated when it is the first in a series on a given technique. Therefore, **uncontrolled unreplicated treatment research** is an original case study on a new treatment technique. Case studies use no control groups or control conditions. Consequently, case studies do not offer the assurance that the clients would not have improved without the treatment under investigation. Chapters 8 and 9 describe methods of uncontrolled case studies. In the group design strategy, it is the typical single-group design that receives treatment preceded by a pretest and followed by a posttest. In single-subject designs, it is the *AB* design in which the target behavior is baserated (*A* condition) and then the treatment is offered (*B* condition). Neither design rules out the extraneous variables.

An unreplicated study does not test the reliability of already reported findings on a treatment technique. It reports new findings, even if they are uncontrolled. Therefore, an uncontrolled unreplicated study is the first case study on a treatment technique. The goal of such a study is to demonstrate improvement in clients who receive a treatment.

Measurement of Improvement

Measuring improvement in clients who receive treatment is an everyday activity of all professionals. Such measures become a part of clinical reports written on clients, but they do not get published. On the other hand, the results of an uncontrolled unreplicated case study may be published in a journal with a view to stimulate additional research on the technique. Improvement is measured against the initial assessment results, pretests, or baselines of target behaviors. When systematic positive changes follow the application of treatment, the researcher then claims improvement.

Case studies may report on a single case or a number of cases. Generally case studies offer more information on the clients served. Studies with a single case or a few cases may provide detailed information on them. Such information may be useful in judging whether the treatment may be applied to other individuals who share similarities with those in the study.

Because improvement offers only uncontrolled data, the researcher should neither claim effectiveness for the procedure nor recommend it for general professional practice because the data may not be reliable. That is, whether the same or similar results would be obtained when the treatment is applied to other clients remains unknown until a replication is made. Although the goal of uncontrolled unreplicated treatment research is to stimulate further research, a common danger is to uncritically assume that the technique is effective. Promoting a widespread professional practice of a technique based on a case study is unethical. Only techniques based on replications and controlled studies may be ethically promoted. To consider using the technique, professionals should wait at least until controlled studies support it. Ideally, they should wait until controlled replications support it.

Uncontrolled and unreplicated case studies do make a significant contribution to treatment research literature. Kazdin (1998) recommended several steps to increase the chances that the reported improvement may be due to treatment in a case study. First, case studies should offer objective data gathered from direct observations; it should not depend on anecdotal accounts to document improvement. Second, assessment of improvement should be frequent, not limited to just a pretest and a posttest. Pretreatment measures should show that the problem was stable and was unlikely to disappear without treatment. Continuous measurement of improvement during treatment sessions will show the course of treatment and the correlated improvement. Third, the improvement demonstrated should be large enough to be clinically significant and immediately follow the application of treatment. Delayed and limited improvements are not as credible as improvements of greater magnitude that appear soon after the application of the technique. Fourth, improvement should be demonstrated in multiple cases. Credibility of improvement demonstrated in multiple *and* heterogeneous cases will inspire greater confidence.

Results of carefully done case studies on treatment can help both professionals and treatment researchers. Professionals can discard treatment techniques that do not produce improvement in case studies. A technique that did not produce improvement in case studies is unlikely to be found effective in experimental studies. Therefore, researchers my find little justification to design an expensive experimental study to evaluate such a technique. If the results of case studies, especially replicated results, are positive, there is a good chance that an experimental study will establish the effect of the treatment.

Measurement of Generalized Consequences of Treatment

Initially, measurement of generalized consequences of a treatment offered to clients also is uncontrolled and unreplicated. The researcher who documents improvement in a case study may proceed to document generalized production of target behaviors in extraclinical situations. For example, a child who learns new language skills under a new treatment procedure may use those clinically learned language skills at home, school, and in other social situations. Similarly, increased fluency in persons who stutter may generalize to home, office, and social situations. A deaf child who learns American Sign Language at school may begin to use the signs at home.

When skills generalize from the clinic or a special education classroom to the natural environment, the clinician cannot claim that such generalized productions were due to treatment. Generalization of treated target skills is usually measured under uncontrolled conditions, even if the treatment was offered in a controlled study. Therefore, generalized production of clinically established behaviors further documents expanded consequences of treatment, but it neither assures that the treatment was effective nor that the treatment was responsible for generalization. Extraneous variables may be responsible for generalized productions in both uncontrolled and controlled studies.

Measurement of Treatment Outcomes

Beyond documenting improvement in clients who receive treatment, a researcher also may measure broad outcomes of clinical interventions. Because outcomes, as defined in this chapter, are an expanded notion of improvement, the first step in measuring outcomes is to document that clinically established skills are produced in natural environmental contexts. For instance, a patient with aphasia whose communication skills have improved under language treatment should use those skills while talking to health-care professionals in the hospital and family members at home. Eventually, generalized productions should be expanded into more complex behaviors. For instance, the same treated patient with aphasia should expand the limited language skills taught in the clinic into longer and more complex productions to meet the demands of varied communication contexts.

Outcome measures go beyond generalized production, however. The clinically established skills should also be maintained over time and across situations. Therefore, measurement of maintenance also is a part of outcomes research.

Outcome measures are uncontrolled documentation of expanded and clinically valid consequences of treatment. As noted previously, they do not help assert a cause–effect relation between the treatment and the changes that followed.

Measurement of Maintenance of Treatment Gains

Beyond documenting generalization and outcomes of treatment consequences, a treatment researcher also may measure maintenance of target skills across time. Professionals, too, may document maintenance of clinically established behaviors. Therefore, measurement of maintenance may be a part of controlled as well as uncontrolled studies. But in either case, and as noted before, the measures of maintenance remain uncontrolled because it is difficult to establish a cause–effect relation between the treatment (controlled or uncontrolled) and maintenance. By definition, maintained behaviors are generalized and expanded behaviors, too. Furthermore, if the measures of maintenance also reflect clinical validity of treatment gains, they then are an index of outcomes as well.

Chapter 9 on single-subject designs describes a few strategies to measure response maintenance. But generally speaking, maintenance is measured periodically after the client has been dismissed from clinical treatment or has completed a treatment research study. What happens to the clinically established skills once the treatment is completed? Most often, this is the kind of question asked in maintenance research. It rarely asks whether treatment was responsible for maintenance of treatment gains. Such a question, as noted before, is difficult to answer.

Uncontrolled Directly Replicated Treatment Research

The reliability of improvement that results from a treatment when first evaluated in a case study is unknown. The clinically significant improvement initially obtained may not be sustained in subsequent case studies. Therefore, clinicians who first reported improvement with a technique need to replicate their case study.

Uncontrolled directly replicated treatment research is a repetition of the original case study by the same investigators in their original setting with new clients who exhibit the same disorder. If the results are similar to those reported in the original study, a successful replication will have been accomplished. A successful replication increases the probability that the results of the original study were reliable. Repeated direct replications will generate more confidence in the results and the technique's ability to produce improvement.

As with the original case studies, successful but uncontrolled direct replications cannot claim treatment effects or a cause–effect relation between treatment and positive changes in clients, although the technique may be considered a good candidate for an experimental evaluation. Besides improvement, uncontrolled direct replications also may document treatment outcomes, generalized consequences of treatment, and maintenance of clinically acquired skills and their expansions. Such replications may suggest that the technique may have generality to new clients, as each direct replication uses new clients.

Uncontrolled Systematically Replicated Treatment Research

Successful direct replications show that a treatment reliably produces improvement in the original setting, when the original clinicians used the technique with new clients. Such replications do not show that other clinicians in other settings may obtain improvement in their clients with the same technique. In other words, the technique's generality to clients served in other clinics by other clinicians still remains unknown.

Uncontrolled systematically replicated treatment research is the repetition of a case study by other clinicians, in new settings, using new clients to establish the generality of improvement. Generally, new clinicians in new settings will use the treatment procedure as described in the original case studies. In such cases, the new clinicians will not change the treatment procedure. If the clinicians are successful in systematically replicating the results of the original case studies, the generality of improvement data begins to emerge.

In some systematic replications, the new clinicians may modify the procedure in light of their clinical experience, theory, or their client characteristics. Such modifications are a part of systematic replications. For instance, clinicians who systematically replicate a case study may offer the treatment more or less frequently than in the original studies. They may change the reinforcement schedule, amount of modeling, feedback for error responses, and so forth. In fact, even the original investigators, after having directly replicated their findings on a treatment, may make systematic modifications in treatment to obtain greater improvement in their clients. When such modifications are made, the replications are systematic even if done by the original investigators.

Besides improvement, uncontrolled systematic replications also may document other types of consequences that follow a treatment's application, including treatment outcomes, generalized consequences of treatment, and maintenance of clinically acquired skills and expansion of those skills. Once again, there would be no justification for drawing a cause–effect relation between these consequences and the treatment.

Systematic replications of treatment in case study formats will greatly enhance the possibility that the treatment will be found effective in experimental studies. In the absence of controlled experimental data on treating certain disorders, clinicians should at least look for a technique that is associated with systematically replicated improvement in case studies.

Controlled Unreplicated Treatment Research

When a treatment is shown to produce improvement in direct or systematic replications, the next logical step is to evaluate it in an experimental study to find out if it is effective. An initial controlled treatment study is the beginning of treatment efficacy research. Therefore, **controlled unreplicated treatment research** is the first experimental study on a new treatment procedure. Although it is preferable to design a controlled study on a technique that is shown to reliably produce improvement, in practice it may not always happen that way. Treatment researchers may design a controlled experimental study to evaluate the effectiveness of a technique even when there are no case studies on it.

Researchers may use either a group or a single-subject experimental design to establish a cause–effect relation between a treatment and the consequences that follow. To demonstrate that it was the treatment and no other variable that produced the consequences, researchers may use the pretest–posttest control group design, described in Chapter 8. This design will effectively rule out extraneous variables and establish a treatment's effects by showing that only those who received the treatment, and not those in the control group, showed positive changes. The participants need to be randomly selected and randomly assigned to the two groups at the beginning of the experiment. Significant changes in the posttest scores observed only for the experimental group will help demonstrate the treatment effectiveness.

Similarly, the *ABAB* design or the multiple baseline design, described in Chapter 9, will help accomplish the same goals within the single-subject strategy. While these designs avoid a control group that does not receive treatment, they use multiple control conditions to show that when the treatment was absent, the consequences, too, were absent in the same individuals. All participants receive treatment in single-subject experiments, although in some designs, participants may receive it in a staggered fashion. In multiple baseline design across subjects, for instance, participants receive treatment in sequence, not simultaneously. Those who have not yet been treated will serve the control function by not showing the treatment effects until they, too, are treated. In the *ABAB* design, the skills to be treated are first baserated (initial *A*), the treatment is then offered (the initial *B*), and the treatment is then briefly withdrawn (the second *A*), and it is finally reinstated (the final *B*) to end the experiment with treatment.

In addition to effectiveness, controlled unreplicated studies also may measure treatment outcomes, generalized consequences of treatment, and maintenance of clinically acquired skills and their expansions. Of all these measures, only the effects observed during the treatment sessions may be causally linked with the treatment. Outcomes, generalized productions, and maintained skills may or may not be due to treatment because other variables may be responsible for them.

When an experimental design is used to evaluate a treatment, the researcher can conclude that the treatment was or was not effective, depending on the data. But in no case can a researcher claim that the results of an initial (unreplicated) study are applicable to other clients, served in other settings, by other clinicians. In fact, the researchers cannot claim that their own future clients will react the same to the treatment. This is because the reliability of the results of a single experiment is unknown, regardless of the sample size. That reliability is established only through replications. Only the replications will tell whether the treatment will be applicable to other clients in the same or different setting.

Controlled Evaluation of Single or Multiple Treatment Effects

Controlled treatment research may evaluate either a single treatment or multiple treatments. The effect a single treatment produces on its own is known as the **independent effect** or **absolute effect.** As noted, this effect is studied within several group and single-subject designs.

Controlled evaluation of multiple treatments require more complex designs. Multiple treatment evaluations seek to assess the relative effects of two or more treatment procedures. **Relative effects** refer to lesser or greater effects of two or more treatments. Whether one treatment is more effective than the other is the main research question to be investigated. Therefore, this kind of research assumes that the independent effects of the multiple treatments under study have been established. If this is indeed the case, then within the group design approach, there usually is no reason to include a control group that does not receive treatment. Each treatment will have been evaluated against a control group in prior studies. Therefore, investigators using the group design approach may select the multigroup pretest–posttest design or the multigroup posttest-only design to evaluate the relative effects of two or more treatments. The number of groups in a study will be the same as the number of treatments being evaluated. Each group will receive a different treatment, as described in Chapter 8.

Within the single-subject approach, relative effects of two or more treatments may be assessed by using the *ABACA/ACABA* design or the alternating treatments design, both described in Chapter 9. In the *ABACA/ ACABA* design, one set of participants experience the *ABACA* sequence of conditions and another set experiences the *ACABA* sequence. In the *ABACA* sequence offered to one set of participants, the initial *A* condition represents the baseline; the *B* condition represents Treatment 1, the second *A* represents withdrawal of treatment to recapture the baseline, and the *C* condition represents Treatment 2. In the *ACABA* sequence offered to another set, the initial *A* condition represents the baseline; the *C* condition represents Treatment 2, the second *A* represents withdrawal of treatment, and the *B* condition represents Treatment 1. In essence, Treatments 1 and 2 are counterbalanced, which means that each appears once in the first place and once in the second place. All participants receive both the treatments.

In the alternating treatments design, also described in Chapter 9, two treatments are alternated across treatment sessions in a semirandomized order. In Session 1, for example, Treatment 1 may be offered and in Session 2, Treatment 2 is offered. From then on, the sequence is semirandomized so that the resulting patterns are not exactly anticipated by the participants. Both the treatments are offered equally often.

Controlled Evaluation of Treatment Interactions

After having established the independent and perhaps relative effects of multiple treatments, researchers may wish to evaluate the combined effects of two or more treatments. When treatments are combined, one might expect an effect that is larger than just the additive effects of those combined. Combined treatment effects that are larger than what might be expected by just adding each treatment's independent effects are known as **interactional effects.** This is an important area of treatment research because clinicians hope to increase the effectiveness of their treatments by combining procedures that enhance the overall effect.

Studying interaction also requires complex designs. Within the group design approach, multiple groups of participants may help evaluate interaction. For instance, in evaluating the independent and interactive effects of two treatments, researchers may form three groups. Group 1 will receive Treatment 1, Group 2 will receive Treatment 2, and Group 3 will receive both the treatments. A much larger effect in Group 3 will indicate a potential interaction and definite clinical benefits of combining the two. To draw valid conclusions, the three groups should be equal on all relevant variables. A randomly drawn and assigned sample will assure that.

The interactional design, described in Chapter 9, is the most commonly used single-subject design in evaluating interactional effects of combined treatments. The design helps assess both the independent and interactional effects of two or more treatments, although studying more than two variables within the design is cumbersome and often impractical. A common variation of the interactional design is described as the *A-B-BC-B-BC/*

A-C-CB-C-CB design in which *B* and *C* are different treatments. To counterbalance the two treatments and their independent positions in the sequence, the *A-B-BC-B-BC* sequence is applied to one set of participants and the *A-C-CB-C-CB* sequence is applied to another set of participants. Note that the first and the single treatment offered is *B* in the former sequence and *C* in the latter sequence. This is the essence of counterbalancing. In each sequence, a treatment is offered alone twice and offered in combination with the other twice. If the combined conditions show greater effects than the single conditions, there is perhaps an interaction. For clinicians, the implication is clear: It is better to combine the two.

Controlled Directly Replicated Treatment Research

The first step in evaluating the general applicability of a treatment procedure that was shown to be effective in an initial experimental study is to conduct controlled direct replications. **Controlled directly replicated treatment research** is the repetition of an original experimental study by the same investigators in their own setting with new clients. The original investigators will apply the experimental treatment in the same manner as before to see if the results of the original experiment can be recaptured. The investigators may use the same experimental design as before, but some investigators may use a different design. For instance, a researcher who had shown a treatment's effectiveness within an *ABAB* design may replicate it within a multiple baseline design. It is important to note that what is replicated is the experimental treatment and its results, not necessarily the experimental design.

Controlled directly replicated studies also may measure additional treatment consequences, including treatment outcomes, generalized consequences of treatment, and maintenance of clinically acquired skills and their expansions. As with the original controlled studies, such replications, cannot claim that these additional consequences were the effects of treatment.

Controlled directly replicated experiments that show that the treatment effects are replicable begin to establish the generality of that treatment's effects. Although more replications are needed, a successful direct replication of a treatment effect might suggest that other replications, too, may be successful. Direct replications only show that the treatment effects are reliable in the original setting, with the original investigators. There is no assurance that the treatment will produce the same positive results in other settings, in the hands of other clinicians. Systematic replications are needed to find out if the treatment will produce the same or similar results in other settings.

Controlled direct replications may involve a single treatment, multiple treatments, or interaction between treatments. The design options remain the same as those in the previous section on controlled unreplicated research.

Controlled Systematically Replicated Treatment Research

The highest level of treatment research evidence is produced by controlled systematic replication of treatment effects. **Controlled systematically replicated treatment research** is the repetition of an experimental treatment study, typically conducted by other investigators in new settings recruiting new clients. Although the highest form of systematic replications will be performed by investigators other than the original researchers in different settings, the original researchers themselves may begin such replications. Selecting new clients, the investigators who have completed direct replications of their prior controlled studies on a treatment may begin to fine-tune the technique to produce better results. In light of the previous findings, they may change some aspect of the procedure to enhance the effectiveness of the technique. The investigators may also wonder if the technique will be effective with clients who are older or younger than those in the original and direct replication series. They may then apply the technique to clients with different age levels to find out. The investigators may sample clients of different gender, ethnocultural group, and even those with a different disorder. For instance, an intervention found to be effective with articulation disorders may be effective with language disorders. All such efforts of the original investigators of a treatment procedure constitute systematic replications, although they are done in the original setting. Replications of this kind show that the treatment is or is not effective with clients who differ from those in the original study on some defined dimension. In essence, such replications help establish generality or the limits of generality of the treatment procedure.

Investigators who replicate studies published by other researchers help expand the scope or define additional limits of generality. When other investigators' replications in new settings are successful, the technique's generality across settings, clients, and clinicians begins to emerge. When multiple investigators in varied settings obtain similar results in controlled studies, the technique's generality is well established.

Investigators who replicate someone else's controlled treatment studies might initially closely follow the original treatment protocol. If they change the treatment procedure in some manner, failure to replicate the original findings will be hard to interpret. A treatment in a systematic replication may fail because of lack of setting generality, clinician generality, client generality, treatment modification, or a combination of these factors. One would not know which one is responsible for the failure. Therefore, it is safer to use the treatment as described in the original reports. Even then, reasons for a failure to replicate may not be clear, but there is at least no confounding from treatment modifications. When a variety of investigators in varied settings have systematically replicated the technique's effects, potential reasons for failure in other studies may be suggested. Possibly, failed replications did not use the technique properly or they included clients with unique characteristics.

If the patterns of failed replications are themselves replicated, limits of a treatment's generality is established. It is important for the clinicians to know to whom the technique applies and to whom it does not. A treatment procedure's limits of generality suggest that the technique is inappropriate for certain clients. For instance, systematic replications of a treatment procedure may consistently fail with certain clients: nonwhite clients, older clients (or younger clients) women (or men), and so forth. Such failed replications that produce a pattern of failure are important studies. The technique can then be withheld from such clients.

In addition to effectiveness, controlled systematically replicated studies may measure treatment outcomes, generalized consequences of treatment, and maintenance of clinically acquired skills and their expansions. As with all forms of controlled research, only the effects observed in the treatment sessions may be causally linked with the treatment. Outcomes, generalized productions, and maintained skills may or may not be due to treatment because other variables may be responsible for them.

The foregoing section emphasizes that generality is not only not achieved by a single study, it is not achieved even by a few replications. Only multiple replications in varied settings with varied clients and clinicians will eventually establish generality as well as its limits. Even a single well-designed study may establish improvement under, or effectiveness for, a treatment technique. Multiple replications conducted over several years are required to establish generality (see Chapter 10 for more on generality and replications).

Controlled systematic replications may address a single treatment, multiple treatments, or interaction between treatments. The same experimental methods described in the section on controlled unreplicated research will be used to replicate multiple treatment effects and interaction between treatments.

SUMMARY

- Treatment research is a variety of clinical research conducted to establish the consequences of treatments. Treatment research may be described as follows:

  — Uncontrolled, which only documents improvement

  — Controlled, which documents treatment effectiveness

  — Directly replicated, which establishes the reliability of improvement or effectiveness

  — Systematically replicated, which extends the generality of improvement or effectiveness

- Treatment produces several types of consequences:
  - Improvement, which is positive change in those who receive it, with no assurance that the treatment caused it
  - Effects, which are demonstrated in experimental studies with the assurance that treatment caused the effects
  - Generalized consequences, which are additional and indirect changes in treated skills
  - Maintained consequences, which are clinically established skills that are durable across time
  - Outcomes, which are generalized, maintained, indirect, and clinically valid consequences of treatment with no assurance that treatment caused them

- All treatment effects studied in experimental research should demonstrate various kinds of validity and generality:
  - Internal validity is the degree of assurance that the treatment, not another variable, produced the measured positive changes in the recipients.
  - Clinical validity is the degree to which the consequences of a treatment are socially and personally meaningful to those who receive it.
  - External validity, also known as generality, is the degree to which the results of a treatment research study may be extended to other people who need the same treatment but did not participate in the study.
  - Statistical generality is the extension of conclusions of a study to all individuals in a population when a study draws a random sample from that population.
  - Logical generality is the degree to which the conclusions of single-subject treatment research may be extended to those who are similar to the individuals in the treatment study.

- The popular distinction between treatment effects and efficacy is methodologically meaningless.

- There are logical and empirical constraints in establishing treatment effects:
  - Logically, one should show that treatment, and no other factor, produced the effects.
  - Empirically, one should arrange conditions to rule out the extraneous variables; those conditions define an experiment.

- Group designs and single-subject designs are the two approaches used to demonstrate treatment effects; the group designs approach in medicine is often described as RCTs with the following characteristics:

  — Participants are randomly assigned to experimental and control groups.

  — Random selection of a sample (a representative smaller group) from a population (a larger group with defined characteristics), though required, is skipped.

  — Theoretically, samples may be drawn by probability or non-probability sampling techniques.

  — Matching subjects is an alternative to sampling.

  — Pretests and posttests are administered to participants in all groups.

  — Either the patients only or both the patients and those who administer treatment and measure its effects may be blinded to the procedures (single or double blinding, respectively).

  — Control groups may receive an established treatment, no treatment, or a placebo.

- Single-subject treatment research uses a small number of participants, with the following characteristics:

  — All participants receive treatment, with no control groups.

  — There are multiple control conditions, including treatment withdrawal, reversal, baselines, simultaneous multibaselines, replications, rapid alternations, and criterion-referenced change.

- Randomized clinical trials and single-subject designs share certain similarities and differ on certain aspects:

  — Both can establish internal validity of experiments.

  — Generality is a matter of replications, not experimental designs; therefore, the claim of statistical generality in RCTs is questionable.

  — All participants in RCTs and single-subject designs are self-selected.

  — Denial of treatment to control groups is ethically questionable, an aspect not found in single-subject designs.

  — Administration of placebo in RCTs is also ethically questionable, an aspect not found in single-subject designs.

- Treatment research in medicine and treatment research in communicative disorders differ on institutional, economic, and scientific grounds:
  - Medical research is conducted in large national and international institutions with a large pool of patients available for research.
  - Medical research receives substantial financial support from global pharmaceutical companies.
  - Compared to that in communicative disorders, treatment in medical research is more standardized, that is, more easily administered by medical personnel in multiple centers and countries.
  - Treatment in communicative disorders is less standardized, requires more training time to have multiple clinicians administer it uniformly, takes longer, and is more labor intensive.
- Treatment research may be classified according to the degree of experimental control (causality) and generality; accordingly, treatment research may be characterized as follows:
  - Uncontrolled unreplicated, which measures improvement, generalized consequences, outcomes, and maintenance
  - Uncontrolled directly replicated, which documents the reliability of findings in the original setting
  - Uncontrolled systematically replicated, which documents improvement in different settings, by different investigators
  - Controlled unreplicated, which establishes the effects of a treatment, relative effects of multiple treatments, or interaction between treatments
  - Controlled directly replicated, which establishes the reliability of treatment effects in the original setting
  - Controlled systematically replicated, which helps extend the treatment to other clients, served in other settings, administered by other clinicians

STUDY GUIDE

1. Define treatment research.

2. What can be claimed through uncontrolled treatment research? What cannot be claimed?

3. What is the method of controlled treatment research?

4. What is replication? Define and distinguish direct and systematic replications.

5. What are the main consequences of treatment?

6. Define and distinguish *improvement* and *effectiveness*.

7. What are the similarities between generalized consequences, maintained consequences, and treatment outcomes?

8. Define and describe internal and external validity of experimental results.

9. What is statistical generality? Under what conditions can this be claimed?

10. Describe clinical validity and point out its importance in treatment research.

11. Define logical generality. What kind of experimental designs can claim this?

12. Define and distinguish the concepts of treatment efficacy versus treatment effectiveness. Is this distinction valid? Why or why not?

13. What are extraneous variables? How are they ruled out?

14. How are causes and effects related? What conditions must be met to claim that *A* is the cause of *B?*

15. What are randomized clinical trials? What kinds of designs are used in them?

16. Describe the various kinds of sampling techniques and point out their strengths and limitations.

17. Describe the two kinds of matching techniques. Which one is better? Which one is more practical?

18. What is the purpose of random assignment of participants? How is this done?

19. Describe the procedures and purposes of blinding in treatment research.

20. What is a placebo? Why is it used in some medical research?

21. Describe the various control mechanism used in single-subject treatment research. How do they help rule out the influence of extraneous variables?

22. Distinguish withdrawal from reversal. Critically evaluate the usefulness of these two control mechanisms.

23. What are baselines? What are baseline criteria?

24. Compare RCTs with single-subject treatment research. Point out their strengths and limitations.

25. Do RCTs and single-subject designs differ in terms of internal validity? Why or why not?

26. Compare single-subject designs and RCTs with regard to statistical generality and clinical validity.

27. Why is the claim of statistical generality for RCTs questionable?

28. What kinds of group research can claim statistical generality?

29. Describe how participants in RCTs are essentially self-selected.

30. Describe the effects of governmental regulation of research on subject selection.

31. What is the effect of self-selection of participants on treatment research?

32. Give an overview of the ethical issues involved in having control groups in treatment research.

33. Compare the advantages and disadvantages of placebo control groups versus no-treatment control groups.

34. Describe the differences and similarities of treatment research in medicine versus treatment research in communicative disorders.

35. How is treatment research classified? Describe the different types of treatment research.

Chapter 5

◆◆◆◆◆◆◆◆◆◆◆◆◆◆◆◆◆◆◆◆◆◆◆◆◆◆◆◆◆◆◆◆◆◆◆◆◆◆

Other Types of Research

- Ex Post Facto Research
- Normative Research
- Standard-Group Comparisons
- Experimental Research
- Clinical and Applied Research
- Sample Surveys
- Relation Between Research Types and Questions
- Summary
- Study Guide

Research in everyday usage includes a variety of activities. A student wishing to buy a computer may research the market, the hardware, the software, the service provided by different dealers, and so on. A couple planning to buy a house may research the housing market, interest rates, and lending institutions. The term *research* in these contexts refers to relatively well-planned and systematic activity.

Scientific research, on the other hand, may require more formal planning, and the questions asked require more technical activities to produce an answer. Nevertheless, scientific research can also be more or less formal and may include a variety of activities designed to obtain different kinds of information or answer different kinds of questions. For example, a speech–language clinician may research the number of children with articulation disorders in a school district. A second clinician may research the typical language behaviors of a group of 5-year-old children. A third clinician may research the conditions under which stuttering began in a group of children. A fourth clinician may research the effects of a treatment procedure on the language skills of persons with aphasia.

Each of the research activities just described has a different question behind it. Different research activities use different methods, generating different results. They will have unique strengths and limitations that determine the kinds of conclusions one can draw from the results. Therefore, it is necessary to understand different types of scientific research so that questions are researched with appropriate methods and the results are interpreted within the scope of those methods.

There are different ways of classifying research, and several classic types are common across classifications. An overview of typical research activities in communicative disorders and related disciplines suggests the following types of research: ex post facto research, normative research, standard-group comparison, experimental research, clinical research, and sample surveys. These research types are not mutually exclusive categories. There are research styles that combine different types or their elements. Chapter 4 considered treatment research, a form of clinical research because of its special relevance to communicative disorders. This chapter describes the other types of research.

EX POST FACTO RESEARCH

Many research studies published in communicative disorders are of the ex post facto type. **Ex post facto research** is a type of research in which a retrospective search of the causes of events is made without an independent variable. As the term suggests, it is an "after the fact" type of research in that the independent variables have occurred in the past and the investigator starts with the effect.

Procedures of Ex Post Facto Research

The case history method used in clinical sciences is an excellent example of ex post facto research. Many disorders or diseases are initially researched through the ex post facto method. In fact, the causes of most human disorders and diseases are not experimentally manipulable. Some experimental research on certain diseases and disorders may be possible only at the subhuman level. However, the results of subhuman experiments may or may not be applicable to human beings. Therefore, much of the research in clinical fields, including medicine, uses the ex post facto method.

In the case history method, the starting point of an investigation is a disease or a disorder. The investigator then proceeds to find out what may have caused the problem. Evidently, the onset has occurred in the past. Therefore, the investigator cannot experimentally manipulate the potential instigating causes and must begin by taking a detailed case history. The case history is a chronology of events that are relevant to the disorder under investigation. The client and other informants (such as parents) may be interviewed. Information on the conditions under which the disorder was first noted is gathered. If events that may be potential causes of the disorder are reported to have occurred, the investigator may conclude that a potential cause–effect relation has been identified.

The retrospective search for causes often is guided by past research and theoretical expectations. The past research may provide some clues to the causes of the problem under study, and the investigator may search the case history for those causes. The investigator may look for causes suggested by deductive theories. Should the case history provide evidence of events suggested as causes by either past research or a current theory, the investigator may conclude that the disorder is due to those events.

Many currently accepted cause–effect relations are based only on ex post facto research at the human level. For example, the relation between smoking and lung cancer is based entirely on ex post facto research. Repeatedly, studies using the case history method have shown that smokers have a higher chance of developing lung cancer than nonsmokers. A majority of people who have developed lung cancer report a history of smoking. On the basis of such observations, it has been concluded that smoking and lung cancer are causally related. Such conclusions have formed a basis for significant social policies such as those requiring warnings on cigarette packages.

In communicative disorders, Johnson's extensive research on the onset of stuttering in young children illustrates the ex post facto variety (Johnson, 1955; Johnson & Associates, 1959). In a series of studies, Johnson and his associates tried to determine the conditions under which stuttering was first noted by the parents of a large number of children who stuttered. With the help of an extensive schedule of interviews, the parents were questioned about such factors as family conditions, the child's health, the child's speech and language development, amounts and types of dysfluencies, and so on.

Similar interview data were also gathered from parents of nonstuttering children.

Johnson made a comparative analysis of the interview information obtained from the parents of children who stuttered and of those who did not. The parents of children who stuttered reported that their children exhibited such dysfluencies as repetitions, interjections, and prolongations, which prompted them to consider their children as stutterers. However, the parents of nonstuttering children also reported that the children had various kinds of dysfluencies in speech. Based on this information, Johnson concluded that *at the time of stuttering onset* children who are thought to stutter speak no differently than those who are considered normal speakers. This became the well-known diagnosogenic theory of stuttering. Essentially, the theory stated that the origin of stuttering was the parental negative evaluation of normal nonfluencies and the mistaken diagnosis of stuttering. Of course, the negative evaluation and the unfavorable diagnosis would soon start the real problem—apprehension, anxiety, struggle, and avoidance reactions developed by the children. For Johnson, dysfluencies themselves were not the major problems. The problems were the events that followed the diagnosis of stuttering based on normal nonfluencies.

Johnson's research and the resulting theory illustrate both the method and the problems of the ex post facto research. It is clear that Johnson's method was retrospective. The identified independent variable was the parental diagnosis of stuttering in the absence of stuttering. One can speculate whether Johnson had that assumption before he started his investigation or whether it was indeed a conclusion based on the interview data. It is clear, however, that the presumed independent variable had occurred in the past. He did not (of course, could not) observe or experimentally manipulate the parental diagnosis that, in his judgment, caused stuttering. Therefore, the cause–effect relation between the parental diagnosis and stuttering was based upon interview information, not upon experimental evidence. In other words, Johnson did not show that no other factor was responsible for stuttering.

Strengths and Weaknesses of Ex Post Facto Research

Ex post facto research (a) is not experimental, because the cause is not introduced or withdrawn (manipulated) and (b) lacks control in that extraneous independent variables are not ruled out. When the observations are ex post facto, the experimenter has no control over the independent variable. Consequently, a direct relation between the presumed cause and effect cannot be established.

Carefully done case histories may reveal that children with language disorders did not receive enough language stimulation, or that they had limited intelligence, or that they experienced certain emotional problems, or that they came from lower socioeconomic strata. Assuming that there are reliable and valid ways of measuring these variables, one can conclude that those variables were indeed observed and measured. However, whether they actually caused the language disorder is a different question. The ex post facto observations that documented the existence of those variables could not have done anything to show conclusively that they were the causes of the language disorder.

The documented observations within the ex post facto method cannot assert cause–effect relations for both empirical and logical reasons. As pointed out earlier, the empirical reasons are a lack of experimental manipulations and an absence of controls to rule out competing hypotheses. The logical reason is that both the effect and the presumed cause are measured at the same time. As a result, even the minimum requirement of a causal relation—causes precede effects—is not fulfilled in ex post facto research because, in most cases, the prior existence of the presumed causal factor is not documented. The presumed causes and their effects are both studied simultaneously.

Statistical correlations often are used in the analysis of the results of ex post facto studies. The analysis might reveal significant correlations between events. However, such correlations do not necessarily suggest causation. Correlations suggest that events tend to coexist or covary, but the cause of one or both of the variables may be some other unobserved factor.

The often cited justification of ex post facto research is that it is the only possible type of research that can be implemented in many important areas of investigation (Kerlinger, 1986). Ethical restrictions prohibit experimental research on human diseases and disorders. The only way, then, is to explore the past history of patients with given diseases and disorders for possible causal factors. In such situations, however, one should be clear about the distinction between the social implications and the scientific implications of ex post facto research. From the standpoint of science, the impracticality of experimentation is beside the point. Weak scientific evidence does not become stronger because better evidence cannot be produced.

Similarly, from the standpoint of social policies designed to protect human lives, the limitations of scientific evidence may be recognized but considered unimportant. In such cases, each society makes an evaluation of the available evidence to support social policies that are best for its people. Scientists would support those policies as long as social and scientific evaluations of research data are not confused. People may justifiably accept the social implications of weak scientific evidence because such a course of action serves their best interests. Relative to questions such as smoking and lung cancer, members of a society may be more willing to take the risk of being scientifically wrong than being prematurely dead.

The scientific evaluation of ex post facto research may be done independent of social policies. The main limitation of ex post facto studies is that it is not possible to explain an event on the basis of their results. The social or personal significance of the results is beside the point. Ideally, ex post facto research should lead to a suggestion of variables that may be verified through other means of investigation. In this sense, it is a desirable exploratory method of research. In practice, however, many investigators whose characteristic research method is ex post facto may not be inclined to find other means of verifying potential causal relations suggested by their method. Disregarding the limitations of the method, explanatory theories may be offered that might enjoy a certain degree of incongruous acceptance in the discipline.

In many cases, the difficulty in conducting better controlled research is somewhat exaggerated. Certainly, Johnson could not have asked parents of fluently speaking children to diagnose stuttering to see what happens; however, it is possible to think of large-scale preventive studies in which parents of high-risk children are asked not to diagnose stuttering and see if imminent stuttering is avoided. Or, by selecting children in the very early stage of stuttering, one can modify the punitive parental behaviors to see what effects follow. With appropriate control measures (such as a control group whose parents are not asked to change their behaviors), it is possible to gather more convincing evidence than that produced by the ex post facto method. In the case of human diseases, similar preventive experimental studies are possible. For example, cholesterol intake of individuals may be differentially monitored and modified to see what health benefits and risks follow. Such naturalistic experiments have been conducted. In addition, when appropriate, animal experimental research might support ex post facto data.

NORMATIVE RESEARCH

Another extremely popular form of research in communicative disorders as well as in child psychology can be called normative research. Traditionally, it is not recognized as a separate type of research, but the enormous amount of effort that goes into this kind of research makes it necessary to consider it separately.

Normative research is defined as the type of research in which the distribution of selected dependent variables across age groups is observed and recorded. For example, the number of phonemes correctly produced (dependent variable) by 2-, 3-, and 4-year-old children may be observed and recorded. The major purpose of normative research is to arrive at norms that are the averaged performance levels of presumably typical reference groups. Normative research seeks to establish behavioral differences across age groups. This type of research is also known as developmental research or descriptive research. It tends to provide descriptive data on typical behaviors of different age groups.

It is generally believed that for clinical disciplines, norms are extremely important. It is argued that norms tell us how children's behaviors change as they grow older and that such information will help us judge whether a given client's behavior is normal or disordered. It is further suggested that unless the clinician knows age-based norms, target behaviors for clinical intervention cannot be determined. For example, the clinician should know the typical language behaviors of 4-year-olds to judge whether a 4-year-old child is delayed in language acquisition. Also, once it is judged that the child has delays (because, perhaps, the child's language approximates that of a 2-year-old), norms are needed to establish the treatment targets. Assuming that the child in the example has all the behaviors of average 2-year-old children, initial target behaviors may be that of average 3-year-olds and eventually that of average 4-year-olds.

The bulk of research in morphology, syntax, phonology, semantics, and pragmatics is normative and theoretical. It is thought that lack of norms in certain aspects of speech and language creates problems for making clinical judgments relative to evaluation and treatment. Therefore, it is considered high-priority research.

Procedures of Normative Research

Normative research typically uses the participant and response sampling procedure to establish the statistically averaged response patterns across age groups. Theoretically, norms are established on randomly selected participants who are representative of the population. Unless the sample is representative, conclusions cannot be extended to all the children in the population. Because the goal of normative research is to determine the typical behaviors of children in the population, not merely that of selected children, normative research must use adequate statistical sampling procedures.

To achieve an adequate statistical sampling, one must meet two conditions. The investigator must have access to the entire population, such as all school-age children with language disorders. Once this type of population has been identified, every member of that population must be willing to participate in the study. These two conditions are important because the random theory is based on the assumption that a representative sample of a population can be drawn only when the population is large and when every member had an equal chance of being selected into the sample. The sample size is related to the size of the population. The larger the population, the bigger the sample size required to represent that population. The sample is typically cross-sectional in that a certain number of participants are drawn from each age level.

After having drawn a random representative sample of the population, the investigator proceeds to sample the behaviors of selected participants. Speech, language, or auditory behaviors are sampled in a somewhat short period of observation. Each participant may be administered a brief test designed to sample the behaviors of interest. Various tests of articulation, language, and hearing ability are used to sample behaviors in normative research.

The researcher makes a statistical analysis of the behaviors sampled across selected age levels. The mean performance levels of each age group are determined along with standard deviations. The mean scores may be statistically transformed into other types of scores to reduce variability across participants and to facilitate comparisons among participants. The means and other kinds of scores typical of the age group are considered the norm for that age group. Children in the population at large are expected to show the same kinds of behaviors as those of the sampled children at specific age levels. In evaluating individual clients, the clinician is expected to use such norms to judge whether a child deviates from the expected (typical) performance levels. The presence of deviation suggests a clinical problem, whereas the degree of deviation determines the severity of the problem.

Strengths and Weaknesses of Normative Research

The strength of normative research is its logical appeal and not its empirical validity. The reasoning that clinicians need to know the typical behaviors of participants in different groups formed on the basis of age, gender, socioeconomic status, or occupational levels is logically consistent with the clinical demands of determining deviations and disorders based on such variables. It is useful to know the typical language behaviors of children of different ages, of male and female participants, and of people in different walks of life; the availability of such knowledge makes the diagnosis of a disorder or deviation less demanding.

It is also useful to know how the dependent variables are distributed in the population. Science starts with the observation of some effects (dependent variables). Before other kinds of research manipulations can be achieved, one must be clear about the dependent variables. Therefore, a good description of speech, language, fluency, vocal, and auditory behaviors across variables that do make a difference in these behaviors would be essential for further empirical research and sound clinical practice.

Most of the serious problems of normative research are empirical. The procedures and assumptions of this type of research seem to lack empirical validity, a problem that has received surprisingly little critical attention in communicative disorders.

The problems inherent in normative research are common to most research studies based on the statistical theory of probability and random sampling from the population. These problems will be discussed in Chapters 7 and 9 and, therefore, will be mentioned only briefly here. The first empirical problem is that true random samples that permit the nationwide use of the resulting normative information are rarely drawn. Most normative studies draw local samples based upon varying degrees of randomization. Therefore, the behavior patterns found across age groups may or may not be representative of the children in the target population. As a result, the major goal of normative research is rarely achieved in practice.

The second empirical problem is also related to the sampling procedure. Normative researchers sample not only participants but also responses under investigation. Because groups of participants are examined at different age levels, most often the investigators are able to obtain only a brief sampling of responses. Whether it is language or articulation, the opportunities to produce specific behaviors are extremely limited. For example, children may be given two or three chances to produce a given phoneme or a grammatical morpheme. When age-based norms are derived from such limited sampling of responses, their reliability is doubtful. Unfortunately, the only kind of sampling the normative researcher typically thinks of is participant sampling, which is done inadequately anyway.

The third empirical problem is a more serious one and involves a logical problem as well. Any population is heterogeneous, not homogeneous; that means that among a large number of persons, there is much variability. This is nothing but the popular notion of individual differences and uniqueness. A good sample, therefore, must be as heterogeneous as the population it seeks to represent. Consequently, the more heterogeneous the sample, the more variable the participant performance. Unfortunately, the more variable the performance, the less meaningful the average (the norm). In other words, even when an investigator achieves a representative random sample, the resulting norms will be highly variable, a contradiction of terms. Therefore, it is likely that the notion of norms is a logical and empirical fallacy.

The fourth empirical problem is probably due to a misapplication of the statistical theory of probability and the random procedure to questions of individual performance. The theory and procedure are designed to extend the results from the sample to the population and not from the sample to an individual. An average performance of a smaller group is supposed to help predict the average performance of the larger group. Within the theory, there is no empirical basis to predict an individual's performance based on a sample study. Disregarding this, clinicians routinely assume that what is true of an averaged sample performance of a group should also be true of an individual client's specific (unaveraged) performance.

The fifth empirical problem of normative research is also a matter of practice. Normative research asks how the behaviors are distributed across certain arbitrarily selected variables such as age; it was never intended to answer the question of why those behaviors are distributed the way they are. In other words, normative research can only describe the events observed; it cannot explain those events. Investigators of normative research do not exert any kind of control on potential independent variables. As such, no matter how extensive, normative research cannot support a theory. It seems that this limitation is also mostly ignored in practice, for most of the theories on how and why children acquire language, semantic notions, pragmatic rules, or phonological systems are based on normative research.

Normative research assumes that the arbitrarily selected variables across which the behaviors seem to show different patterns are indeed the independent variables. For example, most investigators of language acquisition explicitly or implicitly assume that age is an independent variable. This commonly held assumption needs a careful look.

Age is a measure of the passage of time relative to the beginnings of some living or nonliving entity. While time is impersonal and physical, age is personal and often biological. As age changes, certain behaviors also change. Most people then assume that age is the cause of those changes. Age is an implicitly or explicitly offered explanation of any kind of behavioral development in most normative research.

It is hard to think that age, which is a personal measure of the passage of time, is an independent variable of anything. If it is, it is a discouraging variable for clinicians who wish to remediate disorders because the only course of action open to them would be to let time pass for the child with communicative disability to show improvement. Of course, once that time had passed the disturbing question of why time did not help the child would have to be stoically ignored. Fortunately, in practice, most clinicians do not believe that age is the independent variable of communicative behaviors. In practice, most clinicians believe that treatment is a more important variable than the mere passage of time.

Age is a convenient term for known and unknown variables that influence observable behaviors as time passes. Some of these variables include biological changes that take place within organisms; others include events in the environment. A better explanation of behaviors might emerge if manipulable independent variables are taken seriously. More important, a better technology of treatment would simultaneously become available. There is some evidence to show that "developmental milestones" of language are susceptible to environmental contingencies that can be experimentally manipulated (Capelli, 1985; De Cesari, 1985). In other words, experimental research on language acquisition is possible, and it offers a more valid means of explaining the language learning process than mere age offers.

If normative research is applied strictly to observe and describe dependent variables, it can serve a meaningful purpose. However, to generate clinically useful data, the normative researchers may have to curtail the overuse of the cross-sectional method, in which the individual behaviors are sampled inadequately. Repeated and more intensive observation of small numbers of children may produce data that are more applicable to individual cases (Brown, 1973). When behaviors are observed more intensively, patterns that may not become apparent under the cursory cross-sectional method may be observed. Such observations would still not explain the behavioral changes but can possibly suggest potential independent variables for further experimental inquiry.

STANDARD-GROUP COMPARISONS

Another type of research not traditionally recognized as a distinct variety can be called standard-group comparison. The standard-group comparison method is a cross between the ex post facto and the normative types of research. Though it is not recognized as a separate type of research, it is necessary to consider it as such because of the sheer volume of this kind of research done in clinical sciences. In communicative disorders, standard-group comparisons are almost as popular as normative research.

Standard-group comparison is a type of research in which groups formed on the basis of one dependent variable are compared on the basis of the same or other dependent variables. An a priori dependent variable serves as an initial basis to form groups, and then the presence or the absence of selected dependent variables across the groups is measured. Typical group comparisons involve two groups that are different on the initial a priori variable. On the subsequent measured dependent variables, the group may or may not be different, though the expectation is that they will be. In many clinical disciplines, including communicative disorders, "clinical" groups are compared with "normal" groups on some measure of one or more dependent variables.

Standard-group comparisons are not the same as the two- (or more) group experimental research. The latter type of research is experimental and is described later. The type of experimental research that involves two or more groups is a more active research arrangement in which an independent variable is manipulated by the experimenter. In the standard-group comparison, there is no manipulation of an independent variable. Only the dependent variables are measured.

Procedures of the Standard-Group Comparison

For the most part, the standard-group comparison is an extension of the logic and methodology of normative research. After having discovered the distribution of certain dependent variables in certain general samples of participants, some clinical researchers move on to find out if the distribution of those variables is in some way different across selected samples of participants. The general sample is the "normal" group, and the special samples selected for comparison are the "clinical" groups.

The clinical groups are formed on the basis of a clinical diagnosis. For example, children with language disorders, patients with aphasia, or persons who stutter can be identified through clinical assessment. Once a clinical group has been formed, the researcher proceeds to form a normal group with no communicative problems. Certain screening procedures may be used to rule out the existence of communicative disorders. The two groups are then compared on selected dependent variables.

There are two strategies of comparing the two groups. In the first strategy, the groups are compared further on the same criterion variable that separated the groups in the first place. In the second strategy, the groups are compared on variables that did not serve as explicit criteria for the initial separation of the groups.

The first strategy is illustrated by studies in which children who have language problems are compared with normal-language children on the age at which they master selected grammatic morphemes. In fact, they may be compared on any or several of the many language measures: grammatical, semantic, or pragmatic variables. It must be noted that comparisons in such instances are made on the same criterion variable that separated the two groups. Language skills separated the two groups to begin with, and it is on the same variable that the two groups are further compared. Similarly, children with phonological disorders may be compared with normally speaking children on certain phonologic variables.

This kind of comparative analysis may lead to a description of further linguistic differences between those who are acquiring language or phonological features normally and those who are not. For example, an investigator might find out that, compared with normally speaking children, children with language disorders do not use certain pragmatic structures or passive sentence forms. Similarly, children with phonological disabilities may be found to be deficient in acquiring certain phonological skills.

In the second strategy, the criterion and the comparison measures are different. Groups are formed on the basis of one variable, and they are compared on the basis of different variables. For example, an investigator may assess the difference in motor performance between persons who stutter and those who do not. The criterion variable in this case is stuttering, which is the basis for forming the two groups. The variable on which they are compared, on the other hand, is entirely different. It is a measure of motor proficiency, which is not the same as stuttering. Later, stuttering and motor proficiency measures may be linked theoretically, but they are different kinds of responses. There are many examples of this kind of comparison. Persons with and without aphasia may be compared on the basis of memory skills or on a test of intelligence. The performance of children with phonological disorders on a motor proficiency test may be compared with that of normally speaking children. A measure of intelligence of normally speaking children may be compared with that of children who have language problems.

In recent years, the standard-group comparison method has been used extensively in the study of neurophysiological differences between persons who stutter and those who do not. These two groups have been reported to be different on several neurophysiological variables. Numerous investigators have made comparative analyses of phonatory reaction times of people who stutter and people who do not. In a majority of studies, adults who stutter have been found to speak more slowly than normal speakers in initiating and terminating phonation upon a signal. Other variables on which people who stutter and people who do not have been compared include phonatory transition between voiced and voiceless sounds, laryngeal muscle activities, dichotic listening tests, and hemispheric processing of linguistic stimuli.

Most of the studies on these and other variables have reported differences between people who stutter and people who do not to varying degrees, with a remarkable extent of individual differences within each group. Many theoretical speculations have flourished on the basis of standard-group comparisons of this kind.

Strengths and Weaknesses of Standard-Group Comparisons

The standard-group comparison can yield useful information regarding the differences between normal and clinical populations. It is necessary to understand the differences between those who have a communicative disorder and those who do not. Furthermore, it is also necessary to understand the difference between particular disorder groups and normal groups. The standard-group comparison studies can describe, for instance, the dependent variables on which the normal and stuttering groups or normal and language-disordered groups differ. The method is useful in identifying and describing dependent variables. Because it is necessary to have clear descriptions of the dependent variables researchers study, the standard-group comparisons serve a useful purpose.

The standard-group comparison method poses no significant problems when it is used to identify and describe dependent variables across clinical and nonclinical groups. Problems arise when the method is misapplied, however. Many investigators show a problematic tendency to explain disorders on the basis of standard-group comparisons. For example, on the basis of standard-group comparisons, stuttering has been explained as a problem of inherent phonatory slowness. In other words, slow phonatory reaction time is treated as the cause of stuttering. However, in a standard-group comparison, there is no independent variable at all. As observed and measured in the studies, the slow phonatory reaction time is a dependent variable, not an independent variable. Therefore, there is no reason to suggest that phonatory slowness is the cause of stuttering. Of course, the cause of phonatory slowness is also not clear. In fact, no causal relation of any kind would be clear in a standard-group comparison, because it is not an experimental procedure. There is no assurance that an unidentified and unobserved variable is the cause of the effect under study. As such, standard-group comparison cannot support theories or explanations.

Some investigators designate the normal group as the control group and the clinical group as the experimental group in a standard-group comparison research. The use of this terminology is misleading because the method is not experimental. Clinical groups are not to be automatically considered experimental groups. Unless a group receives a treatment variable, it is not an experimental group.

EXPERIMENTAL RESEARCH

The most powerful strategy available to discover functional relations among events is experimental research. This type of research shares many characteristics with other types. The formulation of a research question, the task of finding a suitable method, systematic observation of the phenomenon under investigation, and analysis and interpretation of data are all common across research types. Experimental research has as its distinguishing feature the experiment. The normative, the ex post facto, and the standard-group comparison types of research do not involve an experiment. Therefore, the term *experiment* is not a synonym of research, although one can find such an inappropriate use of that term in the literature. An experiment is only a part of a series of technical operations in some research studies.

An **experiment** can be defined as a series of controlled conditions of dynamic arrangement in which one or more independent variables are manipulated and the effects of such manipulations on the dependent variable are measured. Alternatively, an experiment is a method of arranging conditions in such a way that a functional (cause–effect) relation between events may be revealed.

In an experiment, the investigator manipulates an independent variable to (a) produce a dependent variable (effect); (b) increase the magnitude of a dependent variable; (c) reduce the magnitude of a dependent variable; or (d) eliminate the dependent variable. Logically, any one of those successful manipulations is evidence of a functional relation between the independent variable and the effect (dependent variable). A combination of such manipulations will further strengthen that evidence. Replications of those functional arrangements and comparable results will enhance the generality of the evidence.

Procedures of Experimental Research

The effect (i.e., the purpose) of an experiment is to reveal a functional relation between two or more events. In this sense, an experiment is more advanced than descriptive research, in which the investigator asks a fundamental question relative to the existence and properties of events. In descriptive research, events are observed systematically and their properties are noted; no variable is manipulated to produce an effect. Descriptive research seeks an answer to the question, "What is it?" An experiment is designed to answer the question of which events are functionally (causally) related to the phenomenon that is known to exist and whose descriptive properties are reasonably well understood. In other words, experimental research seeks to explain an event by discovering its causal variables. Therefore, experimental research is essential for constructing deductive and inductive theories.

There is no experiment without the manipulation of one or more independent variables. An experiment is the most active of the research arrangements because it seeks not only to observe a phenomenon, like many other types of research, but also to control that phenomenon. The term *control* in this context simply means that some change in the phenomenon has been effected. The experimenter, however, cannot exert a direct control over the phenomenon. The only means of affecting the event is to gain control over its independent variable(s). This is true of applied situations as well. A physician, for example, cannot directly manipulate a disease. The disease is brought under control only through effective treatment. A speech–language pathologist cannot directly affect aphasia; it can be affected only through certain treatment techniques.

An independent variable is manipulated in many ways. An independent variable is manipulated when it is introduced, increased or decreased in magnitude, withdrawn, or reintroduced. For example, in assessing the effect of white noise on stuttering, the experimenter may first establish the baseline of stuttering and then introduce noise through headphones while the participant who stutters is talking. The experimenter will continue to measure the rate of stuttering. The level of noise may be increased or decreased in appropriate experimental conditions. In subsequent conditions, the noise may be withdrawn to observe the effects on stuttering. Finally, the noise may be reintroduced to find out if the original effects can be replicated. Alternatively, the investigator may introduce the noise to one group of persons who stutter and withhold it from another group.

Two independent variables are manipulated when one of them is introduced and another is later added, subsequently subtracted, then added a second time, and so on. For example, in assessing the effects of providing both feedback on performance levels and verbal praise for correct articulation, one may start with giving only neutral feedback to the participant. In the next experimental condition, verbal praise may be added to feedback. In the subsequent condition, the verbal praise may be withdrawn, leaving only the feedback as the independent variable. In a final condition, the verbal praise may be reintroduced. Throughout, the correct production of target phonemes is measured to assess the effects of the experimental manipulations. There are other and more complex manipulations of independent variables, but these help illustrate the basic strategy.

A critical aspect of experimental manipulations is that they must be done under controlled conditions. **Controlled experimental conditions** exist when it is possible to rule out the influence of potential independent variables not under investigation. This means that most events (including improvement in a clinical condition) have multiple causes, and in any given experiment, the investigators are interested in only one or a few of them. Therefore, the investigators need to demonstrate that the other potential causes, typically called **extraneous variables,** did not create the event. When the extraneous variables are ruled out, the effects observed on the dependent variable can be attributed to the independent variable being manipulated by the experimenter because no other variables were present. In effect, under controlled conditions, the experimenter isolates a cause–effect relation.

In many respects, conditions are controlled to simplify the typically complicated empirical relations that exist in nature. Normally, multiple controlling variables (causes) may be simultaneously active, though not to the same extent. When different variables are allowed to exert their varying and as yet undetermined influence on the dependent variables, no specific empirical relation can be isolated.

Physically isolated and specially constructed laboratories often are used in creating controlled conditions. The need for such physical control measures varies across disciplines and with the nature of the problems under investigation. Generally speaking, a certain degree of control over the physical setup is necessary in all types of experimental research. But the setup can be more or less structured depending on the nature and stage of research. For example, an experiment on auditory perception might need a highly controlled experimental setup (a soundproof booth). A clinical experiment in which a certain language treatment procedure is evaluated may initially need a controlled physical setup, but in the later stages—in which generalization to the natural environment is evaluated—the setup must be more natural. In all cases, the extraneous independent variables must be controlled.

It is somewhat difficult to control independent variables in natural settings, but it can be done. Experiments on the effects of teaching methods evaluated in regular classrooms, those on child social behaviors conducted in playgrounds, or those on different modes of teaching sign language in special education classrooms illustrate naturalistic experiments. Experiments conducted in naturalistic settings are sometimes called **field experiments.**

In addition to physical control measures, an experiment should also include control measures designed to minimize the influence of other variables related to the participants themselves. An investigator must make sure that other events in the lives of the participants were not responsible for the changes observed in the dependent variable. In many cases, biological events such as those included under the term *maturation* must also be ruled out. For example, a clinician who evaluates the effects of a language treatment program must show that no other treatment was simultaneously applied and that maturational factors were not responsible for the eventual gains in the participants' language behaviors. There are two basic approaches to rule out such extraneous variables: the between-groups strategy and the single-subject strategy.

In the between-groups strategy, two comparable groups are formed on the basis of random selection and assignment. One of the groups, the experimental group, receives treatment, whereas the other group, the control group, does not. If the desirable changes are seen only in the experimental group, both the extraneous environmental and possible biological variables are ruled out. The only reason the experimental group showed changes is that its members received the treatment.

In the single-subject strategy, the participants are exposed to different conditions of the experiment, and the differences in their response rates under those different conditions are taken as evidence of the effect of the independent variable under study. Typically, there is no control group that does not receive treatment in a single-subject strategy. These two strategies of designing experiments are described and evaluated in Chapters 7 through 10.

Basic and Applied Experimental Research

Experimental research has two varieties: basic and applied. **Basic research** is often theoretical, and the problems addressed might not have immediate practical implications. **Applied research** is practical, designed to solve immediate problems.

It is sometimes assumed that experimental research is always basic and laboratory oriented whereas applied research does not use experimental methods. This notion is strengthened by the view that basic research finds out answers to important questions and applied research simply exploits those answers in solving practical problems. This is a mistaken notion. Both basic and applied research can use the same experimental methods. When related applied and basic research are equally experimental, a useful interaction results. Such an interaction can speed up the process of finding solutions to practical problems.

In some cases, it may take a long time for the basic researcher to give answers to applied questions. In other cases, there may be no basic science that would ask and answer the same questions that have to be answered by the applied scientist. To a certain extent, this seems to be the case with communicative disorders. In the area of language, speech–language pathologists have often looked to linguistics for a variety of answers. But by its very nature, linguistics is not likely to ask such questions as whether language treatment procedure *A* is more effective than procedure *B*. Linguistics and other nonclinical disciplines may be able to describe potential dependent variables but may not give any clues as to what independent variables may be necessary to change those dependent variables. That is the task of specialists in communicative disorders. See Chapter 4 for more on using experimental research to evaluate clinical treatment methods and educational teaching methods.

A prudent applied or clinical scientist learns to do at least some of the basic research to take care of his or her own business. Contrary to popular notions, experiment is the most needed operation in an applied science. Based on whatever information is made available by basic researchers, an applied scientist may begin to experiment to find out answers to practical questions. Interestingly enough, applied or clinical experimental research not only can help solve practical problems but also can generate new knowledge that can influence basic sciences. In essence, an experiment is a method to answer certain types of questions, and those types of questions must be answered in applied sciences as well.

The question of applied experimental research will be discussed in the section on applied and clinical research.

Strengths and Weaknesses of Experimental Research

It is sometimes argued that in behavioral sciences, experimental research is artificial, too mechanistic, and therefore inappropriate (Bannister, 1966; Gadlin & Ingle, 1975). Specially created and fully controlled experimental situations are so far removed from the social settings in which behaviors naturally occur that the results may not have much validity. The experimental investigator tends to isolate an independent variable responsible for the effect under study. However, under natural conditions, single variables may not be responsible for specific effects. For these and other reasons, the experimental results may not be relevant to the behavioral events taking place in the natural world.

The argument that experimental research is too mechanistic for human behavioral sciences is an old one. There is a long-held belief that the scientific approach may be appropriate for physical phenomena but not for human phenomena. It is further believed that the mechanistic approach of science will dehumanize the human species. The origin of such beliefs is in the ancient philosophical position that human beings are unique in the scheme of the universe. Although Darwin did much to dispel this cherished sense of self-importance, some of the prejudices against the science of human behavior have persisted and have appeared and reappeared in various disguises.

Another weakness of experimental research, according to some critics, is that the effects of independent variables manipulated in human experiments are very weak (Kerlinger, 1986). Many times, controlled experiments manage to demonstrate only small changes in the dependent variables, whereas the same variables in real-life situations may produce very large effects. For example, expansion of children's utterances in a laboratory study may result in only small increases in language complexity, but the same variable in real life may produce larger effects.

None of those criticisms of experimental research seem to be valid. That independent variables are isolated is a strength, not a weakness, of experimental research. Only by isolating the effects of a variable can an experimenter observe functional relations between variables. Real-life situations are typically confounded, making it difficult to determine specific cause–effect relations. That in natural situations variables are multitude and the relations complex is not contradicted by technical isolation of specific causes. The need to isolate and individually analyze the different causes of a complex event arises from logical as well as technological considerations. After having analyzed the isolated effects of major factors, the scientist proceeds to analyze the interactive effects of those multiple factors. Such analytical steps are taken to eventually obtain an integrated picture of the phenomenon under investigation. In this way, a better approximation of the reality is achieved through laboratory research than through rational arguments.

The critics of the experimental method do not suggest an effective alternative to an analytical approach to determining functional relations. If isolated functional relations are unreal, then the complex, real, but hopelessly confounded relations do not permit any conclusions. In addition, many events cannot be held for observation in their totality. Often, there is no technological means of experimentally manipulating a multitudinal complex. Besides, some apparently complex situations may hold only a few causal factors while the rest of the multitude may be a collection of covariables with very little functional significance.

The objection that the experimental approach is too mechanistic may be consistent with certain scholastic traditions but is not consistent with any empirical evidence. Science neither glorifies nor degrades its subject matter. Human behavior will not be transformed into mechanical events because the methods of science have been used in studying it. For example, when scientists gain a better understanding of the language learning process through application of the experimental procedure, human language will not turn into machine language. Behaviors or feelings called *love* or *cooperation* will remain the same even after scientists have experimentally analyzed them.

The final criticism—that compared to situations in real life, experiments tend to produce relatively weak effects of independent variables—probably applies to some research traditions. However, this problem is not inherent in the experimental approach itself. Experiments can and have produced large effects significant in natural settings, but the traditional statistical approaches to experimentation have asserted that large effects are not necessary to draw valid conclusions. *Statistically significant* small effects are considered sufficient to permit statements of cause–effect relations. The experimental tradition can be completely divorced from this statistical philosophy. There is nothing in the logic or the tactics of the experimental method that would prevent the production of larger effects of independent variables.

The strengths of experimental research are the strengths of science itself. Experimental research is the most appropriate method to isolate a cause–effect relation. Clinically and educationally, it is the only method to firmly establish the effects of treatment and teaching methods. Many other types of research can suggest possibilities of causal relations, but only the experimental approach can confirm them. Therefore, in developing theories and testing empirical hypotheses, no other research type matches the power of experimental research. Because a theory is both a description and an explanation of some natural phenomenon, investigators need the experimental procedure to rule out alternative explanations and hypotheses. Types of research such as the ex post facto and the normative may suggest hypotheses and theories, but typically, the same piece of research may suggest several rival hypotheses without testing their relative validity. Only experimental research can examine alternative hypotheses and theories, supporting one while ruling out the others.

CLINICAL AND APPLIED RESEARCH

Clinical and applied research often are contrasted with basic or experimental research. Clinical and applied research are thought to be qualitatively different from experimental research. However, only a few contrasts are valid because basic/experimental and applied/clinical research have much in common.

Clinical and applied research both address questions of immediate practical significance. They are designed to solve pressing physical, social, or personal problems. While experimental research may yield data that may be used in the future to solve some practical problems, clinical and applied research seek solutions to current problems. Basic experimental research may be theoretical or may be designed to find order and uniformity in natural events; it may seek to explain events, understand their causes, and predict their occurrences. Clinical and applied research, on the other hand, may seek to modify undesirable effects that have already taken place, improve certain existing conditions, or prevent certain unfavorable consequences. Research studies aimed at treating language disorders, improving an articulation treatment program, researching more effective ways of teaching American Sign Language, or developing better ways of teaching arithmetic skills to people with mental retardation illustrate these kinds of applied or clinical efforts.

Clinical research is defined as investigations that are connected with diseases and disorders of living organisms. Therefore, as in medicine, many research studies in communicative disorders should be clinical. Research aimed at understanding and treating various disorders of communication is necessarily clinical.

The distinction between applied research and clinical research is not crucial except that in many cases **applied research** may be nonclinical as defined here. For example, research aimed at reducing energy conservation in homes is applied but not clinical. Similarly, research aimed at building better bridges or safer highways is applied without being clinical. However, both clinical and applied research try to solve problems, and in this overriding sense they are the same. Therefore, in this book, the terms *clinical research* and *applied research* will be used interchangeably and will be distinguished only when necessary.

Clinical research uses the same basic procedures as the other types of research; its procedures are not necessarily unique. Depending on the particular clinical study, the method may be descriptive or experimental.

Descriptive and Experimental Clinical Research

Clinical research can be either descriptive or experimental. One of the popular misconceptions is that clinical research is always descriptive and, therefore, less exacting. However, clinical research is not necessarily less exacting than basic research. If, in practice, much of the clinical research is informal and less exacting, it is because some researchers believe that it should be this way.

Generally speaking, nonexperimental research can be less demanding than experimental research; however, when clinicians begin to ask experimental questions, they will have to be as rigorous as the basic scientists. For example, the research question of whether school teachers and speech–language pathologists differ in their attitudes toward stuttering is answered without an experiment. No variables need to be controlled to answer it. The researcher is interested in some existing differences in the two groups; he or she is not asking whether something can be done to change anything. On the other hand, to answer the question of whether articulation disorders are affected by Treatment *A* or Treatment *B* or with a combination of *A* and *B*, the clinician needs the experimental method in which the disorders are changed. Because the changes in articulation should be demonstrated under controlled conditions to rule out the influence of other potential independent (treatment) variables, the method is as demanding as that of basic experimental research.

In the early stage of clinical research, the concern is to establish the dependent variables. In other words, the clinician first needs to know the effects well. It often is the stage of descriptive research. The behaviors or disorders, their form and frequency, and their variations over time or conditions are described. Once the dependent variables have been clearly established, the question of causes emerges, demanding experimental analysis. In essence, after having clearly described the effects, the clinical scientist proceeds to find out their causes through experimental research.

The clinical investigator may search for instigating or maintaining causes. In communicative disorders, experimental analysis typically involves maintaining causes, not instigating causes. An experimental analysis of stuttering or an articulation disorder, for example, would be concerned with potential independent variables that decrease those behaviors while increasing their counterparts: fluency and appropriate articulation. The brain damage that resulted in aphasia may be the original cause, but it is not accessible for experimental analysis, whereas the patient's verbal behavior is. Similarly, several causes of hearing loss are not accessible. In such cases, the educator or the audiologist can only manipulate the communicative behaviors of people with hearing impairment.

Importance of Experimental–Clinical Research

In communicative disorders, experimental–clinical research is essential in three areas of investigation. First, it is essential in generating basic knowledge about the acquisition, production, and maintenance of various aspects of communication. Clinicians need to know the neurophysiological, genetic, environmental, and other factors that are functionally (causally) involved in the processes of speech. Other methods of research can suggest possibilities that remain speculative. But the experimental method can produce more definitive evidence on the independent variables that may be responsible for normal communicative behaviors. One limitation is that some kinds of independent variables are more easily investigated through experimental research than are others. For example, environmental variables are more easily built into experimental designs than genetic or neurophysiologic variables.

Second, the experimental method is essential in gaining an understanding of the factors that lead to disordered communication of various kinds. The method can isolate the factors involved in the production of disordered communication. Once again, the experimental method can be more effective in isolating environmental independent variables of disordered communication than genetic or neurophysiologic variables.

Third, experimental research is essential in evaluating the effects of various treatment programs designed to remediate disorders of communication. Even routine clinical treatment is more like experimental research than normative research. Treatment, by definition, is an operation designed to change a clinical condition. By modifying an independent variable, the scientist modifies some effect, and by manipulating the treatment variable, the clinician also modifies the disorder or disease. The only difference between routine clinical treatment and experimental research is that the former may lack controls for extraneous variables. Such controls are essential in experimental research. However, when the question is whether a given treatment procedure is effective, clinicians need the experimental methodology, which is no less exacting than that used in basic research. See Chapter 4 for an application of experimental methods in treatment evaluation.

Because it is very important to evaluate the effects of treatment procedures used in clinical sciences, the meager amount of experimental research done in communicative disorders is distressing. It appears that, compared with other types of research, controlled evaluation of treatment is of low priority. Ex post facto, normative, and survey research, along with standard-group comparisons combined with speculatively theoretical research papers, far exceed the number of experimental reports in most issues of journals on communicative disorders. Annually, very few experimental treatment evaluation studies are published in professional and scientific journals. In language and phonology, most studies are either normatively descriptive or categorically theoretical. Categorically theoretical papers usually suggest various ways of categorizing the dependent variables (language or phonological classificatory schemes).

Clinical investigators justify nonexperimental research on the basis that first they need descriptive evidence. The belief is that one needs to prepare for experimental research. As noted before, this justification is valid to a certain extent. However, from a technical standpoint, experimental research has been possible for a long time. Therefore, it appears as though communicative disorders is endlessly preparing itself for the much-needed experimental research.

Instead of experimentally demonstrating the effects of treatment programs, investigators who do not appreciate the experimental method often resort to offering speculative "recommendations" for treatment. When such recommendations are incorporated into existing therapeutic procedures, needless diversity of questionable treatment practices results. In such cases, clinicians do not know whether the incorporated recommendations contribute anything to therapeutic success. Therefore, experimental research is as crucial to a clinical science as it is to basic science.

When experimental data are lacking, theoretical speculations flourish. Such speculations create vigorous debates and controversies fueled not by evidence but by rational arguments, intuition, and subjective opinions. A desirable side effect of experimental-clinical research is a mitigation of such endless and useless debates and controversies. Experimental research may not settle all arguments, but at least it will force the debaters out of their armchairs and into the clinical laboratories so that, instead of offering arguments, specialists can collect and offer data that matter.

Epidemiological Research

The variety of clinical research known as epidemiological research is mostly nonexperimental, although some authors include experimental treatment research under the category of epidemiological research. **Epidemiology** is defined as the science of the frequency and distribution of diseases, injury, and health-related behaviors and events to determine their potential causes with the goal of designing programs to control and prevent their development and spread in human populations. The term is derived from *epidemics*, the outbreak of deadly diseases or other health-related events. Epidemiological research has greatly improved human health and community sanitary standards. Through the epidemiological research on diseases and their distribution, modern societies have developed means of transporting clean drinking water, mechanisms of sewage treatment, and refrigeration of food and beverage.

Studying incidence and prevalence of diseases, disorders, and other health-affecting events is a major effort of epidemiologists. **Incidence** refers to the events that happen over time or the occurrence of an event in a specified duration of time. For instance, to say that the incidence of stuttering in most societies is 1% means that 1% of any nonstuttering population may develop stuttering. The **prevalence** of a disease refers to the proportion of a population that already has a disease or a disorder. To say that there are 500 children who stutter in a given school district is to make a statement of prevalence. Through the study of incidence and prevalence epidemiologists establish patterns of distribution of specified diseases and disorders in human populations.

A pattern of distribution of a disease may suggest or hint at conditions under which the disease appears and develops. Such conditions are of great interest to epidemiologists. In the past, they were concerned with conditions under which epidemic diseases such as plague and cholera would occur. Modern-day epidemiologists are concerned with the distribution of a wider variety of factors such as heart diseases, various forms of cancer, acquired immunodeficiency syndrome, criminal behavior of youths, child abuse, domestic violence, drug abuse, teen smoking, exercise behavior, and dietary habits. Once the distribution is known, epidemiologists search for potential causes that may be controlled or eliminated to reduce the frequency of the disease or disorder. Even controlled experimental evaluation of various treatment and public health programs are epidemiological in nature.

Epidemiology is now a vast field of research with varied research topics and methods (Hennekens & Buring, 1987; Rothman & Greenland, 1998b). Only a few major epidemiological research methods are highlighted here. Epidemiological research may be experimental or nonexperimental. Experimental research in epidemiology includes controlled treatment evaluations, field studies, or community intervention. **Controlled treatment evaluations** are the same as randomized clinical trials described in Chapter 4. As noted in that chapter, experimental and control groups are used to evaluate the effects of various treatment procedures on patients with specific diseases or disorders. **Field trials,** on the other hand, are conducted on healthy persons to evaluate the effectiveness of health promotion or disease prevention programs. Such programs often are conducted in natural settings because healthy people do not seek treatment in clinics and hospitals. For example, there have been large-scale field trials to evaluate the effects of vitamins and diet in reducing mortality due to heart disease or cancer or in reducing the frequency of the common cold. Experimental evaluation of various vaccines or cholesterol-lowering drugs (sometimes controlled with placebo) also are field studies. In essence, both randomized clinical trials and field studies use the group design strategy described in Chapter 8.

Community intervention is a type of experimental epidemiological research in which the participants are not individuals (as they are in clinical and field trials) but whole communities of people living in a certain geographic area. For instance, as part of a program to reduce the incidence of dental caries in a community, the community's water supply may be treated with fluoride. Note that the treatment is aimed not at a particular individual but the entire community. Another community whose water is not fluoridated may be selected as a control. Police may institute a program to reduce the number of red-light runners or drunk drivers; the program is exposed to all in the community simultaneously.

Nonexperimental research in epidemiology includes several methods, but I shall highlight only cohort studies and case-control studies (Rothman & Greenland, 1998b). Most nonexperimental epidemiological studies may be retrospective or prospective. **Retrospective studies** are those in which a disease or a condition is already evident and perhaps has been for some time. In **prospective studies,** some subjects are known to have been exposed to the risk factor, but the clinical condition has not yet appeared. For instance, children who have had early traumatic brain injury and those without a history of such injury may be two groups of cohorts. In this case, traumatic brain injury is the risk factor for developing learning disabilities later in school. In a retrospective study, children who are already in grade schools and who already have learning disabilities may be compared with those who do not have the history and are doing well in the schools. In a prospective cohort study, observation of both the groups will start before any evidence of learning disability emerges; the investigators observe its emergence.

Cohort studies involve a group of people who have a common characteristic or face a similar risk for developing a disease. For example, children who have a family history of language disorders constitute a cohort. They share a family history and possibly are at risk for developing language disorders. All adults with a parental history of premature death due to heart disease are another cohort.

A study may involve more than one cohort. Two groups, one exposed to a risk factor (e.g., family history of learning disabilities) and the other unexposed to the same risk factor (e.g., no family history of learning disabilities) constitute two cohorts. One or more cohorts may be observed for a relatively long duration to determine the incidence of a disorder, disease, or health-related event. For instance, two cohorts, one with and one without a family history of learning disabilities, may be followed for several years of schooling to determine the effect of the exposure (family history) on the incidence of learning disabilities in children.

Case-control studies involve a clinical group (case) that has a disorder and a control group that does not. These studies are similar to standard-group comparisons described earlier. Case-control studies also are similar to cohort studies in that the cases and controls are cohort groups. The main difference between the two types of studies is this: in the cohort method, none of the cohorts yet exhibit the clinical condition, although some may be at risk; in the case-control method, one group already exhibits the clinical condition and is being compared with another that does not.

Typically retrospective, case-control studies compare the history of the two groups and any other current information that might contribute to an understanding of why the cases manifest the diseases while the controls do not. The investigator may collect data from interviews, case histories (cases), biographical information (controls), questionnaires, and previously recorded laboratory measures, clinical findings, and diagnostic and treatment data to see if the cases and controls differ systematically on some variable or variables. The difference found may be hypothetically linked to the clinical condition.

Case control is a commonly used clinical research method. An investigator, for instance, might select people who have had a recent stroke and compare them with healthy individuals with no history of strokes. The case-control research methods may reveal that there were systematic differences between the two groups on two variables: diet and exercise. These two variables then might be related to the incidence of strokes in the cases, and presumably in the population. Johnson's diagnosogenic theory of stuttering may be described as a case-control epidemiological study (Johnson & Associates, 1959). After studying parental attitudes toward fluency and stuttering in parents of stuttering (case) and nonstuttering (control) children, he concluded that parents who are excessively concerned with fluency and who diagnose stuttering on the basis of normal nonfluencies in their children actually cause stuttering.

Strengths and Limitations of Clinical and Applied Research

Clinical and applied research offer many advantages to individuals and society. These two types of research are the main means by which science helps solve practical problems, improve individual living conditions and general social conditions, reduce disease frequencies, promote health and fitness, and find new treatment procedures for illnesses. Clinical and applied research studies always address socially and personally significant problems. The best kinds of research studies in this category build on basic research and thus help extend its usefulness. Therefore, clinical and applied research are valuable for society.

Compared to nonclinical basic research, clinical research has its limitations. Clinical research is sometimes more difficult to implement than nonclinical research. Clinical research raises many ethical concerns. Sampling a sufficient number of participants for clinical research can be difficult. In group experimental designs, achieving sampling equivalence between the experimental and control groups also may be difficult. In nonexperimental clinical or applied research, it is difficult to draw firm conclusions about cause–effect relations. Many of the strengths and limitations of clinical and applied research are discussed and elaborated in Chapters 4, 8, and 9.

SAMPLE SURVEYS

Surveys assess some characteristics of a group of people or a particular society. Like normative research, surveys try to determine the distribution of certain variables in the population. For example, a survey researcher might be interested in finding out the attitudes of teachers toward students with hearing impairment in certain elementary schools. Another investigator might be interested in the most frequently used stuttering therapy procedure in university clinics. Yet another researcher may wish to assess the opinions of school administrators regarding the necessity of speech–language services in schools under their administration. Research concerns such as these require the survey method.

Technically, surveys try to find out how variables such as attitudes, opinions, and certain social or personal practices are distributed in the population. However, rarely can a surveyor assess the entire population. The typical strategy is to draw a representative sample of the population and find out its members' reactions to a set of questions designed to evoke answers of interest. Therefore, scientific surveys often are called sample surveys.

Surveys are routinely used in assessing public opinions and attitudes of various kinds. Some of the well-known surveys include Gallup polls, Harris polls, and those that are conducted by television networks and national newspapers. Most of the attitudes and opinions assessed in these polls are related in some way to political, social, or economic issues. Predicting voter behavior, for example, is a regular form of survey research. Assessment of people's attitudes toward contemplated legislation and economic policies is also done frequently. The need for such sample surveys is so great that many commercial firms specialize in conducting them.

In academic and clinical fields, surveys might address questions regarding the distribution of certain variables either in the population at large or in specific groups. A professional organization may wish to find out how many people know about speech–language pathologists. In this case, knowledge, defined in some operational way, is the dependent variable, the distribution of which in the general population is measured in a survey. Similarly, when a speech–language pathologist wishes to determine the number of persons who have aphasia in a given town, the dependent variable is aphasia, the distribution of which in the population is assessed.

The results of surveys are only as valid as the sampling technique used in them. Technically, a random sample is needed to accurately assess the dependent variable. A nonrepresentative sample will lead to invalid conclusions. The issues surrounding the random theory are discussed elsewhere in the book. It is sufficient to note here that all sampling techniques have a margin of error. Currently, the typical national sampling of citizens of voting age in the United States involves about 1,500 individuals. It may carry a sampling error of 4 to 6 percentage points. For example, assuming a 5%

sampling error, when a survey reports that 34% of the voting-age population favor a tax reform package, the actual percentage in the population may be anywhere between 29% and 39%.

Strengths and Limitations of Sample Surveys

It is necessary to understand what surveys can and cannot do. Surveys can help formulate certain professional and social policies. They let us know what people are thinking on certain issues or what kind of actions the people think they might take in certain situations. For example, it may be important to know whether school administrators might support more speech–language pathology positions in the schools.

Surveys, however, cannot answer questions of causality because of lack of experimental manipulation. For example, a survey might show that a certain procedure is widely used in the treatment of persons with a laryngectomy, but it cannot determine whether the technique is indeed effective. Such a survey reflects only a current practice, not its effectiveness or validity. As in normative research, when the question concerns the distribution of the dependent variables, surveys are useful, but when the questions concern functional relations between events, they are not.

The best surveys with adequate random samples can help predict group behaviors but not the behaviors of an individual. One might find out, for example, that a given stuttering treatment is used by a majority of clinicians. However, from this survey information, one cannot answer the question of whether a given clinician is using the technique. Similarly, an opinion survey may show that a given candidate is likely to be elected by a majority of voters, but this is of no help in predicting the voting behavior of an individual citizen.

An additional limitation of surveys is that they tend to focus on "soft" dependent variables. Attitudes and opinions are the most frequently sampled dependent variables in a survey research. However, in most cases, attitudes and opinions themselves are of little interest to the survey researcher, who in fact tries to predict actions or behaviors of individuals in populations. The researcher infers certain imminent actions from the people to whom the conclusions of the sample survey are extended. However, there is very little assurance that presumed attitudes and opinions always translate into actions. In some limited instances, opinions and attitudes may accurately reflect a group behavior. For example, just before the polls open, or during the polling hours, an accurate sampling of voters may reflect actual voting behaviors. In such cases, a television network may be able to declare a winner a few minutes or a few hours ahead of the official announcement. Such accurate but competitive predictions may have commercial advantages, but their scientific utility is limited.

RELATION BETWEEN RESEARCH TYPES AND QUESTIONS

Six major types of research have been discussed in this chapter: ex post facto, normative, standard-group comparison, experimental, clinical, and survey. It must be clear to the reader that each research type handles a unique type of research question. The nature of the question determines the type of method used.

Research types are not entirely matters of methods, however. They reflect both methodological and philosophical stances. As noted earlier, each type of research is capable of answering certain kinds of questions. Therefore, the kinds of methods used depend on the kinds of questions asked, and a researcher can use different methods to answer different kinds of questions. In practice, however, most researchers develop a tendency to investigate certain types of questions. A majority of those who are typically interested in normative research in language development, for example, may not be inclined to ask questions that require experimental analysis. Those who wish to determine the independent variables of their dependent variables rarely indulge in normative research.

Broadly speaking, the six research types can be grouped into three categories. The first category contains the ex post facto type of research, which can answer questions regarding potential relations between events that have passed. In ex post facto research, the investigator infers a cause of an effect from a knowledge of past events. It may be noted that evaluation research is essentially ex post facto in that it tries to establish whether certain events took place (process) and whether certain other events followed (impact).

The second category contains the normative, standard-group comparisons and survey types of research, which are capable of answering questions concerning "the way things are." All three types of research in the second category are concerned with the distribution of dependent variables in the population. There are philosophical and other differences between the three types within this category. Normative research is based on the philosophy of developmentalism and seeks to establish typical performances of defined groups. Standard-group comparisons are made to find differences between identified groups. Both normative and standard-group comparisons are thought to help determine boundaries of normal and disordered or deviant behaviors.

The third category contains experimental research of all varieties: laboratory, clinical, and nonclinical. Experimental research does not search for causal relations in the past, nor does it simply ask a question about the way things are. It creates conditions under which expected or unexpected things may happen. What happens when an independent variable is manipulated under controlled conditions is the concern of experimental research. Therefore, research questions about cause–effect relations in which the experimenter must have a reasonable degree of confidence dictate the use of the experimental method.

Many beginning researchers often wonder what type of research they should do. Instead, they should wonder about the types of questions they would like to investigate. Within their limitations, all types of research contribute something to the knowledge base. Some types of research, however, do more than others in helping researchers understand the events they study. The experimental method does the most in helping scientists both understand the events and gain control over those events. Understanding and controlling events are the essence of science, regardless of such qualifications as applied, clinical, and basic.

SUMMARY

TABLE 5.1
Summary of Research Types and Their Strengths and Weaknesses

Type of Research	Strengths	Weaknesses
Ex post facto: Retrospective study of events; case studies	Can describe an effect and suggest potential causes in the past Sometimes the only possible research type	Cannot isolate causes or explain effects Not experimental
Normative research: Studies the distribution of behaviors across age groups	Can describe behaviors specific to age groups Helps establish norms	Cannot specify causes Not experimental Cannot explain behaviors
Standard-group comparison: Study of clinical versus non-clinical groups	Can describe differences Helps distinguish clinical groups	Cannot specify causes Not experimental Cannot explain effects
Experimental research: Assessment of cause–effect relations	Can isolate cause–effect relations Can explain events and support theories	Cannot be extended to all kinds of problems Criticized as mechanistic and artificial
Clinical and applied research: Designed to solve practical problems	The experimental type can isolate causes, explain events, assess treatment effects	The descriptive type cannot isolate causes, explain events, or assess treatment effects
Sample survey: Study of opinions and attitudes through random samples	Helps determine dispositions of large groups of people	Cannot isolate causes Cannot explain events Not experimental

STUDY GUIDE _____

1. Define ex post facto research. Describe its procedures.

2. You are seeing a client with a sensorineural hearing loss. Design an ex post facto study to identify some of the potential causal variables. Describe possible independent variables and the procedures of uncovering them. Specify the limitations of this kind of study.

3. Justify the need for ex post facto studies in clinical disciplines.

4. What are the logic and the procedures of normative research?

5. Suppose you wish to establish the stages by which children learn to produce the regular and irregular plural forms with 80% accuracy. You also wish to have a local representative sample. Design a study to accomplish your objectives.

6. Summarize the strengths and limitations of normative research.

7. Is chronological age an independent variable? Why or why not?

8. Describe the method of standard-group comparison. It is similar to what other type of research?

9. Select a clinical group and design a standard-group comparison study. Describe fully the dependent variables, assigned variables, and measurement procedures.

10. Justify the statement that standard-group comparisons cannot establish cause–effect relations.

11. Define experimental research. Describe its procedures.

12. Suppose you wish to experimentally evaluate the effects of an articulation treatment procedure. Describe a hypothetical treatment procedure and design an experimental study to evaluate its effects.

13. Specify the criticisms of experimental research. How would you refute those criticisms?

14. Distinguish between clinical and applied research.

15. Summarize the importance of experimental–clinical research.

16. Define and describe epidemiology.

17. Compare the cohort study method with the case-control method. Define both and give examples.

18. What is the purpose of sample surveys? Write two research questions that can be answered by the survey research.

19. What are the limitations of survey research?

20. Justify the statement that each research type handles a unique type of research question. Suggest two different types of research questions and methods for answering them. Give examples.

Chapter 6

◆◆◆◆◆◆◆◆◆◆◆◆◆◆◆◆◆◆◆◆◆◆◆◆◆◆◆◆◆◆◆

Observation and Measurement

- Observation and Measurement
- Philosophies of Measurement
- Traditional Levels of Measurement
- Some Measures of Communicative Behaviors
- Client-Assisted Measurement
- Indirect Measures: Self-Reports
- The Observer in the Measurement Process
- Mechanical Aids to Observation and Measurement
- Reliability of Measurement
- Summary
- Study Guide

Observation and measurement are two basic scientific activities. The beginnings of observation are in the sensory experiences generated by some natural phenomena. When people see, hear, touch, and smell things, people may wonder about things' characteristics and causes. They may then take a closer, more systematic look at the event. Observation is, at the simplest level, looking at something and describing what is seen. Other senses, including hearing, touch, smell, and taste also may be involved in observation. In essence, observation is establishing a sensory contact with an event and then making a report on that experience. In this sense, observation is an everyday activity.

Compared with everyday observation, **scientific observation** is more systematic, thorough, and objective. Scientific observation is *systematic* because it is structured and the results of observations are carefully recorded. The observation is *thorough* in that the scientist attempts to observe as many instances and as many aspects of a phenomenon as possible. It is *objective* in that the results of observation may be publicly verifiable because different observers can try to achieve the same or similar results.

Scientific observation is rooted in empiricism. Normally, scientists do not take seriously events that do not generate sensory consequences. Exceptions emerge when indirect evidence and theory suggest the existence of a phenomenon though there are not yet direct sensory consequences. The existence of a phenomenon that cannot be measured may be temporarily postulated when many strong empirical reasons support it. In many cases, instruments allow for the observation of events that do not generate sensory stimulation. The issue of mechanical aids to observation will be addressed in a later section.

OBSERVATION AND MEASUREMENT

Scientific observation is essential for measuring a phenomenon. Without systematic measurement, a scientist cannot go much beyond observation. For example, to experiment, the event should be measured before, during, and after the introduction of the independent variable. Changes in events should be documented through measurement.

Measurement has been defined variously as "assignment of numbers to represent properties" (N. Campbell, 1952, p. 110) and as "assignment of numerals to objects or events according to rules" (Stevens, 1951, p. 1). In essence, **measurement** quantifies observed objects, events, and their mathematical properties. This is done according to a standard set of rules that define units of measurement (Johnston & Pennypacker, 1993).

Quantified observations are the measured value of an event, object, or its property. Technically, what is measured is not the event, object, or its property, but some dimensional quantity. Frequency of an event, for example, is a **dimensional quantity** because standard number units can be assigned to that frequency; other dimensional quantities of behavioral events include duration, latency, and interresponse time.

PHILOSOPHIES OF MEASUREMENT

Social and psychological sciences have evolved a philosophy of measurement that is different from that of natural sciences (Johnston & Pennypacker, 1993). Natural sciences have found that absolute and standard units of measurement are essential to objective quantification of observations. Johnston and Pennypacker (1993) have called this kind of measurement **idemnotic,** that is, the units of measurement have a standard and absolute meaning. Idemnotic units of measurement are independent of the measured phenomenon. Without idemnotic measurement, natural scientists would not have achieved the level of precision and objectivity for which they are well known.

To the contrary, social and psychological sciences often do not measure the dimensional quantities of events using absolute and standard units of measurements. Instead, they measure those quantities in relative standards that are defined within the confines of the variability of the phenomenon under investigation. Johnston and Pennypacker (1993) have called this type of measurement **vaganotic,** meaning the units of measurement vary.

In vaganotic measurement, standards of measurement keep changing depending on the amount by which a phenomenon varies. For example, a rating scale developed to measure the severity of stuttering typically yields different values depending upon the amount of variability found in different groups of people who stutter. Different rating scales designed to measure the same stuttering severity yield different values when used on the same clients. Similarly, rating scales developed to measure different disorders will result in vastly different values.

Social and psychological sciences often measure dimensional quantities indirectly. Instead of directly observing behaviors, social or psychological scientists may sample participants' verbal statements (or those of others who are supposed to know). For example, a supervisor may fill out a questionnaire on the productivity of his or her employee. The investigator will use the questionnaire responses as though they were direct observational values of productive behaviors themselves. However, the investigator will not have directly observed and counted productive behavior with a standard and absolute system of numbers.

The proverbially derogative statement, "By taking a new job, he raised the IQ of the people he left and the people he joined," illustrates this philosophy of relative and indirect measurement defined in terms of the variability of the phenomenon being measured. Nobody's intelligence was increased or decreased by a person's move, but because the variability changed, the assumption is that the measured value also changed. If one were to assume that a given student on a university campus is as intelligent as the "average student" on that campus, then that student's intelligence will continuously change, depending on which university he or she attends. Compared to a group of persons who are clinically anxious, I may have less anxiety, but compared to someone who is unusually calm, I may have more anxiety. All along, my level of anxiety may not have changed, but the relative scale used to measure it assumes that it has.

Johnston and Pennypacker (1993) have traced the history of vaganotic and idemnotic measurement. In the 17th and 18th centuries, mathematicians and scientists were concerned with the variability in measured values of a given phenomenon. When a natural phenomenon is measured repeatedly, the values are typically not constant. The question, then, is what is the "true" value of the phenomenon? This concern eventually led to the development of modern statistics in the works of Adolphe Quetelet (1796–1874). Quetelet proposed that such human characteristics as height vary only because nature missed the ideal. What nature missed could be calculated by measuring the heights of many individuals. In effect, when repeated measures are plotted, the result is a normal curve, which to many suggests the ideal in the form of a mean. Thus, the nonexistent average person, created to neutralize the measures of variability in people, gave not only a stable measure of persons but also the concept of an ideal person.

It was Francis Galton (1822–1911) who believed that mental abilities are also distributed normally and that the distribution of measured values across a vast number of participants would suggest the ideal (the average). Soon, Binet (1857–1911) and Cattell (1860–1944) developed tests of intelligence, and the tradition of vaganotic measurement based on the variability of the phenomenon measured became firmly established in psychology and social sciences. The tradition was strengthened by the development of statistical techniques designed to infer the true value of a population from the measured sample values.

Although psychology and social sciences use indirect and relative systems of measurement, the radical behaviorism of Skinner has shown that the use of absolute and standard units of measurement is possible in the study of human behavior. Skinner (1953) avoided indirect and statistically based measurement of behavior by defining his dependent variable as the rate (frequency) of observable and directly measurable responses of an organism. When the occurrence of a given response of a class of responses is counted, a direct and absolute number system is used. For example, when a clinician counts the number of times a child produces the regular plural morpheme *s* in a segment of conversational speech, an absolute value of frequency is established. The value would not be relative to the variability found in the phenomenon of plural *s* usage. To the contrary, the normative statement, "On the average, 5-year-olds produce the plural *s* with *x* percent accuracy," is relative to the variability found in that phenomenon.

The measurement philosophy and the nature of a subject matter interact in a curious manner. A measurement philosophy can influence the way a subject matter is conceptualized and researched. To a certain extent, intelligence and personality were conceptualized as they were because of the measurement philosophy and technique adopted by those interested in mental measurement. In turn, the way a phenomenon is conceptualized determines to some extent how it can be measured. If variability is believed to be intrinsic to the behaving organism—as with the statistical approach—then group designs and statistical methods of neutralizing variability are necessary techniques of research. On the other hand, if it is believed that variability is extrinsic to the behaving organism, it becomes a subject of experimental analysis. The measurement procedure adopted in this case would not be solely determined by the variability of behaviors.

TRADITIONAL LEVELS OF MEASUREMENT

Social and psychological scientists typically describe what are known as *levels of measurement.* These levels are an integral part of the indirect and relative measurement strategy. Some of the levels are closely related to statistical scaling techniques.

Typically, four levels of measurement are described: nominal, ordinal, interval, and ratio. In **nominal measurement,** numbers assigned to an event or object simply help distinguish one event or object from the other; the numbers have no mathematical meaning. Therefore, the numbers are much like proper names; hence, the term *nominal.* Nominal measurement yields categorical data: 1 may stand for the female participant and 0 for the male participant. What is "measured" is simply given a parallel symbol system, which may consist of numbers without their mathematical meanings. Questionnaires that evoke *yes* or *no* responses illustrate nominal measurement, as do telephone numbers and numbers assigned to football players. Diagnostic categories such as stuttering and aphasia are clinical examples of nominal measurement.

Nominal measurement is described as the crudest or the simplest of the measurement levels. It is probably no measurement at all. It does not measure a dimensional quantity, and it does not serve any purpose other than distinguishing one set of observations from another. It does not accomplish anything that a name would not, and naming a thing is not the same as measuring it.

Ordinal measurement assumes that the property being measured is continuous, not categorical; relative concepts such as *greater than* and *less than* are used in ordinal measurement. It is usually accomplished by rank-ordering events, objects, or properties because of their graded increases or decreases. For example, a school that graduates the most straight-A students may be assigned the rank number 1, and the school that graduates the lowest number of straight-A students is assigned the last rank. In rank-ordering students on the basis of their Graduate Record Examination scores, admission officers use ordinal measurement. Ranks only tell that one student has scored more or less on the examination in relation to students with higher or lower ranks. Ranked values do not tell how much more they scored, nor do they indicate an absence of the quality measured. In other words, there are no absolute numbers and there is no zero that indicates the total absence of the measured property.

The frequently used 5-point Lickert-type rating scale consists of ordinal measurement. When a person expresses *strong disagreement, disagreement, neutral, agreement,* or *strong agreement,* the opinion on the issue in question is measured on an ordinal scale. The categories of judgments can be given numbers to derive numerical values. For instance, *strong agreement* may be given a scale value of 1 and *strong disagreement* a scale value of 5. However, such numbers and their corresponding categories do not have mathematical meaning. Also, the intervals between numbers or categories are unknown and probably not equal. For example, one cannot assume that *strong agreement* is twice as strong as *agreement.* Therefore, numbers assigned to ordinal categories cannot be added or subtracted.

Ordinal scales at best provide indirect and subjective measures of properties measured. They are greatly influenced by the uncontrolled, momentary, and subjective judgments of the observer. There is no standard unit of measurement. This type of measurement is commonly used in the assessment of such subjective and highly variable intervening variables as attitudes and opinions.

Interval measurement is an improvement over ordinal measurement in that the numerical distinctions of the scale do suggest similar distinctions in the measured property; that is, the difference between 1 and 2 on an interval scale would be the same as the difference between 3 and 4. As noted before, there is no such assurance in an ordinal scale. The interval scale has a zero, but it is arbitrary. The zero does not mean the absence of the measured property. Therefore, the scale values of an interval scale, though of known, equal intervals, cannot be added or subtracted.

Measurement of temperature and calendar time are examples of interval scales. On either the centigrade or Fahrenheit scales, zero does not mean an absence of temperature. The beginning of the Christian calendar is also arbitrary. If four clients' stuttering is measured on an interval scale, the client who is assigned a score of 4 stutters twice as severely as the client who receives a 2. Again, because of a lack of zero, the numbers are not additive or subtractive.

Ratio measurement, the final level of measurement, has all the properties of the earlier levels and also has a zero that represents an absence of the property being measured. Ratio measurement uses the number system in its mathematical sense. It is possible to count, add, and subtract the values of a ratio scale. Most measures in the natural sciences are on this scale; most of those in the social sciences are not. However, when the dependent variable is the frequency of discrete events, it is possible to use the ratio measurement. The frequency of a given discrete response can be measured with real numbers. A zero response rate means that the organism did not respond.

SOME MEASURES OF COMMUNICATIVE BEHAVIORS

Communicative behaviors can be observed, measured, and recorded in different ways. The kinds of measures used depend on the definition of the communicative behavior targeted for measurement. Some definitions allow direct measurement whereas others permit only indirect and inferential measurement. For example, language may be defined either as linguistic competence or as the production of various language responses. Linguistic competence cannot be measured directly; it is inferred from other kinds of data. The production of particular responses, on the other hand, is directly measurable. Generally speaking, a phenomenon can be measured more directly if it is defined operationally. **Operational definitions** are descriptions of procedures involved in measuring an event; for example, the term *articulatory proficiency* does not define anything operationally, but the statement *production of /s/ in initial positions of 10 words at 90% accuracy* does.

The following sections describe seven types of measures that are relevant for most clinical research in communication sciences and disorders: frequency, duration, interresponse time, latency, time sampling, momentary time sampling, and verbal interaction sampling.

Frequency Measures

The **frequency** with which a behavior is exhibited under specified stimulus conditions is one of the most useful and objective of the measured values of communicative behaviors. This measure often is used in clinical research.

Frequency measures can be used in counting the number of times a client produces language responses of particular classes, the number of sounds misarticulated, the number and types of dysfluencies, the number of pitch breaks, and other such communicative behaviors. To establish frequency measures of various speech and language behaviors, the observer often should count also the number of **contextually correlated behaviors,** that is, behaviors that occur only in certain contexts such as the number of syllables or words spoken. For example, speech sounds, dysfluencies, and so forth normally occur only in the context of syllable and word production.

The measurement of the frequency of communicative behaviors poses a special problem. Communicative behaviors are discriminated. In other words, their production is not reflexive and automatic but context dependent. Therefore, in measuring the frequency of communicative behaviors, the investigator should first arrange the discriminative stimulus conditions that set the stage for the particular kinds of behaviors targeted for observation and measurement. Various kinds of stimulus pictures, objects, topic cards, and conversational devices help evoke communicative behaviors.

In establishing the frequency measure of specific speech–language behaviors, the investigator should take into consideration the number of opportunities afforded those behaviors in a given period of observation. For example, in the measurement of the frequency of grammatical features, the number of discriminated opportunities to produce those features should be considered. Brown (1973) has described such opportunities as **obligatory contexts,** which are the structural contexts of phrases and sentences in which the use of a particular grammatical feature is dictated by the rules of a given language. For example, the regular plural inflection would be obligatory in the context of "I see two frogs here." The concept of obligatory contexts can be used in measuring semantic and pragmatic response classes as well.

The productions of specific sounds also have their discriminated opportunities. An omission is suggested when a child does not produce the /s/ at the beginning of the word *soup* because of the obligatory context for that production. The number of syllables or words spoken may be the discriminated opportunities for the production of dysfluencies. Speech itself is the discriminated opportunity for various voice qualities.

When the discriminated opportunities and the number of opportunities in which the behavior under observation appears are both measured, a percent-correct response rate can be derived. This rate can be calculated for most of the communicative behaviors whose frequency can be measured. The percentage of (correct) articulation of a given sound in a given word position and that of dysfluencies are among the commonly reported frequency-based measures in research studies. Studies on language have also frequently reported percent-correct measures of productions of various grammatical features and vocabulary items.

Frequency measure, though simple, direct, and objective, may not be practical in measuring all kinds of communicative behaviors. Frequency measure is most appropriate for behaviors that are of relatively low rate and have a clear beginning and end. In other words, the behaviors should be discrete and should be a part of other behaviors. Many speech and language behaviors fulfill these two criteria. Grammatical features, for example, are used in the context of other behaviors and are therefore of relatively low rate. They also are discrete behaviors in the sense that their onset and termination can be easily determined.

Some nondiscrete communicative behaviors of high rate are not appropriately measured by frequency count. For example, some voice qualities such as hoarseness or harshness may not be most efficiently counted according to their rate. A pervasive hoarseness of voice (high rate) that does not have a discernible beginning or end (except for the speech–silence dichotomy) should be measured some other way.

Another limitation of frequency count is that it may not be a comprehensive measure of certain behaviors. Mere frequency count may miss other equally significant dimensional quantities of a behavior. Other important dimensional qualities, such as the duration of certain behaviors, may be missed in the frequency count. For instance, a frequency measure of dysfluencies may not necessarily reflect their durational quantity. Theoretically, dysfluencies of low frequency may be of relatively long duration, and those of high frequency may be of short duration. This theoretical possibility has not been observed in a majority of people who stutter, however. In most cases, low frequency of dysfluencies is associated with relatively shorter duration and vice versa. But in those exceptional cases where frequency and duration are unrelated or opposite to each other, both measures should be obtained.

Procedures of counting the frequency of a behavior may be simple or complex. Many speech–language behaviors can be counted with the help of various kinds of counters. In most clinical sessions, behavioral frequency can be counted with certain kinds of marks on a piece of paper. Speech–language behaviors, because of their transitory nature, require some form of recording before they can be reliably counted. Audio or video recordings often are necessary to count speech–language behaviors. In most cases, the recorded behaviors should be reviewed repeatedly to obtain accurate measures.

Durational Measures

The **duration** over which a specified behavior is sustained can be a useful measure. It is especially useful in the case of continuous behaviors. The total number of seconds or minutes for which the behavior is sustained is usually measured and compared against the total duration of time for which the observation was made. For example, a clinician may record the duration for which a client maintains an inappropriately high pitch within a 30-minute conversational speech. In this case, the percentage of time spent exhibiting the appropriate pitch also can be calculated.

Duration, being a temporal measure of behavior, gives a different kind of information than does frequency. Frequency, which shows the number of times a behavior is exhibited, gives no clues to the length of behavioral episodes. As pointed out earlier, duration of dysfluencies is an important dimensional quantity. It can be of both empirical and theoretical significance in a research study. In communicative disorders, most vocal qualities are better measured for their duration. If talking behavior (a global measure of language use) is the subject of experimental manipulation, the time spent talking (instead of specific language behaviors) may be a more appropriate measure.

The durational measure can be impractical with many behaviors. Duration is a valid measure of behaviors that have an appreciable temporal dimension. It is true that all behaviors have a temporal dimension, but depending on the purposes of a study, measurement of duration may or may not be essential or practical. For example, in the measurement of grammatical features or semantic notions, the interest may be in frequency and not duration. How many times a child produces the present progressive -*ing* in a conversational sample may be of greater interest than the duration of -*ing* productions.

In clinical research, duration measures are less frequently used than frequency measures because extremely brief durations of behaviors are hard to measure without sophisticated instrumentation. The duration should be noticeable in order for durational measures to be used in routine clinical research. For example, sound or silent prolongations of stuttering persons have a noticeable durational dimension, whereas *schwa* interjections do not. Therefore, measurement of duration is relatively easy in the case of prolongations and difficult in the case of interjections.

In clinical research, durations that can be measured with a stopwatch may be reported more frequently than those that require complex instrumentation. Clinical target responses of extremely brief durations are better measured for their frequency. Generally speaking, without instrumentation, durational measures are harder to record than are frequency measures.

Whenever possible, durational measures should be combined with frequency measures. Together, they give a better measure of behaviors. In some cases, a pure duration measure can be meaningless unless the frequency measure is also reported. For example, it may be misleading to report merely the mean duration of sound prolongations in stuttering. For this observation to be meaningful, the frequency of such prolongations also should be reported.

Interresponse Time Measures

Another time-based measure of behaviors is the **interresponse time measure:** the duration that lapses between any two discrete responses or other events. Interresponse time can be a useful measure in some kinds of research. For example, in clinical studies that are concerned with too-sparse response rates, the clinician might be interested in decreasing the interresponse time.

Clinically, interresponse time may be a function of the rate at which the clinician presents the training stimuli. For example, a clinician may present language or articulation stimulus cards at a faster or slower rate, generating a shorter or longer interresponse time. When the rate of stimulus presentation is changed, the interresponse time also may change. Other treatment variables may affect interresponse time. One can investigate such variables with a view to increasing the response rate and decreasing the time spent not giving the target response.

It is obvious that interresponse time is closely related to the frequency of responses. A high response frequency is likely to be associated with short interresponse durations; a low response frequency is likely to generate long interresponse durations. Therefore, it is meaningful to report the frequency measure along with the interresponse durations.

Latency Measures

Another temporal measure of behavior is the latency measure or reaction time. Latency measure differs from duration measure in that it is not a measure of time for which a response was sustained. **Latency** is the time that lapses between the termination of an environmental event (often a stimulus) and the onset of a response. The time it takes for an organism to respond after stimulation is sometimes taken as a reflection of learning: the faster the reaction time, the stronger the learning. Whether this is valid or not, reaction time can be an indirect measure of frequency; other things being equal, the greater the latency, the lower the frequency of responses per unit of time.

Latency is an important aspect of communicative behavior. In conversational speech, the listener and the speaker alternate their roles. Each provides certain verbal and nonverbal signals to the other person to switch the role (initiate or terminate responses). Therefore, latency measures may be necessary in an analysis of conversational speech. In clinical research, a client's response latency can be a useful dependent variable in that shorter latencies often are one of the targets of treatment. A delayed response may be as good as no response, and often it is scored as such. Decreasing the latency, then, becomes a primary target of treatment.

A few seconds of reaction time is considered typical in clinical situations. Most clinicians allow up to 5 seconds for the client to respond. If the response latency is too long, the clinician tends to shape progressively shorter latencies.

Latency has been a dependent variable in several studies on the vocal behaviors of people who stutter. Two latency measures have been researched extensively: the voice initiation time (VIT) and the voice termination time (VTT). Several kinds of stimuli can be used to initiate or terminate a vocal response, although auditory stimuli have been used most frequently. In using an auditory tone as the stimulus, the experimenter may instruct the participant to initiate a vocal response such as /a/ as soon as the tone is heard and terminate the response as soon as the tone ceases. The actual time that elapses between the onset of the tone and the onset of the vocal response is the VIT. The time that elapses between the termination of the tone and that of the response is the VTT. Studies of this kind have generally shown that the reaction time of people who stutter is somewhat slower than that of people who do not stutter, and that reaction time tends to improve with practice (Bloodstein, 1995).

Time Sampling Measures

Time sampling measures gauge time intervals during which behaviors selected for observation occurred. Time sampling should not be confused with the response duration measure, which is also based on time. In time sampling, time refers to periods during which the occurrence of a behavior is observed and recorded; in duration measurement, the length of a response is recorded.

In time sampling, the investigator observes a behavior during selected intervals of time. The intervals may be of short duration: a few seconds to a few minutes. An entire treatment session of 45 minutes may be subdivided into 5-minute blocks. During each block, whether or not a specified behavior occurred is recorded. During the observational interval, multiple occurrences of the same behavior are not distinguished; the behavior is scored only once during the interval. The duration of the response is also ignored.

The observational periods may be consecutive or may be interspersed with nonobservational periods. This method requires intense observation because during the interval or period of observation, the investigator should pay continuous attention to the participant being observed. For example, a special educator might observe a child for 10 minutes, divided into 10-second intervals. During the interval, whether the child exhibits a given target behavior such as quiet sitting or reading is noted. At the end of the interval the presence or the absence of the behavior is recorded. Similarly, in an assessment of mother–child interactions, an investigator may use time sampling to observe specific communicative behaviors (such as conversational turn taking) during selected intervals.

Time sampling, because it generates categorical data (presence or absence), may not accurately reflect the frequency of measured behaviors. It is most useful in measuring behaviors that do not have a clear beginning or end. The results of time sampling are analyzed in terms of the number of intervals during which the behavior occurred against the number of intervals in which the behavior was absent.

Momentary Time Sampling

When it is known that a behavior is somewhat constant or of high frequency, continuous observation and measurement may not be necessary. It may be sufficient to observe the behavior periodically and record its occurrence. This method of periodically observing and recording the occurrence of a behavior is known as **momentary time sampling** or *spot checking*.

In momentary time sampling of behaviors, the investigator predetermines the times at which the behavior will be checked. Some kind of signaling device, such as a timer or a wrist alarm, may set the occasion to observe the behavior. As soon as the timer goes off, the investigator looks at the participant and determines whether he or she is exhibiting the target behavior. The behavior is scored as present or absent at the moment of observation. A percentage is then calculated by dividing the number of momentary samples during which the behavior was present by the total number of samples and multiplying the quotient by 100. For example, at 30-minute intervals that are set off by a wrist alarm, a special educator may observe a child to see if he or she is sitting quietly. Assuming that over a few days the specialist had 38 total spot checks and the behavior was scored as present in 24 of them, the percentage of time-sampled value would be 63 ($24 \div 38 \times 100 = 63$).

One advantage of momentary time sampling is that it does not require continuous observation of the target behavior. Clinicians and classroom teachers working with groups are not able to observe a particular client or child constantly. And yet, clinicians and teachers need to measure and monitor various behaviors of the individuals in the group. In such cases, momentary sampling can be useful. Momentary time sampling can be appropriate to measure various noncooperative behaviors of specific children in a group therapy session. At predetermined times, the clinician can check a particular client to see if the client is exhibiting nonattending, off-seat, or any other undesirable behavior.

Verbal Interaction Sampling

Most of the measures considered so far are suitable for measuring behaviors that are relatively independent, discrete, and exhibited by one or a few individuals. The various language productions of one or a few individuals may be measured for their frequency, duration, and interresponse time. Many of these measures may be obtained through either time sampling or momentary time sampling. However, verbal behavior presents the need for another kind of measure, which has been used only in recent years. It is the measure of **verbal interaction**—the typical or atypical communicative exchanges between individuals.

Ethologists and animal psychologists have observed social interactions between members of groups of animals either in natural habitats or laboratories. In this method of observation, sometimes called **sequence sampling**, a sequence of behaviors of multiple individuals is recorded (Altman, 1974). In some respects, the problem faced by the speech–language pathologist is similar to that of the ethologist and the animal psychologist interested in patterns of social behaviors. Communicative behaviors are essentially social interactions. Studied in natural settings, communicative behaviors involve an interaction in which multiple sequences of verbal behaviors can be simultaneously active.

The term **dyadic interaction** refers to communicative exchanges between two persons. This kind of interaction is often used to describe the kind of behavior that is sampled in what I have called here verbal interaction. In many cases, verbal interaction is dyadic. Much of the current research in normal and disordered communication is concerned with interaction between two individuals, often a child and his or her mother or other caregiver. Nonetheless, verbal behaviors are not always dyadic. An analysis of verbal interaction between three or more individuals has barely begun, but it can be expected to be an important part of language analysis. Therefore, the term verbal interaction sampling may be more suitable to describe a method of observation designed to measure interactive verbal behaviors of multiple individuals. The term does not restrict, on a priori grounds, the number of individuals involved in verbal interactions.

In verbal interaction sampling, two or more individuals' verbal behaviors are sampled. Interactions are usually arranged for the specific purpose of observation, and in this sense they may not be as naturalistic as everyday conversations; however, every attempt is made to make the interaction as natural as possible. A mother and a child, for example, may be asked to talk to each other in their usual manner. A variety of play materials, pictures, and other stimulus items may be provided to stimulate verbal interaction. This kind of observation may be made at the participants' home or in a research laboratory.

The actual measures obtained through verbal interaction sampling depend upon the research questions and theoretical orientations of the researcher. For the most part, the frequency of a variety of types of verbal responses is noted. For example, the number of requests, comments, and topic initiations the child and the mother make may be observed and recorded. Verbal interaction sampling also may be used to observe other conversational skills, including turn taking and topic maintenance.

The frequency, duration, interresponse time, latency, time sampling, momentary time sampling, and verbal interaction sampling measures all require direct observation of the behavior to be measured. When necessary, the conditions of behavioral occurrence should be carefully arranged, and the observer or a mechanical device should be present to record the dimensional quantity of the measured behavior. Any of these measures can be obtained in experimental or nonexperimental research conducted in naturalistic settings or laboratories.

Measures obtained by investigators are preferable to those obtained by participants themselves. However, in clinical research, it is sometimes necessary to obtain the measures of behaviors in the client's natural environment in the absence of the clinical investigator. In such cases, client-assisted measurement may be used.

CLIENT-ASSISTED MEASUREMENT

In **client-assisted measurement,** the client performs some important task necessary to document the occurrence of the behavior being measured. The clinical investigator is not present while the behavior of interest is naturally occurring. The client can record his or her own behavior with audio or video recording devices and submit the records to the clinician. It is the clinician who measures the frequency or other dimensional quantity of the target behavior from the submitted recordings.

This kind of measurement is especially important in establishing a reliable frequency of the target behaviors in the natural environment before, during, and after treatment. It is possible that no amount of direct measurement in the clinic or laboratory will fully and accurately reflect the communicative behaviors of clients in the home, school, office, and supermarket. When the concern is the assessment of treatment effects sustained in such natural environments, client-assisted measurement is necessary.

Client-assisted measures may be preferred even when the clinical investigator can be present in a client's everyday situation to measure the target behaviors, because the presence of the clinician may affect the frequency of measured behaviors. Usually, the effect is positive; the clinician is a discriminative stimulus for the treated behaviors. Because the clinician is not a permanent part of the client's natural environment, a more valid measure of the target behavior can be recorded only when the clinician is absent.

The client should be trained to record his or her behavior in natural settings. Most clients should be trained in the correct use of a tape recorder or a video recorder. In communicative disorders, clients often are asked to record their conversational speech at home or in other situations. They should be given detailed instructions on how to arrange the conversational situations. The conversational speech should be natural (habitual) and should be long enough to permit reliable measures of the dependent variables targeted for treatment. Possibly, the conversations with different individuals may have to be recorded at different times of the day. Typically, repeated recordings are needed.

When both are obtained, direct and client-assisted measures can give a more comprehensive and reliable picture of the dependent variables. However, some investigators also may use another kind of measurement in which the dependent variable is neither observed as it occurs nor measured through client-submitted recordings. This is the indirect measurement of behaviors.

INDIRECT MEASURES: SELF-REPORTS

Indirect measures are those obtained without the experimenter coming into contact with the dependent variable in vivo or after the fact. There is no direct observation of the event being measured. In obtaining self-reports, the investigator asks clients to describe their behaviors. The participant can report orally or in writing, and the format of the report may be more or less standardized.

The most commonly used self-reports are questionnaires of various kinds. Questionnaires of personality, attitudes, interests, fears, anxieties, and avoidance reactions are frequently used in clinical research. Most of these questionnaires are used by clinical psychologists and psychiatrists in the assessment of behavior disorders. In communicative disorders, attitudinal scales to measure the reactions of people who stutter to various speech situations are used by some researchers and clinicians. Also available are various rating scales that seek information from persons who stutter regarding their fluency and dysfluency levels in many speaking situations. Other questionnaires may measure attitudes and reactions of parents, teachers, or employers toward various speech–language disorders. Speech and hearing centers may seek the reaction of their patrons regarding the services offered.

The validity of questionnaire measures depends upon the correspondence between what the participants report and the actual behavior that is being reported on. If there is a good correspondence, self-reports may be valid. However, the approach assumes that the participants themselves are reliable and keen observers of their own behaviors, a questionable assumption at best.

A distinction should be made between those self-reports that seek information from the client on specific behaviors exhibited in situations that are not easily accessible to direct observation and those that seek to assess internal states such as attitudes and personality traits. A person who stutters, for example, may be asked to compare the extent of his or her dysfluencies at home and at work. When this client reports more dysfluency at home than at work, one might take it as a reasonably valid statement. However, if the investigator then assumes that the person has a negative attitude toward the workplace, he or she is going beyond reported observations. Therefore, self-reports that simply supply additional information on behaviors exhibited in extraclinical situations are more useful than those that seek to measure internal states or inferred entities.

However, accepting even those self-reports that simply describe behaviors exhibited in extraclinical situations can be problematic. One cannot be sure that a participant's reports are reliable. Therefore, self-reports of clients are an inadequate substitute for direct observation. Client-assisted observation is preferable to self-reports.

Self-reports are an indispensable method in the case of some dependent variables, however. When an investigator is concerned with what the client thinks and feels, verbal or written reports are the only means of assessment. For example, in assessing a patient who is obsessive, the clinician has to ask the patient to describe his or her obsessive thoughts and feelings. In communicative disorders, it is possible that a clinician is interested in the feelings and thoughts associated with a speech or language disorder. In such cases, self-reports provide the only means of assessment. The clinician then should exercise caution in interpreting self-reports because the dependent variables may not have been quantified objectively.

THE OBSERVER IN THE MEASUREMENT PROCESS

The process of observation has two important components: the phenomenon being observed and the individual who observes it. The scientist–observer is supposed to record the events impartially, without injecting his or her own prejudices and biases. Sometimes the mere fact of observation may change the phenomenon. However, the reactivity of dependent variables is not as major a problem in communicative disorders as it is in such fields as social psychology.

Two issues often are raised in the discussion of the human observer: observer bias and the training of the observer. The first, **observer bias,** refers to a potential tendency on the part of the observer to produce data that might support his or her preconceived ideas about the phenomenon being observed. Subtle changes in the method, duration, and intensity of observation can distort data. For example, if a child is known to talk more at home but less at school, the investigator who spends more time observing the behavior at home may introduce subtle bias into the data. In another example, the short-term effects of treatment may be more impressive than the long-term effects, and an observation may be terminated before the data show a decline. The percentage of dysfluencies calculated on the basis of the number of syllables spoken may give a different picture than that based on the number of words spoken.

Faulty analysis of results and improper conclusions drawn from data also may be due to observer biases. However, this is not a significant problem when the data resulting from the observations are clearly separated from the inferences and conclusions. It is only when the observer records inferences instead of the dimensional quantities of events that this problem becomes serious. For example, when a clinician records that "the client was aggressive on five occasions during the treatment session," independent observers have no data to judge the client behaviors. On the other hand, if the clinician records the observable actions (five times the client hit another person) instead of inferring what the actions mean, then the independent observers can come to their own conclusions.

Observer bias is not a problem restricted to the person doing the observation. It is also a matter of the way the dependent variables are conceptualized. Bias is inevitable when the dependent variables are poorly conceptualized, and methods of observing them should of necessity be indirect. In essence, indirect measurements and vague dependent variables create opportunities for observer bias. When discrete responses are dependent variables, observer bias can be minimal or, at the least, when it does occur, external observers can rectify it.

The second issue, **observer training,** is much more important because proper training can help generate reliable and valid data with minimal or no observer bias. As pointed out by Johnston and Pennypacker (1993), observation is a response of the scientist, and objective (bias-free) observation is strictly under the control of the event being observed, not the preconceived ideas of the investigator. Like any other complex response, the act of observation is a learned skill and improves with experience.

In communicative disorders, the training of observers has received little systematic attention. Many investigators hire research assistants who may be only minimally trained in observational skills. Some of these assistants are graduate students who at best receive some instructions on what to look for and how to record what is being measured. Graduate students may consider themselves "experienced" if they have had an opportunity to watch a senior investigator make some scientific observations.

To make scientific observations, the observer (a) should be clear about the topographical aspects of the event, (b) should know the dimensional quantity selected for observation, (c) should be aware of the rough limits of variability of the phenomenon, (d) should have observed and recorded along with an experienced, reliable observer before working on his or her own, (e) should have mastered the technical aspects of observing and measuring, and (f) should have the disposition of a scientist. These conditions will not guarantee reliable and objective observations, but in their absence, measurement is questionable.

First, the observer should have a thorough knowledge of the form of the response targeted for observation. The observer should know what the behavior looks and sounds like. A person who is unsure of the topography of the response under observation is not likely to record its occurrence consistently, if at all. For example, a student who is not sure of the structure of a verb phrase will not be able to observe and record its occurrence in a language sample. Observers who do not know the form of various dysfluencies cannot be expected to count their frequency. Students who do not know how a vocal fry sounds will not be able to indicate its presence or frequency.

One can be relatively sure of the response topography when it is conceptualized directly and defined operationally. In the self-or-other training process, dependent variables that are unobservable internal events ("cognitive reorganization," for example) often are inferred, not directly observed. Inference is not observation, and if the act of observation itself requires inference, then training objective observational skills is especially difficult.

Second, a clear understanding of the dimensional quantity selected for observation is essential, and observer training should be specific to that. What aspect of the event should be observed and measured? Is it the duration, the frequency, or some other dimensional quantity? Are there multiple dimensions, such as duration and frequency, that should be measured simultaneously? How should repetitions of the same response topography be recorded? For example, when a person who stutters says, "I stu-stu-stu-stutter," the same response topography is repeated three times. Is this scored as one instance of syllable repetition or three? (Most researchers would count this as one instance of part-word repetition).

Third, the observer should have some idea about the limits within which the phenomenon under observation can vary. Repeated events do show some variability in their topography. Sound prolongations may be relatively long or short, or they may be produced with greater or less muscular effort (force). But they are all still counted as sound prolongations only. The same morphological feature may be used in inflecting a word, or it may be a part of a phrase or a sentence. The hypernasality of a client may be more pronounced on certain speech sounds and less on others. But such variations may not be considered significant in measuring the presence of hypernasality.

Fourth, an observer should first observe and record the same event along with an experienced observer. This is probably the most important aspect of actual training in observation. It is not sufficient for the awe-struck student to merely watch the senior scientist's smooth observational skills. The student observer should observe and record the behavior along with the more experienced observer. The two (or more) persons should measure the same event simultaneously but independently of each other.

Contingent feedback is an essential part of this phase of training. The student and the scientist should compare their measured values and discuss the differences. It often is necessary to talk about the differences as soon as an instance of observational act is completed. This is more efficient when the behaviors to be observed are recorded. While measuring behaviors from audio- or videotapes, the scientist and the student observer can freeze the event to discuss the behavior and its dimensional quantity being measured. The student in this process should receive contingent corrective and informative feedback on all aspects of measurement.

Fifth, when instruments are used in observing and measuring a behavior, the observer should have the necessary technical skills to operate the instruments. The use of relatively simple instruments such as tape recorders necessitates some training and skill. Complex instruments require much more training time, and the student observer should be sure of operating them correctly. The observer should also be able to recognize malfunctions of instruments.

Sixth, the observer should have the behavioral disposition of a scientist. The observer should separate observations from opinions, data from inferences. During the act of observation, the observer should not be interpreting the phenomenon. The sole purpose during observation and measurement is to record the selected dimensional quantity of the event under study. Interpretations and inferences come later. They are offered in such clear distinction with measured values that other observers can make their own interpretations and inferences.

The training of observers is difficult and tedious, but it is the first step in the training of scientists. I have had the experience of training undergraduate and graduate students in measuring stuttering, defined as specific dysfluencies whose measured dimensional quantity is frequency. Instructors who have done this know that teaching students to observe and measure behaviors reliably takes several sessions. Accurate observational behavior should be shaped with contingent feedback in a series of small steps.

MECHANICAL AIDS TO OBSERVATION AND MEASUREMENT

Mechanical devices are instruments that extend, sharpen, or otherwise enhance the power of human sensory observation. Objects or events that are too small can be enlarged so that they can be seen, measured, and recorded.

Objects or events that are too far away to be seen may be visually brought closer for more detailed observation. Events or processes that do not normally generate sensory consequences also can be tracked and recorded by machines or instruments. Instruments also can magnify processes that are too subtle to be measured by human observers. All of these instruments are valuable tools in scientific observation and measurement.

Mechanical instruments can be simple or complex. A hand-held counter may be useful in recording the frequency of many communicative behaviors. A tape recorder or a video recorder can give scientists a somewhat permanent record of fleeting and temporary behavioral processes. Such records can be used to observe a phenomenon repeatedly for training observers and obtaining more accurate measures. Various electronic response-monitoring devices, such as operant programming devices, can help record responses mechanically and deliver response consequences contingently and automatically.

A variety of mechanical devices simply give the scientist access to what should be measured. For example, a **fiberoptic scope** can be used to view the laryngeal area directly; it does not measure or record any of the laryngeal behaviors. However, a fiberoptic scope can be a part of a video recording system. In this case, the video camera and the recording and monitoring system can make it possible to see the generally inaccessible laryngeal mechanism and record different laryngeal behaviors under different conditions of stimulation and experimentation.

Several other instruments help measure various neurobehavioral processes. **Electromyography,** for example, measures electrical activity in muscles. It can be used in basic research designed to analyze muscle activities in speech production. Electromyography also can be used in evaluating the effects of treatments on the muscles of speech with corresponding changes in some perceived aspect of speech. They are useful in biofeedback research with persons with stuttering, cerebral palsy, and voice disorders. A **kymograph** measures specific muscle activity (nonelectrical) involved in breathing.

Various instruments directly track the electrical impulses of muscles and nerves. With suitable recording devices, one can obtain a permanent recording of the electrical activities of different neuromuscular systems. **Electroencephalography** measures the electrical activity of the brain, picked up by surface electrodes placed on the scalp. Different patterns of discharge are indicative of different kinds of neurobehavioral activity, including linguistic and nonlinguistic activities. Equipment to measure the **galvanic skin reflex** or response (GSR) can help measure the resistance the skin normally offers to the electrical conductance. This resistance is reduced under conditions of emotional arousal. Therefore, GSR is typically taken as a physiological measure of emotion.

Cineradiography is one of the techniques used in recent years to measure various parameters of the movement-related variables involved in speech production. The technique helps measure the movements of the muscles of the jaw, tongue, and larynx in the production of speech. Such movements cannot be measured precisely without cineradiography, which films the entire sequence of action with X-rays.

The parameters of airflow involved in speech production can be measured by a **pneumotachograph. Oscilloscopes** make speech visible by displaying various wave patterns associated with differential speech forms on a television-like screen.

A variety of other instruments are available for the researcher in speech–language pathology. Recent advances in computer technology have provided additional mechanical capabilities in the measurement, monitoring, and modification of speech–language behaviors that cannot otherwise be measured precisely. This section is not intended as an introduction to instrumentation used in studying normal speech and speech pathology. When a particular research investigation requires the mechanical tracking of an independent variable, the investigator should use the instrument that will permit an accurate and reliable measurement of the variable (Baken & Orlikoff, 2000; Borden, Harris, & Raphael, 2003; Cudahy, 1988; Curtis & Schultz, 1986; Silverman, 1998). The main point to be noted here is that mechanical devices are aids to systematic observation and measurement of dependent variables targeted for scientific investigation.

Instruments are devices that help observe and record phenomena. However, in most cases, the human observer should also exercise his or her judgment in the use of instruments and in the evaluation of observations recorded by instruments. An adequate level of technical training in the use of instruments is necessary. The instruments themselves should be reliable so that they are not a source of internal invalidity of research data.

RELIABILITY OF MEASUREMENT

The results of measurement are subject to certain kinds of evaluations. Measured values are useful only to the extent that they are adequate for the purposes of a scientific investigation. Measured values of phenomena are evaluated mainly for their reliability and validity. This section is concerned with the concept and procedures of reliability.

The concept of reliability can be understood in different ways. In everyday language, a person is said to be reliable if his or her behavior is consistent across situations and time. Therefore, consistency with which something occurs or something is measured suggests reliability. Stability also means reliability—if a person's behavior is unstable, it is not reliable. In a restricted sense, predictability also suggests reliability—you can predict an event if it is known to be reliable. Unpredictable events are also unreliable. Dependability is yet another term that implies reliability—dependable phenomena are stable, predictable, and reliable.

Reliability refers to consistency among repeated observations of the same phenomenon. When the measurement of an event is repeated, the measured values should be comparable. If they differ widely, then the measurement is not reliable. When events are measured repeatedly, values are not likely to be the same. Chance fluctuations in the phenomenon and subtle variations in the measurement procedures can cause different values. Nevertheless, to be considered reliable, the divergence in the values of repeated measures should remain within certain limits. These limits are usually arbitrarily defined.

Reliability should not be confused with accuracy. While reliability refers to the degree of consistency between two or more observations of the same event, accuracy refers to the extent to which the measured values reflect the event being measured. For example, if the measurement of language behaviors in a group of children reflects the true performance of those children, one can say that the measurement was accurate. An unreliable measurement may still be accurate in the sense that it reflects the truly fluctuating response of some participants. A reliable measure may not be accurate in that its repeated values are comparable but the values do not reflect the actual performance of the participants studied.

Repeated observation is the key to establishing reliability. The same event is observed more than once either by the same individual or by different individuals. There is a measure of **intraobserver reliability** when the same person measures the same phenomenon repeatedly and a measure of **interobserver reliability** when the same phenomenon is measured by different observers.

In most cases, intraobserver reliability does not pose serious problems. Generally speaking, an observer, even while not measuring something accurately, can be consistent with himself or herself. The same constant mistakes made in the measurement process can result in acceptable reliability of measures. Therefore, intraobserver reliability is typically not reported in research studies. However, it often is required in theses and dissertations. When the research question itself concerns the reliability of measurement of some specific phenomenon, both kinds of reliability may be important.

Interobserver reliability is a crucial element of scientific measurement. Without an acceptable level of interobserver reliability, the results of a study cannot be accepted. Interobserver reliability is one means of convincing the audience that the data are objective. Objectivity in science is realized only by an agreement among different observers regarding the measured values (not opinions) of a given phenomenon. Therefore, interobserver reliability is one of the criteria used in the evaluation of scientific data.

Assessing Interobserver Reliability

There are three general methods of estimating the reliability of research data. The first method, sometimes referred to as the **unit-by-unit agreement ratio,** requires that two observers agree on the individual instances of the response being measured. For example, if two observers measure the frequency of the correct production of /s/ in a speech sample, they both should agree on the particular instance of /s/ production to score agreement. In measuring stuttering, the two observers should agree on specific instances of stuttering and their locations.

Compared to agreement based on total scores of two observers, the unit-by-unit agreement ratios is a much more stringent method of scoring agreement. Research has shown that in the measurement of stuttering, two observers can more easily agree on the total number of instances of stuttering in a sample while disagreeing widely on specific instances of stuttering.

The procedure for estimating the unit-by-unit agreement ratio is as follows. First, the number of units (e.g., measured responses and events) on which both the observers agreed is determined (*A*). Next, the total number of units on which the observers disagreed is obtained (*D*). Finally, the following formula is applied to obtain the agreement index. It is usually expressed as a percentage:

$$\text{unit-by-unit agreement index} = \frac{A}{A + D} \times 100$$

Suppose the two observers scored 37 responses as correct and 22 responses as incorrect. The agreement index in this case would be 63% (37 + 22 = 59; 37 ÷ 59 × 100 = 63%). This index has been used extensively in clinical research involving various kinds of communicative behaviors.

The unit-by-unit agreement index is most useful when responses are scored on discrete trials or time intervals. In the measurement of stuttering, Young's work (1969a, 1969b, 1975) pointed out the importance of the unit-by-unit analysis. He also developed the following formula to calculate the unit-by-unit agreement index when three or more observers are involved:

$$\text{agreement index} = [1/(n - 1)] \, [(T/Td) - 1]$$

n = number of observers

T = total number of words marked as stuttered

Td = total number of different words marked as stuttered

Young's (1975) formula has been frequently used in assessing interobserver agreement involving more than two observers. It is especially useful in assessing the effects of technical training programs designed to enhance reliable measurement skills in student clinicians (Gittleman-Foster, 1983).

The second method uses statistical correlations to calculate interobserver agreement. A correlation, such as the Pearson product–moment coefficient, indicates the degree of covariation between any two sets of measures. In calculating interobserver reliability with this method, scores or measures of one observer are correlated with those of another observer. In calculating correlation coefficients of reliability, each observer should supply several measures. That is, each observer should observe the responses on different occasions, trials, sessions, and so on. For example, the observers may score the correct productions of /s/ in a total of seven sessions. Each observer supplies a total score for each session. This yields seven pairs of scores. These pairs can be correlated to obtain a measure of reliability.

The method of scoring unit-by-unit agreement ratio can be contrasted with the correlational method of scoring agreement. The **correlational method**—a statistical index of covariance among events—gives only a global notion of reliability; in this method, the two observers may score comparable numbers of correctly produced /s/, but they may have disagreed on many individual instances. In other words, there may have been many /s/ productions scored as wrong by one observer and correct as another observer, but because both scored about the same total number of correct and incorrect responses, the resulting reliability index may be spuriously high. Generally speaking, a high correlation results as long as the total scores of the two observers are not too divergent. Such high correlations can mask the fact that the two observers agreed only on very few individual instances of responses. It is known that the unit-by-unit method of scoring agreement is a more accurate method of estimating reliability than the correlational method.

The third method, infrequently used, is called a **frequency ratio;** in this method, the smaller of the two observations is divided by the larger and the resulting quotient is multiplied by 100 to express the ratio as a percentage. Each observer's total number of observations is used in this calculation. Suppose that one observer scored 22 correct productions of /s/ and the other observer scored 16. The frequency ratio for this would be 73% ($16 \div 22 \times 100 = 73\%$). Because of its global nature of assessment of reliability, the method is less preferable to the unit-by-unit procedure.

If desired, the original unit-by-unit interobserver agreement formula can be used to calculate the intraobserver agreement as well. In this case, the units (response instances) on which the investigator agreed on both the occasions of measurement are first determined. Then the instances on which the two measurements of the investigator disagreed are determined. The same formula is then applied to derive the intraobserver agreement index. The Young formula should not be used to measure intraobserver agreement because it is meant only for multiple observers.

Reliability of Tests Versus That of Research Data

The reliability of a standardized test should be distinguished from that of research data. Different procedural details are involved in establishing the reliability of standardized tests. These procedures will not be discussed here and the student is referred to other sources (Kerlinger, 1986; Roseberry-McKibbin & Hegde, 2000).

The reliability of a standardized test may show that when the original sample of participants is tested and retested, the scores are comparable. This is generally taken to mean that any time the test is used to measure other individuals' behaviors, the resulting measures are automatically reliable. This is one of the most questionable assumptions associated with the popular practice of using standardized tests to measure behaviors. From the standpoint of scientific data, reliability is established for the particular measures; it is not inferred from the reliability established elsewhere, by someone else, and in measuring other individuals' behaviors.

The reliability in research is data specific, whereas the reliability of standardized tests is instrument specific. Like a well-calibrated audiometer, the test may be said to be reliable. But the reliability of hearing thresholds reported in a research study may be questionable. That is, even when an audiometer is reliable, certain measured hearing thresholds may not be. Therefore, in scientific research, regardless of the previously demonstrated reliability of measuring instruments, the reliability of specific observations across the experimental conditions should be evaluated and reported.

SUMMARY

- Observation and measurement are two basic scientific activities. In observation, an observer makes a systematic report on some sensory experience. In measurement, an observer assigns numbers to properties of events.

- Idemnotic measurement, used in natural sciences, has absolute and standard units. Vaganotic measurement, more often used in social and psychological sciences, uses relative standards based on variability in the measured units.

- There are four traditional levels of measurement:
  — In nominal measurement, events are distinguished with numbers without mathematical properties.
  — In ordinal measurement, categories are relative and may involve ranking.
  — In interval measurement, units of measures do suggest corresponding and constant differences, but there is no zero.
  — In ratio measurement, all numbers have mathematical properties and there is a zero.

- Measures of communicative behaviors include the following:
  — Frequency—a measure of the number of times a discrete event occurs
  — Duration—a measure of the time interval for which a response is sustained

— Interpersonal response time—a measure of time that lapses between responses

— Latency—a measure of reaction time

— Time sampling—a measure of time periods during which the occurrence or nonoccurrence of a behavior is recorded

— Momentary time sampling—periodic observation and recording of the occurrence of behaviors

— Verbal interaction sampling—measuring the communicative behaviors of two or more persons

• In client-assisted measurement, the client records behaviors in natural settings and the clinician scores them.

• Self-reports are indirect measures of behaviors supplied by the participants themselves.

• In covert measurement, persons whose behaviors are measured are not aware of that fact. It is an ethically questionable procedure.

• Subjective bias of an observer may influence the results of observation. Thorough education and training of scientific observers minimizes such bias. To make scientific observations, the observer

— should be clear about the topographical aspects of the event;

— should know the dimensional quantity selected for observation;

— should be aware of the rough limits of variability of the phenomenon;

— should have observed and recorded along with an experienced (reliable) observer before working on his or her own;

— should have mastered the technical aspects of observing and measuring; and

— should have the disposition of a scientist.

• Mechanical aids of observation extend, sharpen, or otherwise enhance the power of human sensory observation.

• The reliability or consistency of repeated measurement is essential in scientific observation.

STUDY GUIDE _____

1. As described in this chapter, what are the two basic activities of science?

2. Describe the characteristics of scientific observation.

3. Describe the relation between empiricism and observation.

4. How did Campbell define measurement? How did Johnston and Pennypacker define it?

5. What is another name for quantified observations?

6. Describe briefly the idemnotic and vaganotic measurement philosophies. Compare and contrast them.

7. A clinician rates the severity of speech–language disorders on a 3-point scale as follows: mild, moderate, and severe. Is this idemnotic or vaganotic measurement? Why?

8. In his study of behavior, what is the absolute and standard unit of measurement adopted by B. F. Skinner?

9. Are the norms of speech–language behaviors based on absolute or relative measurement? Why?

10. A research clinician assigns a number to each of the 10 participants with aphasia in an experiment. What kind of measurement is this (nominal, ordinal, interval, or ratio)?

11. Roger Brown has rank-ordered 14 grammatical morphemes according to the order in which the children he studied mastered them. What kind of measurement is this?

12. A researcher sent out a questionnaire to measure the attitudes of people who stutter about speaking situations. The questionnaire asked participants to respond to items such as, "My wife (or husband) makes telephone calls on my behalf" with such response options as "always, usually, infrequently, rarely, or never." What kind of measurement is this? What are its limitations?

13. In what sense is the interval measurement an improvement over the ordinal measurement?

14. Give an example of a frequency measure in speech, language, or hearing. Describe how you obtain the measure.

15. Taking the example of dysfluencies in conversational speech, show how a given measure of dysfluencies can be converted into a percentage value.

16. What are some of the difficulties faced in obtaining reliable and valid frequency measures of most communicative behaviors?

17. What are the general limitations of the frequency measure?

18. Define a durational measure and give an example. What kinds of behaviors are best measured with this procedure?

19. In routine clinical sessions, how would you measure hypernasality in conversational speech? What kind of scores or values would you derive from your measurement procedure?

20. When would you use the interresponse time measure in clinical research? Give an example.

21. What are latency measures? In one of the ASHA journals, find a study that measured the latency of a particular behavior. How was it done?

22. How would you use time sampling in measuring specified language responses produced in conversational speech?

23. How do you score the multiple occurrences of nonattending behavior of a child within blocks of time scheduled to measure that behavior? Are they counted once or as many times as the behavior occurs?

24. Give an example to illustrate the statement that time sampling generates categorical data.

25. Describe the momentary time-sampling technique. Is this procedure suitable for high- or low-frequency behavior? Give an example from a group therapy situation.

26. Describe the potential of verbal interaction sampling procedure in conducting experimental studies of mother–child interaction and interaction between three or more individuals.

27. Specify the need for, and the importance of, client-assisted measurement in clinical research.

28. What are indirect measures? What are some of the frequently used indirect measurement tools?

29. What are the indirect measurement tools that focus on internal states? What are some of the problems associated with them?

30. What are some of the sources of observer bias?

31. What are the requirements of objective scientific observation? Summarize the six conditions that were described in the text.

32. What is the function of mechanical aids to observation? Do they negate the need for human observation and judgment? Justify your answer.

33. How is cineradiography used in research involving speech production? Find a description in a published study that used cineradiography.

34. What is the instrument used to measure the parameters of airflow?

35. Define reliability. Distinguish it from accuracy of measurement.

36. Describe interobserver and intraobserver reliability. Which one is generally more important in research?

37. What is the unit-by-unit agreement index? Why is it better than a global measure of reliability?

38. Two clinicians measuring the number of correct and incorrect articulations of selected phonemes by a child have scored the following: 63 correct and 45 incorrect. Calculate the unit-by-unit interobserver agreement index for these scores.

39. Specify Young's formula for calculating the agreement index when three or more observers are involved.

40. Describe how a statistical correlation can be used to assess reliability. What is its most significant limitation? Illustrate your answer with an example.

41. What is the difference between the reliability of standardized tests and that of research data?

PART II

◆◆◆◆◆◆◆◆◆◆◆◆◆◆◆◆◆◆◆◆◆◆◆

Clinical Research Designs

Chapter 7

◆◆◆◆◆◆◆◆◆◆◆◆◆◆◆◆◆◆◆◆◆◆◆◆◆◆◆◆◆◆◆◆◆◆

Research Designs:
An Introduction

Whether the investigator will produce reliable and valid data on the researched question will depend mostly on the design used in the study. In the following chapters, the two major kinds of research designs are considered. This chapter provides necessary background information about research designs, including definitions, descriptions, and purposes.

WHAT ARE RESEARCH DESIGNS?

The definition of a research design depends on the type of research. Although in a general sense, research design refers to the methods and procedures of an investigation, the precise definition of it depends on whether the research is experimental or descriptive. In nonexperimental (e.g., descriptive, normative) studies, a research design is the overall plan of an investigation. The plan describes the research question or questions, the methods of observation and measurement, the different conditions of observation, procedures of collecting data, and the method of data analysis. Many investigators use the term *design* in this general sense.

A more technical definition of a research design applies only to experimental research. Technically, a **research design** may be defined as a structure of temporospatial arrangements within which the selected variables are controlled, manipulated, and measured. An alternative technical definition is that research designs are a scientist's arrangement to reveal a cause–effect relation. In these definitions, design refers to certain technical operations an investigator performs under specified conditions or arrangements to reveal a cause–effect relation between events selected for observation. In this technical sense, a research design can be found only in experimental research in which variables are controlled, manipulated, and measured.

It is useful to consider the various elements of our technical definition of an experimental research design. A design is basically a structure within which certain operations are performed to see what happens. It is an arrangement of conditions for observation, manipulation, and measurement of variables selected for investigation. For example, a design structure may arrange conditions of pretests or baselines, experimental manipulations, withdrawal of those manipulations, and posttests or probes of the dependent variables. Thus, each arrangement within the structure serves a particular purpose while making it possible to observe and measure the dependent variable. This is what is meant by the structure or the arrangement of conditions of a study.

A design structure is more or less flexible depending upon the philosophy on which it is based. Some research designs are less flexible; once selected, design changes during the implementation of the study are considered undesirable. Other research designs allow changes in the course of a study if data warrant them. Typically, group designs of research, described in Chapter 8, have more rigid structures than the single-subject designs described in Chapter 9.

The arrangements of a design allow the researcher to *control variables*. Controlling the variables is a significant part of any experimental research. Variables should be controlled when a researcher wishes to establish a functional (cause–effect) relation between events. The researcher should make sure that the independent variables not under observation do not influence the dependent variable. A good research design makes it possible for the experimenter to rule out the influence of such extraneous variables. This is generally what is meant by controlling the variables.

A design also is a framework within which to manipulate the independent variable selected for the study. An independent variable is manipulated when it is introduced, withheld, varied in magnitude, withdrawn, or reintroduced to see if corresponding changes occur in the dependent variable. For example, in the initial stage of a study, an independent variable—say, a new form of treatment for a speech disorder—is typically not introduced while taking pretest or baseline measure of the disorder (dependent variable). In the next condition, the treatment is introduced. There may be a group of participants who do not receive treatment. Alternatively, the same participants who receive treatment in one condition may be observed in a no-treatment condition. Such manipulations can demonstrate the effects of an independent variable on a dependent variable.

Finally, a design is a condition that allows systematic observation and measurement of the variables of interest. In most research studies, the focus is on the dependent variable, though the measurement of the independent variable also is important. The variables may be measured for their frequency, duration, latency, amplitude, intensity, and so forth. For example, the number of times an independent variable, such as a reinforcer, is delivered in a treatment condition may be measured. In a drug evaluation experiment, the dosage and its frequency are measured throughout the study. Dependent variables such as the production of a plural morpheme or a phoneme may be measured for their frequency. Dysfluencies in speech may be measured for their frequency, duration, or both. Most responses given in relation to a specific stimulus may be measured for latency. Acoustic signals may be measured for their amplitude and intensity.

STRUCTURE AND LOGIC OF EXPERIMENTAL DESIGNS

An adequate understanding of experimental designs involves a full consideration of the logic and the empirical processes of science and research. As was noted in Chapter 2, the scientist's task is to find order in, and functional relations between, natural phenomena. However, order and causal relations are more often concealed than revealed in nature. Therefore, science is a search for something that is not so readily seen. Nature is a complex flux of multitudinous events that are in a constant state of change, variability, and transformation. Events in nature may be independent, correlated, causally related, or interactive.

Science seeks to determine whether certain events are independent or related and, if related, what exactly the type of relation is. Events are **independent** when they are not causally related. Independent events do have their causes, but the observations made have not captured them. Events are **correlated** when they vary together. Two correlated events may increase or decrease at the same time or vary in opposite directions. They may be doing this because of an unobserved third factor that is the cause of both the events; in such cases, because the cause is not observed, one might erroneously think that the correlated events also are causally connected. Two correlated events may indeed be **causally related** in that one is the effect of the other. Finally, several events may produce the same effect, and all of them may be simultaneously present. When multiple variables are simultaneously active, they may interact with each other. **Interactive** variables are those that come together and produce an effect that is larger than the added effect of those events: the whole is greater than the sum of the parts.

A scientist who discovers that certain events are independent, correlated, causally related, or interactive is said to have found *order* in nature. Order may be discovered in a small part of nature, but no part of nature is insignificant. The process of such a discovery is called an experiment, and how that experiment is temporospatially arranged is its design.

An experimental design should be arranged in such a way that if there is a relation between the two events, it will be revealed somewhat clearly because such a relation is anything but clear in the natural flux. In fact, the typically concealing nature can also be misleading, suggesting relations that are not real. Of course, nature does nothing of this sort, but it may certainly seem so for those studying natural phenomena. An experimental design is the scientist's method of uncovering relations against a background of events that vary. The challenge the scientist faces is that a systematic relation lies in the process of what may appear to be chaotic and confusing variability. In some cases, the logic and the structure of a design permit the scientist to observe a relation between events in spite of their variability and the variability of surrounding and correlated events. In other cases, designs make it possible to reduce the variability and thus see the effects of manipulated independent variables on selected dependent variables. In this sense, variability and how to control it are important aspects of experiments and their designs. Therefore, scientists should take a closer look at the issue of variability and how it is handled in experimental designs.

VARIABILITY: SOME PHILOSOPHICAL CONSIDERATIONS

Variability characterizes practically everything humans experience. Physical and chemical events vary constantly, and natural scientists have always tried to analyze the sources of this variability. When biological events began to be studied more closely with the methods of science, the same variability seen in physical and chemical phenomena became apparent. Eventually, it became evident that animal and human behaviors also are highly variable under natural conditions.

The fact of variability, however, is not purely a scientific discovery. Philosophers, poets, and theologians as well as ordinary persons have been aware of variability in physical, biological, and behavioral phenomena. While the statement that all natural phenomena, including biological and behavioral phenomena, are variable has never been especially controversial, how to explain it and technically handle it have been controversial. The controversy has been most intense with respect to human behavioral variability. The variability of physical events may create methodological problems for the scientist who wishes to control such variability, but it does not seem to raise many philosophical concerns in people who are not natural scientists. Variability may be viewed more as a technical problem the scientists should handle. However, the fact of human behavioral variability has been a matter of philosophical, theological, and scientific controversy.

Historically, there have been two distinct approaches to the question of variability in general and of human behavior in particular (Barlow & Hersen, 1984; Johnston & Pennypacker, 1993; Sidman, 1960). One view, the older of the two, holds that variability is intrinsic to the events that vary. The other, more recent view is that behavioral variability is due to external factors that can be controlled.

Intrinsic Variability

The concept of **intrinsic variability** holds that variability is due to internal or inherent factors, not external factors. Assumptions of intrinsic variability have played an important role in the extrascientific understanding of human behavior. Certain traditions of philosophy and theology have asserted that behavior springs from within the individual and, therefore, is not controlled by external events. Internal causes have taken many shapes, the most famous of which is probably the concept of free will. Behaviors vary across time, situations, and individuals. A given individual's behavior also varies across time and situations as well as within them. Traditionally, this is explained by pointing out that people behave differently because of their free will. The popular notion of free will is based on the assumption that physical events may have external causes, but an extension of such a concept to human behavior would violate the notion of freedom of action. In essence, the view of intrinsic variability holds that behavioral variability has unique sources and, therefore, is not the same as the variability of physical phenomena.

Unfortunately, the concept of intrinsic variability has played a significant role in the purportedly "scientific" study of human behavior as well. In this context, the mind has been an important internal source of behavior.

This theory proposes that people behave differently because each person has his or her own mind. Some speculative neurological theorizing has also buttressed this notion, but these theories have replaced the mind with the brain as the intrinsic source of action and behavior. Psychoanalysis and other kinds of psychological theories also are full of intrinsic causes of behavior and its variability. Unconscious forces of motivation, such as the id, ego, superego, self-image, and self-confidence, have been considered intrinsic sources of behavior. It has been hypothesized that the acquisition of language has been made possible by innate ideas and innate knowledge of universal grammar.

The question of variability and the hypothesis of intrinsic causes of behavior may seem separate, but they are closely related. The assumption of intrinsic variability of behavior becomes inevitable when the presumed sources of behavioral control are inaccessible. Most hypothesized intrinsic causes of behavior are indeed inaccessible. It is believed that inaccessible entities such as the mind, soul, free will, unconscious forces, and innate knowledge that are thought to cause behaviors also should be responsible for the variability of those behaviors.

The concepts of intrinsic causes and intrinsic variability of behavior converge to produce a significant effect on the experimental strategy. Obviously, variability that is intrinsic to the behaving organisms cannot be controlled. Therefore, experimental attempts at reducing or eliminating variability would be futile. Consequently, the experimenter has no choice but to accept variability as inevitable and uncontrollable. Nonetheless, the scientist should reduce variability to find cause–effect relations between variables. It is hard to identify the causes of events that vary randomly. Therefore, when the assumption of uncontrollable intrinsic variability is made, researchers should find ways of working around it.

The traditional answer to the problem of behavioral variability in social and behavioral research has been to use large numbers of participants and determine the average performance of the group. Statisticians recommend that the greater the variability, the larger the number of participants needed to show the effect of an independent variable. Obviously, the mean performance of a large number of participants does not fluctuate, simply because it is a single measure. It is the behavior of individuals in the group that fluctuates, but a mean is no reflection of this fact. When this mean is used as the primary measure of the dependent variable in the inferential statistical analysis, it is supposed that somehow the problem of variability has been handled satisfactorily.

The amount of deviation from the mean shown by individuals (standard deviation) does affect the eventual inferential statistical analysis of the data. However, when a large sample is drawn to overcome the problem of variability, one also is sampling a larger amount of variability. The statistical answer to this problem is to require only a greatly reduced magnitude of the effect of the independent variable before the investigator can conclude that the cause manipulated in an experiment had an effect over and beyond chance. For instance, when experimentally evaluating a new treatment program with a large number of clients, the researcher might accept favorable but small effects as significant.

In essence, the traditional research strategies based on the theory of probability and inferential statistics handle variability by ignoring it. Individual variability is minimized post hoc by the averaging method and by accepting only small effects of the independent variables. Typically, such effects are wrested by complex statistical analyses.

It is a common practice in social and psychological sciences to think of variability (the more frequently used term is *variance)* as random fluctuations that the investigator can handle only through statistical methods of averaging group performance data and inferential techniques (Christensen, 1980; Kerlinger, 1986). For the purposes of statistical analyses, variability of participants within a group is considered error variance, which typically includes unexplained (and uninteresting!) individual differences, fluctuations in the behaviors introduced by random variables, and errors of measurement. The kind of variability introduced by the independent variable is called **systematic variance.** Yet another kind of variance is described as **extraneous variance,** which is the amount of variability introduced by independent variables that are not being manipulated or measured by the investigator. Within this framework, an experimental design is expected to enhance systematic variance, minimize error variance, and control extraneous variance. These recommendations are not controversial except for the way the basic variability of behaviors is handled.

Extrinsic Variability

The concept of **extrinsic variability** holds that behavioral variability is extrinsic to the behaving organisms (Barlow & Hersen, 1984; Johnston & Pennypacker, 1993; Sidman, 1960). Much behavioral variability is not a property of either the behavior or the organism but is imposed by external factors. Behavior varies because the factors responsible for it vary, and many of those factors are in the environment. Evidently, this view of variability seriously questions the traditional assumption that free will, soul, mind, and such other intrinsic entities are the causes of behaviors. According to the philosophy of extrinsic variability, behavior is a function of the individual's past history and the present environmental events to which he or she is exposed. Therefore, behavioral variability is not unique; it is a part of the scheme of natural events.

Extrinsic variability does not imply that variables within the organism exert no influence on behaviors. Internal physiological states (such as thirst and hunger) and changes over time (maturation) have certain effects on behaviors. The integrity of neuromuscular systems also is an internal factor that influences behaviors. Similarly, genetic factors set limits on the behavioral variability imposed by natural or experimentally created environmental events. Nonetheless, the assumption of extrinsic variability suggests that most of those sources of variability, when studied appropriately, lead to a better understanding of behaviors than the assumption that variability is a property of behavior itself.

It is clear that the two views of intrinsic and extrinsic variability have profound but contradictory philosophic implications. From the standpoint of experimental methodology, the ultimate truth or falsity of the two assumptions is not of immediate concern. Whether behavioral variability is intrinsic or extrinsic is an empirical question that will require lengthy experimental research. However, whether systematic attempts to produce that answer will be made at all depends upon the assumption of extrinsic, not intrinsic, variability. This is not one of those situations in which contradictory views are both testable and either view has the same chance of producing a valid answer.

If all scientists took the position that behavioral variability is intrinsic, then there would be no reason to design experiments in which such variability is experimentally analyzed, for the assumption is inconsistent with such experimentation. The assumption of intrinsic variability precludes experimental analysis of the sources of behavioral variability. After having placed (intrinsic) variability outside the scope of experimental analysis, researchers will continue to use statistical means of handling it.

A position most valid from an empirical standpoint is to treat all variability as extrinsic at least tentatively, so that experimental analysis of variability may be attempted. Sustained experimental analysis will reduce the territory held by variability that is supposed to be intrinsic. Every time a source of behavioral variability is identified, a chance to control it presents itself. As Sidman pointed out, "Each time such control is achieved, intrinsic variability loses another prop" (1960, p. 143).

Such an approach to variability has a chance of showing that it is difficult to control some sources of variability. This difficulty may be due to the limitations of experimental techniques. Improvements in those techniques may help control that variability. Or, the approach may show the limits beyond which individual variability cannot be controlled. In either case, only the assumption of extrinsic variability can lead us in the direction of self-corrective data. As such, the assumption of extrinsic variability has a chance of disproving itself because the assumption keeps pushing experimental manipulations that, under some circumstances, produce negative evidence. On the other hand, the assumption of intrinsic variability may not correct itself because once assumed, it does not encourage experimentation on controlling behavioral variability.

EXPERIMENTAL DESIGNS: MEANS OF CONTROLLING VARIABILITY

The two philosophical positions on variability often are associated with two kinds of experimental designs: between-groups design and single-subject design. Generally, the group design approach tends to be based on the assumption of intrinsic variability. The single-subject designs are more often based on the assumption of extrinsic variability. But it should be noted that both the approaches to designing experiments recognize the need to control variability; they differ only in terms of what kinds of variability should be controlled and in what manner.

Group designs, even with the assumption of intrinsic variability, include mechanisms to control and isolate the variability produced by independent variables. This approach recognizes the need to control variability produced by factors not under observation (extraneous variability). There is no significant conceptual difference between the group and the single-subject designs on these issues, although there are some methodological differences which will be addressed in later chapters. The difference between the two approaches lies mostly in how the background variability created by differences in the individual response rates is handled and also in how the variability produced by the experimental variable is analyzed.

The effects of all experiments are analyzed against a certain amount of background variability. Suppose, for example, that an investigator wishes to evaluate the effect of a new stuttering treatment program. If the basic two-group design is selected, the investigator forms an experimental and a control group of people who stutter using the random procedure. After taking pretest measures of stuttering in both groups, the investigator treats the participants only in the experimental group. At the completion of the treatment program, the investigator gives a posttest to both the groups. To find out if the treatment was effective, he or she statistically analyzes the pretest and posttest measures of the two groups.

The control group helps rule out the influence of extraneous independent variables. If the mean performance of the control group did not change significantly from the pretest to the posttest, but the mean performance of the experimental group did show such changes, then it is concluded that extraneous variables were controlled. However, this evaluation of the effect of the treatment variable is made, of necessity, against the background of random (hence, uncontrolled) variability. In a group design, the larger the individual differences within the groups, the greater the background variability. As noted before, much of this variability is handled statistically with the help of the arithmetic mean.

The effect of the treatment also is handled statistically. The difference in the performance of the two groups is evaluated on the basis of the mean, which ignores individual differences in response to treatment. Thus, in a group design, both the background and the systematic variability are evaluated nonexperimentally.

On the other hand, the investigator who selects a single-subject design to evaluate the same stuttering treatment program will not try to draw a random sample of participants. Available people who stutter will be used in the study, but each participant will be described in detail. The stuttering behaviors will be baserated until some criterion of stability is reached. The baseline helps reduce the intrasubject variability before the introduction of treatment. The treatment is then introduced and continued until it produces an effect. Subsequently, the treatment may be withdrawn to return the rate of stuttering to its baseline. Finally, the treatment may be reapplied to replicate the treatment effects. In this procedure, no effort is made to average individual performances to show some kind of stability before, during, or after treatment. Variability is handled on an individual basis. As long as the behavior continues to be variable, baselines are extended. It is generally found that when conditions are controlled, sooner or later the behavior stabilizes. Obviously, this approach to pretreatment variability is very different from that found in group designs in which a single pretest measure (arithmetic mean) represents stability.

The treatment effect within a single-subject design is not evaluated by statistical means. The assumption is that when the effects are large enough to be evaluated by visual inspection, there is no need for statistical analysis, which typically tries to identify relatively small effects against a background of uncontrolled variability. Such large effects of the treatment variable neutralize the issue of intersubject variability found in group designs.

Within the single-subject approach, when individual behaviors vary greatly, either during baselines or during treatment, the experimenter may then proceed to find out why (Sidman, 1960). In other words, the variability itself becomes an object of experimental inquiry. Investigators may be willing to postpone their study of the original problem and begin the new task of tracking the intrasubject variability. It may be found, for example, that the variability found in the frequency of stuttering exhibited by a client during baseline sessions is due to the client's participation in rather traumatic staff meetings held every other day. Many clients' variable response rates in treatment sessions may be a reaction to various uncontrolled factors that the clinicians dump under "a good day" and "a bad day."

Regardless of philosophical and methodological differences on the issue of variability, it is clear that experimental designs should address them; after all, a design is a way of controlling some kind of variability while creating another kind of variability. It should control the variability found within and across individuals, and it should produce a large enough variability that can be attributed to the effect of the independent variable. It should be noted that a change in the behavior when treatment is introduced also is variability, but it is the type of variability the experimenter hopes to see and takes every step to create.

VALIDITY OF EXPERIMENTAL OPERATIONS

By allowing the researcher to control and create variability, experimental designs help identify functional relations between variables. The task of an experimental design is to isolate a cause–effect relation between events.

In human clinical and nonclinical research, the demonstration of a cause–effect relation is made with the help of selected individuals, whether in a few individuals as in a single-subject design, or in groups of subjects as in a group design. This raises two closely related questions. The first question is whether, in the individuals who served as participants in a given experiment, the cause–effect relation was demonstrated convincingly. This is the question of internal validity. The second question is whether the demonstrated cause–effect relations can be generalized to individuals who have not participated in the experiment. This is the question of external validity or generality of findings.

The validity of experimental operations refers to the confidence with which the experimenter's claim of a cause–effect relation can be accepted by other scientists. In nontechnical terms, the results of an experiment are valid when the observed cause of an event is not mistaken. When the results are not valid, conclusions drawn from the study may not apply to the individuals who served in the experiment or to those who did not. In other words, there is neither internal nor external validity.

The validity of experimental operations should be distinguished from the validity of measured values of the dependent variables. The **validity of measured values** is the degree to which the measurement of the dependent variable is indeed the best possible reflection of the true value of that variable. The **validity of experimental operations,** on the other hand, is the degree to which the overall experimental arrangements, manipulations, and control procedures lead to valid conclusions. As such, the validity of measured values has a narrower scope than the validity of experimental operations. In a sense, the validity of measures of dependent variables is a part of the validity of experimental operations.

Internal Validity

To achieve internal validity, the investigator should make sure that during the experimental operations, only the independent variable selected for the study was present and that any of the other potential independent variables were not. When the selected independent variable produces acceptable changes in the dependent variable in the absence of other potential variables that could have produced the same results, the data are said to have internal validity. Therefore, **internal validity** is the degree to which the data reflect a true cause–effect relation. Thus, the major concern is to make sure that the variables other than the one selected for study were appropriately controlled for in the design.

In some individual participants, variables that affect the dependent variable may require special analysis. Historically, though, several common factors that affect internal validity across experiments have been recognized. These factors also are described as threats to internal validity or sources of internal invalidity.

Most of the sources of internal invalidity can be found in poor research designs. In fully understanding the discussion of the factors that affect internal invalidity in the following section, it is necessary to keep in perspective a prototype of a poor design in which those factors can easily come to play. Such a design is illustrated in the traditional case studies used frequently in clinical research. For example, a clinician may measure (pretest) language disorder (the dependent variable) in a group of children and then subject them to a new treatment program whose effect is being evaluated. After several months of treatment, the children's language behaviors may be evaluated again. This posttest may show that the children's language behaviors have improved significantly. The investigator may then conclude that the new treatment program was responsible for the changes observed in the dependent variable. However, as discussed in the next section, there are several factors that can affect internal validity in a study such as this.

History

The participants' life events that may be totally or partially responsible for the changes recorded in the dependent variable after the introduction of the independent variable are referred to as **history.** A design that does not rule out the influence of those events cannot demonstrate that the treatment variable had an effect on the dependent variable. In other words, history is a source of internal invalidity in such a design.

In our prototypic example of language treatment research, it is possible that the treatment was totally or partially ineffective. A variety of extraneous factors not monitored by the clinician may have been totally or partially responsible for the results. For example, the classroom teacher may have started a language-stimulation program for the same children receiving treatment from the clinician, and this program may have been responsible for the improvement in children's language. Or the parents, after having discussed their children's language problem with the clinician, may have begun to talk more to their children or read more stories to them at bedtime. Such changes in the parents' behavior may have caused improvement in the children's language. Because the case study method did not rule out such extraneous variables, the clinician cannot conclude that there was a functional relation between the treatment variable and the changes in the language of the children.

It should be noted that the term *history*, though used to describe the effects of extraneous variables, may not be the most appropriate term. It does not refer to the events that have taken place in the past but to events that are contemporaneous with the experimental manipulations.

In the group design strategy, the influence of history is controlled by showing those who do not receive treatment do not show significant changes in the dependent variable. When a control group—also exposed to factors of history—does not show changes, then history is ruled out as a potential variable responsible for changes shown by the experimental group. In the single-subject strategy, after exposing participants to treatment, the experimenter may withdraw treatment and reintroduce it later. If the behavior changed under treatment, returned to the baseline when treatment was withdrawn, and changed again when treatment was reintroduced, the investigator probably will conclude that the factors of history were not responsible for the observed changes.

Maturation

When experiments take much time to conduct, changes taking place within the participants themselves may produce some effect on the dependent variable. In some cases, such changes may account for the entire effect supposedly produced by the independent variable manipulated by the experimenter.

Maturation refers to biological and other kinds of unidentified changes that take place in participants simply as a result of the passage of time. To what extent mere passage of time can produce effects on behaviors is not always clear, however. Obviously, maturation is indexed by the age of the participants. The discussion of normative research in Chapter 4 noted the issue of age as an independent variable. In evaluating maturation as a potential independent variable, the reader should consider all the problems that were identified in that discussion. It is quite possible that maturation and history are not as distinct as they are generally thought to be. Possibly, events in the lives of the participants while they are supposed to be maturing may be responsible for the changes that are attributed to maturation.

In our prototypic example of research, during the time required to complete the experimental language treatment, maturational changes can be expected to have taken place. Those changes may have been responsible for the improved language in the children.

In both the single-subject and group design strategies, the problem of maturation is handled in the same way as the problem of history. Either a control group or a no-treatment condition that follows treatment can rule out the influence of maturation. It can be expected that the members of the control group who do not change over time experience the same amount of maturation as the members of the experimental group. Similarly, participants who change once when the treatment is introduced but change again when it is withdrawn indicate that maturation is not responsible for the changes in the dependent variable. The logic is that when maturation is given a chance and fails to show its effects, the only effect seen is that of the independent variable manipulated by the experimenter.

Testing

As a source of internal invalidity, **testing** means that a dependent variable changes simply because it has been measured more than once. Pretests and posttests may be sufficient to introduce some change in the dependent variable. In such cases, the experimenter's conclusion that the treatment variable of the study was responsible for the changes recorded on the posttest may be erroneous.

Some behaviors are known to change somewhat when repeatedly tested or measured. Measures of behaviors that change as a function of repeated testing are known as **reactive measures.** Scores obtained through questionnaires designed to measure attitudes, opinions, feeling states, personal adjustment, and personality are known to be notoriously reactive. People answering a questionnaire on their attitudes toward racial minorities, for example, may show significant changes when retested even though nothing has been done to change such attitudes.

Because most experiments involve repeated measurement of the dependent variable, one should make sure that testing is not a source of control exerted on the behavior. One way of handling the problem of testing is not to use reactive measures at all. As measures of behaviors, opinions, attitudes, and personality are weak and inferential at best. Whenever possible, it is better to measure behaviors directly. For example, one may either ask a person to fill out a questionnaire on movie-going behavior or measure the frequency with which that person goes to the movies. Obviously, a score on the latter measure is difficult to obtain, but the more easily accomplished score on the questionnaire may be useless. Also, the actual behavioral measure is less reactive than the questionnaire measure. An employer who has never hired a member of a minority group is not likely to suddenly hire one simply because his or her attitudes showed reactive changes on an attitude scale.

Reactive measures are not as bothersome in single-subject designs as in group designs. Single-subject designs do involve repeated measures—in fact, more so than the group designs. For the most part, single-subject designs avoid the use of indirect and reactive measures of behaviors. Group designs have a method of handling testing effects by adding a group that does not receive the pretest, but only receives the posttest. This design, known as the Solomon four-group design (Solomon, 1949), is described in Chapter 8.

Instrumentation

Problems with measuring instruments that negatively affect internal validity are grouped under **instrumentation.** This factor includes not only mechanical instruments that might deteriorate or improve between pretests and posttests but also the changes that may take place in human beings who serve as judges, raters, and observers. In much social and psychological research, persons with varying degrees of expertise observe, score, and measure behaviors. Of course, human observation and measurement is basic to all sciences, but the experimenters' reliance on others to make measurements for them is more extensive in social and psychological research.

An instrument that was in normal working condition at the beginning of a study may develop problems by the time the posttest is made. Or an instrument that already had some problems from the beginning may have been corrected just before the posttest. In cases such as these, the pretests and posttests would not reflect the actual effects of the experimental manipulations. Suppose that in a study of the effects of some medical or surgical intervention procedure designed to improve a certain type of hearing loss the audiologist used a defective audiometer to establish the initial hearing thresholds of the participants. Possibly, because of the mechanical defect, all participants' thresholds were 10 decibels higher than their actual level of hearing. Also suppose that as a matter of routine maintenance procedures, the audiometer was serviced and calibrated just before the posttests. Unaware of the history of the instrument, the audiologist may measure the hearing in the participants after the completion of the medical or surgical treatment. Thresholds on this posttest are likely to show at least a 10 dB improvement over the pretest, but this finding is entirely invalid. In the same study, an audiometer that was working normally but had deteriorated by the posttest would have led to an opposite finding, also equally invalid.

Judges who observe and score behaviors may induce invalidity of findings in several ways. When a group of speech pathologists is used to rate the severity of stuttering before and after some form of experimental treatment, the persons in the group may change their idea as to what constitutes different levels of severity between the pretests and posttests. The criteria used by individual judges may become more or less stringent. The observers may get bored during the posttest. The judges also can become more experienced in measuring stuttering, so they may now score more stutterings because some were missed during the pretest observations.

As a clinical supervisor, I have seen beginning clinicians who scored more and more stuttering behaviors as therapy progressed during the first few weeks. At one time, a very disconcerted student clinician came to my office and showed me this kind of data. This first-time clinician had her worst fears confirmed: Her therapy was making the client stutter more, although the client's fluency seemed to have improved. Her measurement procedures were then analyzed, and it was found that she was gradually becoming more deft at observing and measuring silent pauses, interjections, and more subtle forms of dysfluencies.

In any type of research, the investigator should make sure that the selected instruments are carefully calibrated and found to be in good working condition. Frequently checking the integrity of mechanical devices throughout the course of an investigation is the most effective method of avoiding validity problems due to mechanical defects. In the case of human observers, adequate training in observation, scoring, and rating before the experiment is started will help avoid validity problems due to errors or changes in judgment. Both inter- and intrajudge reliability should be assured. See Chapter 6 for a discussion of observer training and reliability.

Statistical Regression

In clinical research, it is not uncommon to select participants who happen to seek clinical services at the time of the study. It is known, however, that many patients and clients seek clinical services at a time when their problem hits a new peak. This is more likely to happen with those disorders that vary across time and situations and hence are somewhat cyclic. Stuttering, for example, can be a cyclic speech disorder. Many chronic medical conditions, too, may vary across time and on occasion be much worse than the usual. Many such diseases and disorders are not likely to stay at their worst level for long. They soon will return to their less severe and more common level. Such a return from an extreme point to an average level is known as **statistical regression** or regression to the mean.

Regression can pose serious problems for internal validity if the clinical condition is at its worst at the beginning of the experiment, but returns to its average level as the experiment progresses. Such an improvement in the clinical condition can give the impression that the treatment is effective. Obviously, such an erroneous conclusion would not have internal validity.

Statistical regression does not mean that every client will improve without treatment. It is simply a change in the extreme scores of a group of participants; when such changes are confused with the treatment effects, a problem of internal invalidity exists.

Theoretically, our prototypical example of language treatment research does not rule out statistical regression. Whether children with language disorders show statistical regression is a different question, however. The problem of regression to the mean is controlled for in the group design by random selection and assignment of participants to an experimental group and a control group. The amount of regression would then be the same in the two groups. Unfortunately, the random procedure is impractical where it is needed the most. In clinical research, finding a population of clients with a given disorder from which a sample can be randomly drawn is not practical.

In single-subject designs, regression is handled by establishing a stable baseline before starting an experimental treatment. For instance, if the frequency of stuttering shows an improving trend that may be due to regression, treatment would not be started until stuttering stabilized. Also, throughout the experiment, the frequency of stuttering would be measured. Furthermore, treatment typically follows a period of no treatment or treatment applied to some competing behavior. These steps help rule out regression.

Subject Selection Bias

Subjective factors that influence the selection of participants in a study, and thus introduce problems of invalidity, are grouped under **subject selection**

bias. Whenever two groups of participants are used in experimental studies, it is possible that the groups were different to begin with. Therefore, the differences found on the posttest may not be due to the treatment but to differences in participants.

The typical answer to the problem of subject selection bias is to use randomly selected and assigned groups or groups that have carefully matched participants. As already noted in previous chapters, random sampling of clinical participants is not always practical. In matching, one should find pairs of participants who are similar on important variables, but clinically, this procedure is about as impractical as the random procedure.

In single-subject designs, subject selection bias is not a major problem because the conclusions are not based upon group comparisons. Whether or not the treatment is effective in individual clients whose characteristics are well described is the question for analysis. Therefore, there is no need to make sure that the participants are similar, even when several participants are used in a single-subject design.

Attrition

Also known as subject mortality, **attrition** is the problem of losing participants in the course of an experiment, which in turn has an effect on the final results as interpreted by the investigator. Attrition of participants is not as uncommon as most investigators wish it to be. Graduate students, who generally secure participants for their theses and dissertations with great difficulty, dread this problem the most. Current ethical guidelines appropriately guarantee the participants' right to withdraw from research with no consequences (see Chapter 16), and some participants exercise this right freely and in the middle of a study.

Attrition can be a serious source of internal invalidity in group designs. Analysis of results based on group averages can be affected markedly by differential attrition of participants. If, in the prototypical study of language treatment, children with more severe language disorders were to drop out during the course of treatment, the mean of the posttest of language behaviors would be higher (better) than that of the pretest. This might then suggest a feigned treatment effect leading to invalid conclusions. When two groups are used, differential subject dropout in the experimental and control groups can create a problem of greater magnitude. More severely affected participants may drop out from the experimental group, whereas less severely affected participants may drop out of the control group. This would create major differences in the pretests and posttests of the two groups even when the treatment is totally ineffective.

Attrition is a problem only when statistical analysis based on group means is used. In the analysis of results, an investigator may take into consideration the participant attrition and also describe individual data. However, these may not be practical when the groups are large. Unfortunately, even when it is possible, such individual-specific discriminated analysis is not a typical part of the practice of group design strategy.

In single-subject designs, attrition is not a factor affecting internal validity. Whenever possible, the participants who drop out are replaced by others. A lack of statistical comparison of groups of participants avoids the problems created by differential attrition. However, the single-subject researcher may face another problem relative to attrition: The study simply may have to be postponed to a later date when one or more participants become available. In the case of participant attrition, the group design strategist runs the risk of drawing invalid conclusions, whereas the single-subject strategist runs the risk of not having a study at all.

Diffusion of Treatment

A factor that affects the internal validity of some single-subject designs has been called **diffusion of treatment,** which is continuation of treatment effects even when the treatment is withdrawn to show a reduction in the effects (Kazdin, 1982). In most single-subject designs, the treatment is introduced once and then withdrawn to show corresponding changes in the behaviors. However, when the treatment is withdrawn, the behaviors may sometimes continue because they have come under the influence of other independent variables or even the same independent variables administered by other persons. Parents or spouses who have observed the investigator reinforce the language responses of a person with aphasia may begin to do the same at home. The family members may do this at a time when the investigator is trying to reduce the target behavior to its original baseline. Consequently, the patient with aphasia may continue to produce the language behaviors. The investigator then cannot conclude that the treatment was effective because the effects continued when they were expected to decline.

Some single-subject designs involve two or more treatments whose relative (not interactive) effects are evaluated. Such designs also may have the problem of diffusion of treatment affecting internal validity. The two or more treatment conditions may not be clearly discriminated. In such cases, the effect of one treatment may influence the effect of another treatment, but such influences may remain obscured.

Diffusion of treatment is not a problem in most group designs of research. Because the participants who receive treatment and those who do not are in different groups, the question of treatment diffusion from one condition or treatment to the other does not arise.

In summary, history, maturation, testing, instrumentation, statistical regression, subject selection bias, attrition, and diffusion of treatment are the eight sources of internal invalidity. These sources must be minimized or eliminated in a controlled experimental study. Critical consumers of research should evaluate each published treatment study for these factors that may invalidate or limit the usefulness of conclusions. It should be noted, though, that designs are not perfect and that they control for these sources with varying degrees of efficiency. Therefore, most designs are likely to have some control problems to varying extents, but these problems should not be serious enough to invalidate the study. A study appearing to have a single potential source of internal invalidity that may or may not have operated is judged differently from the one with multiple sources, each posing a definite and serious threat to internal validity.

GENERALITY (EXTERNAL VALIDITY)

Unlike internal validity, generality (external validity) is not always a matter of the experimental design itself. Generality is a matter of the extent to which the investigator can extend or generalize the results to other situations, participants, experimenters, and so forth. One may have internal validity but may not be sure of generality. The investigator may be confident that external variables have been ruled out and that the demonstrated relation between the dependent variable and the independent variable is valid within the confines of the study. However, the extent to which the results can be generalized, which is of course the question of external validity, may not be clear.

In many books and articles, discussions of external validity, generality, or both can be confusing. Three sources have contributed to an elaboration of these concepts. One of the traditional sources of discussion on external validity is the group design strategy, with its emphasis on statistical inference. The second source of information is the single-subject design strategy. The third source is applied behavioral research, with its explicit clinical concerns. As a result of these converging approaches and sources, various terms and concepts are used in discussing external validity. An attempt is made here to provide an integrated view of this important concept.

Types and Limitations of Generality

The major concern of the group design approach to generality has been the extent to which the results of a study based on a sample of participants can be extended to the population from which the sample was drawn. Within the group design strategy, random sampling and assignment of participants and inferential statistical techniques help achieve population generality.

The single-subject design strategy has faced the problem of external validity from a different standpoint. Because the strategy does not draw a sample of participants from a population, extending the results of a particular study to a population is not of immediate concern. However, the strategy has faced a different kind of problem: extending the results from a single participant or a few participants to other similar individuals. When the single-subject strategy began to be used more frequently in applied research, additional concerns emerged. For example, if a behavioral technique is demonstrated to be effective in the treatment of some problem behavior, can the technique be effective with other problem behaviors? Will the technique be equally effective in other clinical or professional settings? Answers to such clinical questions have helped identify additional sources of generality.

In this chapter and elsewhere in the book, the terms *generality* and *external validity* will mean the same. In some respects, the concept of generality is more transparent than external validity and can include various forms of clinical generalities. Therefore, the term generality is preferred. What follows is a description of two major types of generality: statistical (inferential) and clinical. The latter includes several subtypes of generality. Clinical validity, a closely related concept, also will be discussed.

Statistical (Inferential) Generality

Relevant mostly to group design studies, **inferential generality** refers to the extension of the conclusions of a study from a randomly drawn sample of participants to the population from which it was drawn. A population is any defined, relatively large group of persons in research studies. For example, all citizens of voting age in a country, all individuals in a state who stutter, all children in the seventh grade in a particular school district, and all children with unrepaired cleft living in a particular city illustrate populations. A **sample** is a smaller number of participants who represent a specific population. The sample should be randomly selected from the population and then randomly divided into two or more groups that participate in an experiment. Typically, one group receives treatment and one other does not. It is assumed that a random sample of a population is as heterogeneous as the population and that it represents the population. Therefore, to investigate a phenomenon found in a population, one need not study the entire population, which would be almost impossible. When it is shown that two events are causally related in a representative sample of participants, it may be concluded that the events are so related in the entire population. Such a conclusion is the essence of inferential generality. This concept of inferential generality is illustrated in Figure 7.1.

Inferential generality is based on inferential techniques of statistics, such as analysis of variance. These techniques are so named because they help infer the values of the dependent variables in the population. In other words, in a treatment research study, the investigator may, with the help of statistical analysis of a random sample study, infer that all those in the population who might receive the same treatment might react similarly to those in the study. Because the population is not tested, generality is a matter of making a valid inference as supported by the theory and technique of statistics.

Two major problems affect inferential generality: lack of random selection of participants and potential interaction between participant characteristics and treatment that is masked in group averages. Random sampling

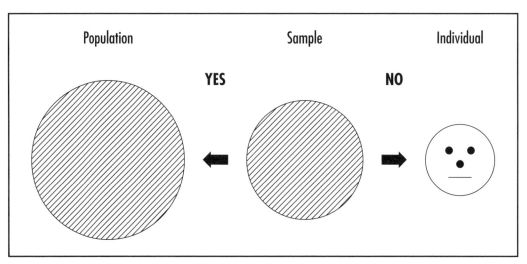

Figure 7.1. The direction of inferential generality—from a random sample to the population. Inferential generality does not permit generalization from the sample to an individual.

is very difficult to accomplish, especially in clinical sciences concerned with the experimental evaluation of treatment procedures. Populations of children with articulation disorders, persons with language disorders, or persons with aphasia typically are not available for the researcher. Moreover, those who are initially selected randomly may not agree to participate because under the current research guidelines, all participants are self-selected (see Chapters 4 and 16 for details on self-selection). Also, those who initially agree to participate may not continue their participation until the end of the study. Consequently, there is no assurance that the results of a group design study can be generalized to the population. Therefore, a serious threat to inferential generality is the lack of random sampling that is so typical of group clinical research.

A randomly drawn sample should also be assigned to the experimental and control groups to make sure that the two groups are equal. This, as noted earlier, is a matter of internal validity. The critical factor for inferential generality is the original sampling of the participants from the population.

The other factor that affects inferential generality, the interaction between participant characteristics and treatment, is related to the method of data analysis. Most group designs average the performance of individual participants to make inferential statistical analyses. Therefore, it is difficult to determine whether all participants behaved the same under the treatment condition or whether individuals with certain characteristics behaved one way and those with other characteristics behaved another way. For example, an experimental study may have demonstrated that a certain treatment is effective, on the average, with a sample of children with articulation disorders. However, it is possible that only those children with mild articulation disorders or high levels of intelligence benefited from the treatment, whereas those with other characteristics may not have shown any improvement. Such interactions between participant characteristics and treatment effects usually are masked in the group performance analyses. Therefore, whether there was an interaction, and if so, its type is usually unknown.

The problem of unknown but possible differential response to treatment by different participants in an experimental group can pose a significant problem for the clinician who wishes to know whether the results can be extended to individual clients with specific characteristics. The clinician can conclude only that, *on the average*, particular sets of clients seem to improve under treatment. It would not be possible to determine whether given individual clients would improve under that treatment. This problem is inherent in most group designs because the direction of inferential generality is from the sample to the population and not from the sample to the individual. Typically, clinicians try to generalize from small groups of clients or individuals to other small groups or individuals. In essence, inferential generality does not serve a clinical science very well.

Clinical Generality

Concerns of clinical researchers have been mainly responsible for delineating several specific forms of generality that apply most forcefully to treatment research. These forms of generality have lacked a common term; therefore, the term *clinical generality* is used here to include various forms of generality that treatment researchers typically try to establish. As defined in Chapter 4, **clinical generality** is the extent to which the conclusions of a study may be generalized to other clinical parameters.

Logical Generality. Because of a lack of random samples, the results of single-subject designs cannot be extended to the population. In other words, the results of particular single-subject design studies do not have inferential generality. However, single-subject designs do not seek inferential generality. Instead, they seek what is known as logical generality (Barlow & Hersen, 1984; Eddington, 1967).

Logical generality is the extension of the results of a study to individuals who are similar to the participants of that study. Because single-subject designs use only a few individuals at a time, the investigator usually gives a thorough description of each of the participants. It should then be possible to tentatively conclude that persons who are similar to those who have served in the study may react to the experimental treatment in the same way as the participants. Logical generality may also be described as generality based on individual profiles. A clinician who wishes to select a treatment for a client may select an experimentally evaluated treatment if the profile of at least one participant in the study matches that of the client. The concept of logical generality is illustrated in Figure 7.2, which also contrasts it with inferential generality.

Logical generality proceeds from a set of selected individuals to a single individual or a few individuals. It is generality from either a homogeneous

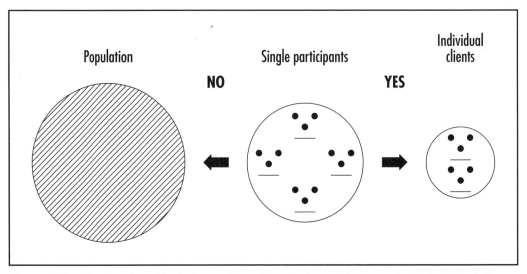

Figure 7.2. The direction of logical generality—from single participants to similar individual clients. Logical generality does not permit generalization from the participants to the population.

or a heterogeneous set of experimental participants to a similar set of individuals who have not been tested yet. For example, an experiment involving a new treatment for persons with dysarthria may be conducted on five individuals whose specific characteristics (client profiles) are described in detail. Practically, five separate experiments, each involving a single participant, are conducted. However, the conditions of the experiment across the participants are the same: baseline, treatment, withdrawal of treatment, and reinstatement of treatment. In making a report on the study, each client's dysarthria and personal and behavioral characteristics (profiles) are fully described. Their behaviors under the conditions of the study are presented and analyzed separately. A clinician reading such a report can conclude when an individual client he or she is working with is like one of those in the experiment who benefited from the experiment. If a participant with a certain profile did not benefit under the experimental treatment, then the clinician would not select that treatment for a client who exhibits a similar profile. Note that in this type of generality, any conclusion regarding how the population of people with dysarthria would react to the same treatment would be inappropriate.

Logical generality can eventually achieve the presumed power of inferential generality through various kinds of replications. If different experiments are performed by different clinicians in a variety of settings involving varied clients with the same disorder, the treatment in question will have been tested across different conditions of generality.

Generality Across Clients. The extent to which the result of a study may be extended to other persons is the **generality across clients.** This type of generality is an important factor in all human research, especially in clinical research. Logical generality is a restricted form of generality. At least in the initial stages of a treatment evaluation, profile matching can be somewhat limited. The clinician might be serving many clients whose profiles do not match those of participants in single-subject experiments. Eventually, what the clinician should look for is generality across clients so that the concern is not to precisely match profiles of clients and experimental participants.

Generality across clients addresses several important questions. If a language treatment is known to be effective with 4-year-old children with specific language disability, will the treatment be equally effective in the treatment of 10-year-old children with similar language problems? Will the treatment be effective with children who have other disabilities, such as developmental disabilities? The treatment may or may not be effective with older or younger children or with those who have other disabilities in addition to language impairment. The results of a treatment study may not be generalized to clients who differ from participants in an experiment. It is precisely in these circumstances that logical generality will not help. Logical generality will support the use of a technique when the participant and client profiles match; it stays neutral when profiles do not match. Research on generality across diverse participants, if successful, will support the application of a technique across different participants whose profiles need not match.

It may appear that inferential generality and generality across clients address the same problem. However, they refer to two related but separate problems. In inferential generality, whether there was an interaction between participant characteristics and the treatment variable may be unknown, and therefore it may not be possible to generalize from the sample to individual clients. The concern in inferential generality is the direction of generality: from the sample to the population, not from the sample to the individual. In generality across clients, the concern is whether the results of an experiment performed on participants whose characteristics are well known can be generalized to clients who have different, but equally well-known, characteristics. The individual participant characteristics are unknown in inferential generality; therefore, the concept permits the extension of conclusion only to the population. It is not critical to determine the characteristics of individual participants in the population.

In generality across clients, the investigator wishes to generalize from one set of known participant characteristics to a different set of known characteristics. For instance, the investigator may have determined that a given treatment is effective with clients who have dysarthria and whose characteristics are well described in the study. Other clinicians can surmise that the treatment may be effective with individuals with the same or similar characteristics, a supposition that is not possible in inferential generality. However, the clinicians would not know whether the treatment would be effective for persons who have dysarthria but who are different from those in the original study. If there is no such generality, then the treatment should be limited to clients of certain characteristics only.

Generality Across Ethnocultural Groups. In recent years, a new concern has emerged about generality of treatment research data. In fact, the concern extends to all kinds of human research, both basic and applied. In applied (clinical) research, the concern extends to the appropriateness of diagnostic categories and assessment techniques. In treatment research, the concern is whether treatment efficacy data have generality across different ethnocultural groups.

Historically, different ethnic groups have not been balanced in most assessment or treatment research. In most countries, the United States included, treatment efficacy data have largely been collected on the ethnic majority (Battle, 2002; Coleman, 2000; Kamhi, Pollock, & Harris, 1996; Kayser, 1998; Payne, 1997; Seymour & Nober, 1998). As the U.S. population has grown more diverse in its ethnocultural composition, the new concern has a new urgency as well. What if the assessment and treatment techniques found to be valid and effective with the majority group just do not work with people of different ethnocultural background? Obviously, this is an important question that practitioners seeking to select procedures that suit the individual client need to ask and answer.

To achieve ethnocultural generality, treatment researchers need to recruit participants more carefully so that the different ethnocultural groups are adequately represented. From a practical standpoint, though, such balancing is not always possible because in some settings, one or a few ethnocultural groups may be all that are available for sampling. Therefore, when studies are published on a given treatment with inadequate balancing of participants from different ethnocultural groups, the practitioner will have to be careful in extending the conclusions to members of unrepresented ethnocultural groups. Meanwhile, other treatment researchers who do have access to certain ethnocultural groups should replicate the findings with members from those groups. Systematic replication, therefore, seems to be the best strategy to establish ethnocultural generality.

The issue of ethnocultural generality of treatment data has received much explicit attention since the 1980s. Nonetheless, classic discussion on generality may subsume this issue. For example, whether treatment data collected on one ethnocultural group may be extended to a different ethnocultural group may be addressed as generality across clients. Lack of generality across clients may be viewed as due to differing ethnocultural background of participants and further analysis may either support or reject this possibility. Even so, in the past, the issue of ethnocultural generality has not been addressed fully or explicitly. In view of its importance, it is essential to consider it as a separate form of generality so that treatment researchers may include different ethnocultural groups in their research.

Generality Across Settings. It is important to establish that the findings of a study conducted in one setting are valid in other settings as well. Of necessity, most research studies are conducted in one or more particular settings. The results may have excellent internal validity. However, it may not be clear that the same results would be obtained if the experiment were to be repeated in other settings, especially in a multitude of settings. **Generality across settings** is the extent to which the results of a study conducted in one or more settings may be extended to many other settings not involved in the original study. Obviously, clinicians look for this important type of generality.

The extent to which a physical setting itself affects the generality of research findings is not always clear. Clinicians sometimes wonder why certain procedures, known to be effective in one professional setting, do not work well in other settings. What works best in a private speech and hearing clinic may not work equally well in a public school setting. Often, the reason why the results of a study are not replicated in another setting is a failure to use the proven procedure in its original form. In any case, if there is no setting generality, additional experimental analyses should be made to determine why. Such analyses may uncover deficiencies in the implementation of the tested technique or suggest ways of improving it so that it can produce more uniform results in different settings.

Generality Across Experimenters.

Sometimes an effect demonstrated by one experimenter may not be obtained by another experimenter or a clinician. The results then do not have **generality across experimenters,** which is the extent to which the results obtained by one investigator may be extended to other investigators who use the same procedure. In clinical research, dramatic effects of certain treatment programs administered by some clinicians may not be replicated by other clinicians.

It is possible that special characteristics, training, and skills of the experimenter contribute to the effects of independent variables manipulated in experiments. However, when such factors are involved, the problem may not be one of experimental design but of who implemented it and in what manner. In other words, designs cannot be blamed if the techniques themselves are used with varying degrees of efficiency and accuracy by different investigators or clinicians. Regardless, the effect on generality is negative.

Discussions on research in social sciences often include a reference to the **Rosenthal effect:** the effect of the experimenter on the dependent variable, much of which is due to the personal characteristics of the experimenter. The physical appearance, race, gender, personal characteristics, and such other variables associated with the investigator as a person may play some role in changing the dependent variable under investigation. However, the actual effects of such variables in treatment research are not well understood.

It is possible that experimenter effects are more troublesome when the independent variable manipulated in a study is relatively weak and the dependent variable measured in the study is an unstable, reactive behavior. Also, when an investigator describes the treatment procedures poorly or incompletely, others who try to replicate the study may, of necessity, modify it in unknown ways. If the results are negative, the investigator may conclude that some personal characteristic of the original investigator was an important variable. But, in fact, the problem might have been that the method itself was not applied as it was in the original study, perhaps because of inadequate descriptions in the original study. When the procedures are clear, variables are strong and nonreactive, and the experimenter is well trained in the methods of the study, these effects should not pose significant problems for experimenter generality. Eventually, all clinical sciences strive to develop treatment techniques whose effects override any personal quality differences except for training and skill.

Generality Across Response Classes. In human and clinical research, a certain independent variable may be demonstrated to have an effect on certain responses. The responses manipulated may belong to a single class, for example, the production of the present progressive *-ing* in sentences. The results may demonstrate that the treatment program was effective in teaching the production of *-ing*. A clinician then may wonder whether the same treatment technique may be used in teaching plural morphemes, passive forms of sentences, correct articulation of phonemes, or sign language. Each of these clinical targets belongs to a separate response class.

A **response class** is a group of responses that share the same causal variables and are used for similar effects. From a practical and teaching standpoint, response classes are groups of responses that may be produced with training of only some of the responses in that group. For instance, in teaching the present progressive *-ing*, one need not use all different forms of sentences in which that structure is used. Teaching a few correct exemplars of *-ing* will result in the generalized production of many different forms of sentences in which the morpheme is correctly used. A different class of response, for instance, the regular plural morpheme, is not affected by the training of the present progressive. The plural morpheme belongs to a separate response class and needs separate training. Therefore, the question of **generality across response classes**—the extent to which the results of one investigation may be extended to responses not investigated—is clinically (as well as theoretically) important (Hegde, 1998a). More often, researchers ask whether a proven technique is useful in treating a disorder that is similar to the one treated in the original investigation. However, one may ask whether the treatment will be effective in treating a very different response— whether, for example, the technique known to be effective in teaching specific language behaviors (one response class) can be used to train mathematical or musical skills (very different response classes).

Generality across response classes is important in clinical research and treatment. Clinicians sometimes assume that a method demonstrated to be successful in the treatment of one disorder of communication may not be effective in the treatment of another disorder. However, clinical evidence shows a considerable degree of generality of treatment variables (Hegde, 1998a). It is important to establish such generality through systematic research because it reduces unnecessary diversity in therapeutic practices.

Clinical Validity

A concept closely related to clinical generality is **clinical validity,** which is the degree to which the treatment effects are socially and personally meaningful. Some treatments may reduce symptoms in clinical settings (e.g., reduced dysfluency rates), but if the effects do not generalize to everyday situations, the clinical reduction will not be of social or personal significance. A child with a language disorder might learn to produce a few morphological structures in the clinic but may still lack language skills necessary to succeed in the classroom. Medically, symptoms of a disease may be reduced, but the patient's general well-being may still be poor. These examples underscore the need to go beyond narrowly defined clinical goals of treatment.

To be socially and personally meaningful, treatment in communicative disorders should achieve broader, lasting, and generalized goals that improve a person's social and personal communication. Furthermore, in the case of children, treatment should enhance academic performance. In the case of working adults, treatment effects should lead to better occupational performance and efficiency. Such broader effects realized through treatment should also last and be sustained across varied circumstances. An effective treatment only means that certain changes were reliably associated with treatment and that without treatment such changes would not have taken place. But an effective treatment may not have been personally and socially significant. Therefore, clinical researchers strive to achieve both effectiveness (internal validity) and clinical validity.

Clinical validity has consequences for generality. If an effective treatment's clinical validity is in doubt, then other clinicians would be unsure as to its application. Therefore, lack of clinical validity will limit wider application of a technique known to be effective. See Chapter 4 for additional comments on clinical validity.

Factors That Affect Generality

The types of generality described so far have their limitations, but they are not by themselves negative or positive factors. All are desirable types of generality that may be achieved to various degrees. However, there are some factors that affect all types of generality and other factors that affect some specific kind of generality.

Pretest and Posttest Sensitization to Treatment

The pretest, or the initial assessment of the dependent variable, may sensitize participants to the treatment in such a way as to enhance the effect of the treatment variable. For example, smokers may become sensitized to the magnitude of their problem when the number of cigarettes smoked is measured prior to implementation of a treatment program. The treatment may have a larger effect in these participants compared with participants who were not pretested and thus were not sensitized to their problem or to the treatment. Therefore, the results may not be generalized to participants who will not be given the same or a similar pretest.

In some research studies, the posttest may also act as a sensitizer of treatment variables. While the pretest may sensitize participants to treatment, the posttest may help demonstrate the effect that would otherwise not have appeared. This can happen because the posttest can help participants recall the information presented in the treatment sessions. For example, questionnaires and interviews designed to find out the effects of a film on attitude change can help the participants simply recall some of the information presented in the film, which may be interpreted as an effect of the film. The posttest of an academic teaching program may have similar effects on the dependent variable.

Sensitization is a more serious problem with reactive variables such as attitudes and opinions. After they are measured, they tend to become more sensitive to techniques designed to change them. The reactive variables then show additional changes simply as a function of the posttest. Rates of actual responses, on the other hand, are less reactive than a participant's verbal statements about those responses.

Sensitization to treatment that limits external validity should not be confused with testing that affects internal validity. Testing that directly changes (to whatever the extent) the dependent variable is a threat to internal validity. In this case, the independent variable may not be responsible for some or all of the changes observed on the posttest. Sensitization, on the other hand, affects the external validity or generality of findings by making the results less relevant to the participants who are not given a pretest. Testing can directly affect the dependent variable, whereas sensitization can make the participants react more favorably to the treatment. What is common to both factors is the reactive dependent variable.

Hawthorne Effect

In social and behavioral research, the knowledge on the part of the participants that they are participating in an experiment may produce an effect in addition to that of the independent variable. The results then may not be extended to participants who do not have such a knowledge. The participants may be aware of the purposes of an experiment and, besides, may know what kinds of responses are expected of them under the different conditions of the study. As a result, they may be more inclined to respond in expected directions. Furthermore, experimental participants may be apprehensive about being evaluated in some way. Such apprehension may also affect the results either positively or negatively. Influences of this kind that limit the generality of research findings are grouped under the **Hawthorne**

effect, which is the extent to which the participants' knowledge that they are participants in an experiment and possibly of expected results affect the actual results.

The well-known *placebo effect* is part of the Hawthorne effect. This effect is evident when participants react to a treatment favorably simply because it is presented as a treatment by experts. The treatment may be totally ineffective, but the participants report otherwise. In drug evaluation experiments, a placebo, which looks like the drug being tested but is actually an inert material, is routinely used to rule out this effect. An effective drug should produce effects over and beyond the placebo effect. The placebo effect can also be troublesome in behavioral treatment programs. When self-report data on the effects of treatments are sought, the clients may report a magnitude of improvement that is greater than that of the actual improvement.

In recent years, the presence of the placebo effect, the extent of the effect, and the ethical issues related to placebo administration in medicine and surgery have all come under close scrutiny. Please see Chapter 4 for a discussion of the issues associated with placebo-controlled randomized clinical trials in medicine and surgery.

Multiple Treatment Interference

In most research studies, the effects of a single independent variable are assessed. However, in some experiments, the effects of multiple independent variables may be investigated. Clinical research of this kind is especially valuable. For example, a clinician may wish to find out if, in the treatment of articulation disorders, immediate feedback on the accuracy of a client's response is more effective than delayed feedback. The two different methods of providing the feedback would be the two treatment variables in the study. When such experiments are conducted, a potential problem is that of **multiple treatment interference,** which is the positive or negative effect of one treatment over the other.

When two or more treatments are applied in sequence to the same participants, the effects of the second treatment may be confounded by those of the first. Also, the overall effect observed in the participants may be at least partly determined by the order in which the multiple treatments were applied. If the same treatments are applied in a different order, the same results may or may not be obtained. This affects the generality of findings. The results may be valid only in terms of the sequence in which the treatments were administered. The generality of the findings with regard to individual treatments would also be unknown.

Multiple treatment interference is a serious problem when the same participants are exposed to different treatments within a single design. Therefore, it often is a problem with certain single-subject and within-subjects group designs. However, this problem can exist within other group designs when the same participants are repeatedly used in several experiments. It is known that often the same college students serve in a multitude of experiments, especially when the students are paid for their participation. The clients of speech and hearing centers may also be repeatedly used in certain experiments, including treatment evaluations. In such cases, the participants' performance on subsequent experiments may be partly determined by their participation in earlier experiments. Therefore, the results of subsequent studies may not have much relevance to participants who do not have the cumulative experience of having participated in many experiments. Multiple treatment interference is further discussed in Chapters 8 and 9.

CONCLUDING REMARKS

Researchers and consumers of research information should be concerned with internal and external validity. Whether the demonstrated relation between variables is valid and whether the same relation would hold in other circumstances are the two most important judgments that investigators and consumers of research should make.

Although researchers may be able to control for some of the factors that threaten external validity in a study, it should be realized that no single study can be said to have all kinds of generality. Generality of research findings is a matter of replication. Unless studies are repeated by other experimenters in different settings using new participants, the eventual generality of experimental findings is not established. There are different procedures of establishing the generality of research data described in Chapter 10.

Before concluding this chapter, a note on the distinction between *generality* and *generalization* is in order. Some investigators use the terms interchangeably. However, this practice is confusing because they are not the same. The discussion so far makes it clear that generality refers to the applicability of research data to participants, responses, settings, experimenters, and so on that were not involved in the original study. It is achieved by the process of repeating the experiments under varied conditions. Generality, therefore, is a result of certain actions, but it is not in itself a behavioral process in the sense that generalization is. **Generalization** refers to a temporary response rate when the process of conditioning is discontinued and the response is allowed to be made. On the other hand, generality does not refer to any response rate; it refers to functional relations between events under new conditions of experimentation.

The act of establishing generality of research findings is a behavioral process, but that is true of the original experiment as well. In this sense, all research activity is behavior, as noted in Chapter 3. There is one sense in which generality and generalization are similar, however. When experiments are repeated and the same functional relation is seen again and again, the scientists are said to have demonstrated generality. It means that as long as the same functional relation is encountered, scientists behave as though the differences in settings, conditions, participants, and other such factors do not matter. The scientists' behavior, then, shows the same properties that characterize generalization. In essence, one can view generality as a functional relation that repeats itself in nature, and one can view generalization (in this particular context) as the behavior of scientists toward generality. A scientist would generalize only when the generality of findings has been demonstrated.

SUMMARY

- Research designs are defined generally as methods of a study and, more technically, as structures of temporospatial arrangements within which the selected variables are controlled, manipulated, and measured.

- Research designs help detect independent, related, correlated, and interactive relation between events. Designs also are a means of controlling variability.

- There are two views on the nature of variability in human behavior:
  - The intrinsic view holds that variability found in behavior is inherent (intrinsic) to human beings and therefore controlled mostly statistically, not experimentally.
  - The extrinsic view holds that much of the variability is due to external factors that may be controlled experimentally, not statistically. The extrinsic view also postulates that variability itself may be a subject for experimental analysis.

- The results of an experiment are subject to an evaluation of their internal validity, generality, and clinical validity.

- Internal validity is the degree to which a design rules out the influence of extraneous variables and thus demonstrates that the independent variable of the study was indeed responsible for the changes in the dependent variable. In treatment research, an internally valid study shows that a treatment was effective. Several factors affect internal validity:
  - History—other events that could produce the same effects as the independent variable
  - Maturation—biological and other kinds of changes that take place within organisms that could produce the same changes as the independent variable
  - Testing—dependent variables that change simply because they are repeatedly measured; such measures are called reactive
  - Instrumentation—data distortions introduced by defective instruments or untrained and biased human observers

— Statistical regression—clients' tendency to seek help when their problems are at their worst and when recruited for a study, and the resulting tendency of the problems to subside to their average levels even without treatment

— Subject selection bias—an investigator's bias in selecting and assigning participants to the experimental and control groups

— Attrition—differential loss of participants in the control and experimental groups that could influence the results

— Diffusion of treatment—treatment effects being maintained when they are expected to decline

• Generality, also called external validity, is the extent to which the conclusions of a study may be extended to new settings, persons (participants), response classes, and investigators.

• Statistical (inferential) generality is the extent to which the conclusions of a study based on a sample of participants may be extended to the population from which the sample was drawn.

• Clinical generality is the extent to which the results of a treatment study maybe extended to other relevant conditions. Forms of clinical validity include logical generality, which is the extent to which the conclusions of a study based on a small number of individuals may be extended to similar individuals; generality across subjects; generality across settings; generality across experimenters; and generality across response classes.

• Clinical validity is the extent to which the treatment effects are socially and personally meaningful.

• Several factors affect generality:

— Pretest–posttest sensitization to treatment—the effects of pretests and posttests that predispose the participants to treatment or its evaluation resulting in greater effects of treatment

— Hawthorne effect—the effects on the results of the participants' knowledge that they are participating in an experiment and what results are expected

— Multiple treatment interference—the mutual influence of multiple treatments that are given to the same individuals

STUDY GUIDE _____

1. What is a general description of research designs?

2. What is the technical description of research designs?

3. What is meant by the manipulation of an independent variable?

4. Why is the concept of variability especially controversial in the study of human behavior?

5. How does the concept of free will relate to variability of behavior?

6. What is intrinsic variability? What are some of the sources of intrinsic variability of human behavior, including language?

7. How do the concepts of intrinsic variability and intrinsic causes of behavior converge to produce a significant effect on experimental strategy?

8. Which one is experimentally more controllable: intrinsic or extrinsic variability?

9. What is the name for the variability induced by the independent variable?

10. What is extraneous variance? Give an example.

11. What is error variance?

12. What is the traditional answer to the problem of behavioral variability in social and behavioral sciences?

13. Define extrinsic variability. What is its relevance to experimental research?

14. Does the concept of extrinsic variability rule out the influence of variables within an organism?

15. What are some of the variables within the organism that influence behavior?

16. A clinician wishes to find out why people who stutter seem to exhibit varying amounts of stuttering on different occasions. How would you try to answer this question on the basis of (a) intrinsic variability and (b) extrinsic variability? What kinds of research will these two assumptions lead to?

17. Which assumption is self-corrective, intrinsic or extrinsic variability?

18. How is variability handled in the group design and the single-subject design strategies?

19. Can variability itself be the object of scientific investigation? Which design strategy is more likely to investigate the causes of variability?

20. Distinguish between internal validity and generality.

21. What is clinical validity? How is it related to generality?

22. What kind of validity is demonstrated by a clinician who convincingly shows that a particular treatment procedure was indeed responsible for changes in the client's communicative behaviors?

23. How is internal validity achieved?

24. What are the factors that adversely affect internal validity?

25. How is maturation controlled for in the group design strategy and in the single-subject design strategy?

26. What are reactive measures? What kinds of dependent variables are most likely to be reactive?

27. What is statistical regression? What kinds of disorders are likely to show this phenomenon?

28. A clinical investigator had 10 subjects in each of two groups (experimental and control). The 20 subjects had a disorder of articulation whose severity varied across individuals. With this example, show how differential participant attrition could invalidate the conclusions based on the group means.

29. Is external validity strictly and always a matter of research designs themselves? Why or why not?

30. Describe the relation between internal validity and generality. Can you have one without the other?

31. Distinguish between inferential and logical generality.

32. Specify the relevance of logical generality to clinical research.

33. Why is inferential generality not achieved in most group design studies?

34. What kinds of generalities are not demonstrated even by an ideal group design study? Why?

35. What is pretest–posttest sensitization to treatment? What kind of validity is affected by this?

36. How is "testing" different from pretest–posttest sensitization?

37. Define the Hawthorne effect.

38. The placebo effect in clinical research is a part of what effect?

39. What research strategy is especially vulnerable to multiple treatment interference?

40. How is generality different from generalization?

Chapter 8

◆◆◆◆◆◆◆◆◆◆◆◆◆◆◆◆◆◆◆◆◆◆◆◆◆◆◆◆◆

The Group Design Strategy

It was noted in Chapters 4 and 7 that there are two basic approaches to designing experiments: the group design and the single-subject design. The relevance of these experimental designs for clinical disciplines is especially great because they are the means by which treatment effects are established. Therefore, I shall describe the group design strategy in this chapter and the single-subject strategy in the next chapter. Together, the two chapters will summarize a variety of designs that are used in investigating experimental research questions.

The group design strategy is well established in psychology and social sciences. The strategy is more commonly used in medical treatment evaluation, although it is being increasingly advocated as the standard of treatment evaluation for all clinical disciplines. Several historical trends have influenced the development and use of the group design strategy.

DEVELOPMENT OF STATISTICAL CONCEPTS AND TECHNIQUES

The **group design strategy** is a method in which statistical means derived from the performances of individuals in two or more groups on one or more dependent variables are compared. The method is now extensively used in experimentally evaluating the effects of new medical and surgical treatment procedures in what are more popularly known as randomized clinical trials, described in Chapter 4.

The group design strategy has its roots in psychobiological measurement, development of statistics, and agricultural research. In fact, the development of statistics is intricately associated with the measurement of human variation—both physical and psychological. Statistical concepts that are fundamental to the group design strategy include the theory of probability and the normal probability curve, random sampling and inferential statistics, statistical significance, and inferential generality.

Theory of Probability and the Normal Probability Curve

The mathematical theory of probability deals with potential occurrences of events versus their actual occurrences. Consequently, probability is expressed in terms of a ratio between possibilities and actualities. In other words, the likelihood of something happening is dependent on all possible occurrences of that event; a single occurrence of an event is a fraction of all such occurrences. The early development of this mathematical theory was rooted in gambling that was popular with the 17th- and 18th-century European aristocrats, especially the French. Known as the "game theory," it tried to predict certain outcomes given all the possible outcomes according to the rules of a game. Subsequently, mathematicians and statisticians took the concept of probability and developed it further (Hacking, 1975; Hald, 1998).

The basic concept of the *theory of probability* is typically described with examples of a coin toss. Given the idea that probability is the actual occurrence of an event among a possible set of such occurrences, a toss of a coin has two possible outcomes: one head or one tails. An actual outcome of a single toss of a coin may be either heads or tails. In other words, statistically, the probability between these two outcomes is exactly the same: There is a 50% chance that it will be tails and an equal chance that it will be heads. This probability is expressed as 1 of 2, ½, or .5, which is typically expressed as $p = .5$ (in which the p stands for probability).

The relevance of the probability theory to any kind of experimentation is simple: What is the probability that the results of an experiment will be the same or similar if the same experiment were to be repeated one or more times? Obviously, one cannot trust a study's results if they are unlikely to be replicated. The goal of all experimentation is to produce results that have a high probability of being replicated, or, in other terms, a high probability of being true. Therefore, group experimental treatment researchers estimate the probability of obtaining the same or similar results when the experiment is repeated. This point will be considered further in a later section about the concept of statistical significance of experimental data.

The development of the concept of the *normal probability curve* has had a significant effect on the eventual group comparison approach in experimental research, including controlled research in medicine, psychology, and education. The credit for developing the concept of the normal curve has been given to the French mathematician and astronomer Pierre Simon Laplace (1749–1827). The normal curve came to be known as the Gaussian distribution or the Gaussian curve mainly because it was Karl Fredrick Gauss (1777–1855), the German mathematician and astronomer, who described how errors in repeated observations of a phenomenon may be symmetrically distributed around a mean or average value. In the bell-shaped normal curve, deviation from the mean value suggests variability in the occurrence of a phenomenon.

Soon the significance of the normal distribution became evident in the works of Adolph Quetelet (1796–1874), the Belgian astronomer and statistician who is often considered the founder of modern statistics (Boring, 1950). Quetelet claimed that data obtained on variations in human characteristics (e.g., height or weight) are normally distributed. Quetelet was probably the first statistician to exalt the mean or the average to the level of an ideal that nature strives and sometimes fails to achieve. His doctrine, *l'homme moyen* (the average man) stated that the average is what nature intends to create and all deviations from the average, including those on the positive side of the mean, are nature's errors.

When psychological testing of human skills and characteristics, especially intelligence, became well established in Britain and the United States after World War II, all individual performances began to be evaluated against the average, giving rise to the notion of the statistical norm. Subsequent developments in agricultural research included the techniques of random sampling and inferential statistics which lead to the group comparison approach in human experimental research.

Random Sampling, Inferential Statistics, and Inferential Generality

Historically, the group design strategy is based on the works of a few individuals who were simultaneously mathematical statisticians, philosophers, psychologists, and biologists of the 19th century. An important event in the development of statistical methods took place in 1901 when Sir Francis Galton (1822–1911) and Karl Pearson (1857–1936) led a few interested persons in establishing a journal called *Biometrika* to publish mathematical and statistical research in psychology and biology. The same year, Pearson established a biometric laboratory at the University College, London (Boring, 1950; Hill, Forbes, Kozak, & McNeill, 2000). Galton's main interest was mental (intellectual) inheritance and Pearson's was mathematical statistics. Galton had already worked out the basic method of a co-relation by way of studying regression to the mean ("regression toward mediocrity" in Galton's words) in physical and mental characteristics across successive generations. Later, Pearson worked out the mathematical details of correlation and another statistician Edgeworth called it the *coefficient of correlation* in 1982. It still is abbreviated as *r*, which stands for Galton's term, *regression*.

Pearson was an avid promoter of the use of statistics in biology and psychology. He was even accused of the belief that statistics can help draw valid conclusions from invalid data, a view repugnant to most experimental scientists (Boring, 1950). His systematic work, however, was more influential than his controversial belief in the power of statistics. His contributions firmly established the statistical approach to research in biology, psychology, most social sciences, and eventually medicine.

It was the work of Sir Ronald A. Fisher (1890–1962) that firmly established the practice of group experimental designs based on statistical analyses (Fisher, 1925, 1942, 1951, 1956). His writings are a classic within this philosophy of research. Fisher believed that statistical techniques and research designs are two aspects of the same whole (Fisher, 1951). He was a brilliant British statistician and geneticist who had an unsatisfactory career for a few years as a teacher in schools and colleges. When in 1919 the famous statistician and geneticist Karl Pearson offered him a job at the prestigious biometrics laboratory named after Galton at London's University College, he rejected it in favor of a statistician's job at an agricultural research station, known as the Rothamsted Experimental Station, some 25 miles north of London (Box, 1978).

From 1999 to 1996, Fisher's job was to analyze archival data on agricultural experimentation that had been collected over a period of 67 years. As he studied old data, he began to formulate new and better methods of data analysis, including analysis of variance and analysis of covariance. Even more important, as he critically evaluated the results of old experiments, he began to think of new methods of data collection—experimental designs. He first developed nonrandomized blocks designs in which multiple treatments are compared with systematic (nonrandom) assignment of treatment. Soon he realized, however, that systematic application of treatment induces a greater degree of error into observations. To reduce such errors, Fisher introduced the concept of randomization of treatments. He would thus let chance decide which plot of land received what kind of seed, how much water, what kind of fertilizer, and so forth, with a condition that all treatment permutations and combinations have an equal chance of appearing in the experimental arrangement. Subsequently, he developed factorial designs (see later in this chapter for varieties of all these designs used in human treatment research). Fisher's first randomized experimental research study was laid out in 1926 in an agricultural plot at Rothamsted. Fisher then went on to design many agricultural experiments to study the interaction between various soil conditions, seed quality, fertilizer, weather, watering practices, and so forth (Box, 1978).

Fisher's method of randomization also was a means to go beyond the actual observations (experimental results) and thus to make his enterprise worthwhile as well as efficient. For Fisher, it was not sufficient to find out that under given conditions a plot of agricultural land yielded more than another. He needed to make the statement that given the same or similar conditions, other plots in other parts of the country could realize the same or similar crop output. Fisher considered all experimental results based on sample observations as an estimation of what happens in the population. He introduced the term *parameters* for the values of variables in the population (Box, 1978). The values of variables actually observed in a sample, which are often such statistics as a mean, are estimates of population parameters. This means that Fisher needed to generalize from what he studied (a small set of observations) to what he did not (a large set of potential observations). As noted in Chapters 4 and 7, to extend the conclusions of a study based on a random sample to a population is to achieve *inferential generality*. Fisher's mathematical analysis convinced him that a random selection of units for observation from a population of potential observations was the initial step in extending the conclusions from a sample of observations to all potential observations. In other words, what can be observed is a sample, but useful conclusions must apply to the population. And to make that extension possible, the sample must represent the population. The only way to make a small sample represent the much larger population is to draw the sample randomly.

Although random selection theoretically helped reduce errors of observation, Fisher still needed tools of analysis that, when applied to the results, would essentially support or refute the hypothesis that a treatment was or was not effective. He reasoned that a treatment is effective if the obtained results, especially the difference in yield between the treated and untreated plots, could not be due to chance. The same reasoning is used in current group treatment research. A treatment or a teaching method is effective only when the observed differences in performance of participants in the experimental (treated) and control (untreated) groups exceed chance occurrences. How can a researcher determine whether the differences in the treated and untreated groups are not due to chance but only to treatment? Fisher's answer was a series of statistical techniques, such as the analysis of variance, which help estimate the probability of obtaining results of the kind demonstrated by an experiment via chance alone. It may be noted parenthetically that it is in Fisher's honor that the statistical outcome of analysis of variance is called the *F* ratio (Kerlinger, 1986), although the original set of ratios were calculated by an Indian statistician named Mahalanobis (Box, 1978). Such techniques of quantitative analyses are known as *inferential statistics* because they help infer the probability of obtaining the same or similar results when the experiment is repeated with samples drawn from the same population.

Research methods Fisher developed in his agricultural fields were later extended to educational, social, psychological, and medical research. It became clear that, just as with agriculture, multiple variables affect human behavior including response to various clinical and educational treatments. The results of all controlled group design studies, including randomized clinical trials in medicine and other health professions described in Chapter 4, are analyzed with inferential statistics. Based on such statistical analysis, researchers can claim that a treatment found effective in a sample of randomly drawn and assigned individuals may be effective with similar persons in the population.

The main concern in the group design strategy is the mean or average outcome of experimental manipulation. The mean is the basic ingredient of all inferential statistical analyses. For Fisher, it was the average yield of a plot treated in some manner that mattered. An individual plant's yield was not of much interest or concern. The same is true of the modern day group treatment researcher. Unlike in the single-subject design, it is the mean group performance that matters the most, not how an individual in a group performs or reacts to treatment.

Statistical Significance

When a statistical analysis is performed on group experimental data, the meaning of the resulting outcome (such as the *F* ratio of analysis of variance) may not be clear. Correct interpretation of inferential statistics required an additional development: the concept of statistical significance. For example, does a given *F* ratio suggest that treatment indeed was effective in the sense that the results could not have been due to chance variations? Significance tests help answer such questions and thus help interpret the meaning of statistical tests. Therefore, **statistical significance** is present when the observed differences in the performances of the experimental and control groups are probably due to treatment (systematic variance) and not chance (random variance). To put it differently, statistical significance of observations based on a sample suggests that the probability of sample statistics being a true estimation of the population parameters is high. Note that the statements of significance are expressed in terms of probability, not certainty.

Statistical significance is typically expressed in levels that suggest different probabilities. Historically, statisticians have adopted two levels of significance: .05 or .01; Fisher was the first to suggest the .05 level (Cochran, 1980). Investigators generally choose one of the two levels, although other levels may be chosen as well. Each statistic is reported as being significant at the chosen level. For instance, when a statistical test is said to be significant at .05 level, it means that there is a 5% chance that the results of the experiment are due to chance and not treatment. Alternatively, it means that there is a 95% chance that results are due to treatment. Note that such statements are based on potential replications and repeated sampling from the same population. In other words, it means that if the study were to be repeated 100 times, each time drawing a different random sample from the same population, the probability of obtaining similar results is 95% in the case of a .05 significance level. A more stringent .01 level of significance means that the results are likely to obtained on 99% of replications.

The adopted level of significance helps evaluate the researcher's hypothesis about cause–effect relations among variables or the effects of treatment or teaching methods. Unlike in the single-subject research strategy, the group design strategy typically involves testing a hypothesis about the nature of the relationship being investigated.

Hypothesis Testing

Consistent with Fisher's advocacy, most group design researchers test hypotheses about the cause–effect relations being tested in experiments. The statistical analyses and the levels of significance described so far are all designed to test hypotheses about the nature of relationship between events examined. When an experiment is performed with two groups and the posttest means of the experimental and control groups differ by some value, two potential explanations may be offered. One is that the observed difference (usually a degree of improvement in the treatment group) may entirely be due to chance and sampling errors. This would then mean that the treatment had no effect. This potential outcome is anticipated in all experiments and expressed in the form of a null hypothesis at the outset. A **null hypothesis,** or the statistical hypothesis, is a statement that asserts that the manipulated independent variable will have no effect on the dependent variable; any difference observed on the posttests of the two groups is due to chance and sampling errors.

An alternative outcome of an experiment—actually a hoped-for outcome—is that the treatment, and no other variable, produced the difference between the two groups: The treatment indeed was effective. This is the **research hypothesis,** which asserts that the planned treatment will be effective. The investigator hopes to sustain the research hypothesis and reject the null via the evidence collected by the planned experiment. Fisher was first to suggest that investigators should state the null hypothesis and then try to reject it by statistical analysis and significance tests. Fisher asserted that "Every experiment may be said to exist only in order to give facts a chance of disproving the null hypothesis" (1951, p. 16). Although this is a questionable assertion because it can be countered that experiments exist to reveal functional relations between phenomena, the idea that experiments are designed to reject the null is now an established practice in group treatment research (see Chapter 3 for an opposing view).

Acceptance of the null hypothesis (the treatment is ineffective) obviously implies that the research hypothesis is false; that is, treatment was ineffective and will be ineffective for the population as well. Rejection of the null hypothesis (the treatment is effective) means that the treatment indeed had an effect in the sample and is likely to have the same or similar effect in the population as well. Because nothing is absolutely certain in science, there is always a chance that the rejection of one hypothesis in favor of the other might be an error. False acceptance of the research hypothesis or false acceptance of the null are the two kinds of errors, known as Type I and Type II errors.

Type I error occurs when the treatment was ineffective, but the researcher concluded that it was effective by rejecting the null hypothesis. In this case, the null hypothesis is true, but the researcher mistakenly rejected it. In Type I error, observed differences are really due to chance, not to treatment. **Type II error** occurs when the treatment was effective, but the researcher concluded that it was not. In this case, the researcher accepted the null hypothesis when it should have been rejected. In Type II error, observed differences are due to the treatment, not to chance, but the investigator interprets them as due to chance. In essence, mistaken rejection of the null is Type I error and mistaken acceptance of the null is Type II error. Conversely, mistaken acceptance of the research hypothesis is Type I error and mistaken rejection of the same is Type II error. Type I error is avoided when a valid null is accepted and Type II error is avoided when an invalid null is rejected. Levels of significance described previously help avoid these errors.

STATISTICS VERSUS RESEARCH DESIGNS

Although group designs are highly statistical in nature, it should be clear that research designs and statistics are not the same. Unfortunately, many books that purportedly deal with research designs do not describe experimental designs to any significant extent. Instead, they describe statistical analyses of data generated by group designs. It is not uncommon for statistical texts to promote the ubiquitous analysis of variance as a research method or design.

This practice promotes the mistaken notion that statistics means research designs.

One should remember that statistics is neither research nor research design but rather a method of analyzing certain kinds of data. McCall cogently made this point as early as 1923, stating that "there are excellent books and courses of instruction dealing with the statistical manipulation of experimental data, but there is little help to be found on the *methods of securing adequate and proper data* [italics added] to which to apply statistical procedures" (p. 23). Designs are methods of collecting adequate data, group designs are only one set of methods, and statistics are but one method of analyzing research data.

The approach taken in this chapter is based on another classic in the field of experimental designs as they are applied in psychology, education, and medicine: Campbell and Stanley's *Experimental and Quasi-Experimental Designs for Research* (1960). This slim volume has helped standardize the thinking on various design strategies and terminology and the overall schemes of describing them.

COMMON CHARACTERISTICS OF GROUP DESIGNS

As noted, the group design strategy, also known as the between-groups strategy, requires the formation of groups on the basis of randomization. Theoretically and ideally, the investigator first identifies a population of potential participants, all of whom are accessible and willing to participate in the study, although this situation usually is not realized in human participants. The required number of participants is then randomly drawn from the population—meaning that each participant has an equal chance of being selected for the study. Once the participants are randomly selected, they are then randomly assigned to the different groups of the study.

The logic of the group design requires that the groups formed for the study be equal on all relevant variables at the beginning of an experiment. This is sometimes referred to as the sampling equivalence of groups. Then the treatment is applied to the experimental group and withheld from the control group. If, as a result of this experimental operation, the groups differ in their performance, the difference is attributed to the independent variable because that was, presumably, the only difference between the groups.

Well-controlled group designs have at least two equivalent groups: the experimental and the control groups. However, an uncontrolled (preexperimental) design may have only one group that receives treatment. Some advanced and complex designs can have more than two groups, and a specially defined control group can receive treatment. As noted in Chapter 4, randomized clinical trials in medicine often include control groups that receive a standard treatment compared against experimental groups that receive new treatments.

In a majority of group designs, investigators measure the dependent variable only on two occasions: once before the independent variable is introduced (pretest) and once after (posttest). The difference between the pretest and posttest scores is an important element of a statistical analysis.

As noted earlier, group designs that have representative samples attempt to establish inferential generality. Whether this is justified is somewhat controversial, and I will address this issue in a later section. In any case, group designs are not expected to help extend the conclusions from a random sample to a single or a few specific individuals. In other words, they do not have logical generality.

Since the publication of D. T. Campbell and Stanley (1966), it is customary for researchers to use diagrams with abbreviations to represent group research designs. For the sake of consistency and clarity, the same system will be used in this chapter in representing various group designs. In these diagrams, the experimental and control groups are represented with E and C, respectively. The measurement of the dependent variable is represented by O, which stands for observation. Pretests and posttests may be indicated by O_1 and O_2, assuming that there were only those two measures in a study. The treatment variable is indicated by X, and the random participant selection by R. In some books, the dependent variable may be represented by Y. In science and mathematics, X is the cause and Y is the effect. The Y is said to be a function of X, which means that X is the cause of Y.

It also is an accepted practice to describe group designs as preexperimental designs, true experimental designs, quasi-experimental designs, and correlational designs. In different books and articles, however, the reader will find differing and sometimes confusing terms in the description of the same research designs. When appropriate, multiple names of the same design will be pointed out.

PREEXPERIMENTAL DESIGNS

Preexperimental designs are commonly used in clinical, educational, social, and psychological research. Although these designs have serious limitations, they are eminently practical. In spite of their limitations, preexperimental designs are useful in applied settings. They often precede experimental research on a treatment.

Several preexperimental group designs are available. Three most commonly used preexperimental designs are the one-shot case study, the one-group pretest–posttest design, and the static-group comparison.

One-Shot Case Study

The one-shot case study is a design in which the treatment is applied to a known clinical group with only a posttest. For instance, to find out the effects of a language treatment procedure, a clinician may select some children who have been diagnosed to have a language disorder and apply the selected treatment procedure. The clinician in this case does not have pretest results and simply assumes that the diagnosis of a language disorder provides a sufficient basis to evaluate the results of treatment. Also missing is a control group. The design is shown in Figure 8.1.

The posttest may contain some measure of the children's language obtained either through a standardized test or a language sample. If the posttest shows no evidence of a language disorder in the group, the clinician may conclude that the treatment was effective.

The greatest weakness of this design is its total lack of control. The absence of a control group makes it difficult to rule out the influence of factors other than the treatment. There is no valid basis to evaluate the changes documented by the posttest because there was no pretest. Whether the children prior to the treatment were indeed not able to produce the language behaviors that were measured on the posttest remains speculative. In fact, the absence of a pretest makes it impossible to say whether there were any changes due to treatment at all. The clinician comes to some sort of conclusion because of the common knowledge that children with language disorders do not produce certain language behaviors, and if they do after treatment, the treatment, therefore, must have been effective.

The one-shot case study is not useful in making valid judgments regarding the effectiveness of treatment variables. In spite of the logical appeal of the treatment program and thoroughness of the posttest, investigators cannot demonstrate a functional relation between the treatment and the target behaviors. Of the factors that affect internal validity, history, maturation, and statistical regression typically invalidate the results of one-shot case studies. Depending on the particular study, other sources of internal invalidity may also be involved.

One-Group Pretest–Posttest Design

The one-group pretest–posttest design is similar to the one-shot case study in that there is no control group. A single group is used in the study. Typical case studies in clinical sciences follow this design format. However, unlike the previous design, this one includes a pretest of the dependent vari-

X	O
Treatment	Posttest

Figure 8.1. The one-shot case study. Note that the design lacks a control group and pretests.

ables. The treatment is introduced after the pretest, and a posttest is conducted to evaluate the effects of the treatment. The difference between the pretest and posttest scores is attributed to the effects of the independent variable. The design is illustrated in Figure 8.2.

To continue with our hypothetical example of language treatment research discussed under the previous design, the clinician using the one-group pretest–posttest design measures the language behaviors of children serving as participants in the study both before and after the treatment. These measures help document the changes in language behaviors that may have taken place during the course of the study.

The results of the one-group pretest–posttest design can be analyzed through statistical methods. The most frequently used technique is the parametric t test for correlated samples. Nonparametric tests may also be used in analyzing the results. Two such tests are the sign test and the Wilcoxon matched-pairs signed-ranks test (Huck, Cormier, & Bounds, 1974).

Although the design is an improvement over the one-shot case study, it still is not able to generate data that can support a functional relation between the changes in the dependent variable and the independent variable. The clinician in our example can be reasonably sure that the language behaviors of children studied did (or did not) change over the course of the experiment. However, he or she will not be able to conclude that the observed changes (the differences between O_1 and O_2) are due to the language treatment program. The design cannot rule out the influence of history, maturation, testing, instrumentation, statistical regression, and differential participant attrition. In essence, the design lacks internal validity.

There is no assurance that a change in the parents' behavior, a new language stimulation program started by the classroom teacher, an unspecified biological change taking place within the children, or a combination of all of these factors was not responsible for improved language in children. Similarly, the pretest itself may have introduced some changes in the language behaviors, or the testing instruments may have been unreliable. Although statistical regression may not be a problem with language disorders, the design itself is not capable of ruling it out. Differential participant attrition can certainly be an additional problem. The posttest scores may be better than the pretest scores simply because more severely affected children may have dropped out during the course of the experiment. However, because the design uses only one group, participant selection bias is not a factor.

O_1	X	O_2
Pretest	Treatment	Posttest

Figure 8.2. The one-group pretest–posttest design. Note that the design lacks a control group.

Static-Group Comparison

Another frequently used preexperimental design is known as the static-group comparison. This design uses two existing groups: one that has already received treatment and another that has not. Because the design does not require the formation of new groups, it is called the static-group comparison method. However, the design does not have pretests of the dependent variables. The design is diagrammed in Figure 8.3. The difference in the dependent variable between the group that has received treatment and the group that has not is attributed to the treatment. For example, a clinician may evaluate a stuttering treatment program offered by a large clinic. The persons with stuttering who just completed the treatment program may be compared with those who are yet to receive the same treatment. No pretest measures are obtained for the "control" group because none are available for the experimental group, which has already received the treatment. The static-group comparison also is involved when the academic performance of students who have gone to junior colleges is compared with the performance of those who started at 4-year colleges. Similarly, children with repaired cleft palate who have had speech therapy may be compared with those who have not. Some measure of speech intelligibility may be the dependent variable. Then the better speech intelligibility found in the experimental group may be attributed to previously received speech therapy.

The results of the static-group comparison are analyzed through a parametric *t* test. Such nonparametric tests as the Mann-Whitney U test and the median test also may be used. A chi-square test also is appropriate (Huck, Cormier, & Bounds, 1974).

In static-group comparisons, the group that does not receive treatment does not help control extraneous variables. The major problem of internal validity faced by this design is that of participant selection bias. The design does not require random selection or assignment of participants into the two groups. Therefore, there is no assurance of random sampling of the two groups before the treatment. For example, people with mild stuttering may have gone through the treatment program, whereas those in the control group may have had more severe stuttering. The experimental group of children with repaired cleft may have had good speech intelligibility all along. The second major problem is that of differential participant attrition.

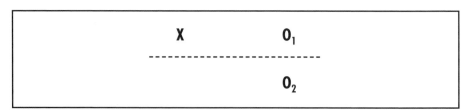

Figure 8.3. The static-group comparison design. Note that the design uses existing groups (not randomly formed) and lacks pretests.

Even when the two groups are identical to begin with, they may become different not because of treatment but because of participant attrition. As such, the static-group comparison cannot rule out the influence of extraneous variables and, therefore, cannot help establish functional relations between variables.

Summary and Summative Evaluation of Preexperimental Designs

Preexperimental designs are those that do not have adequate controls to rule out extraneous independent variables. Consequently, they lack internal validity. The one-shot case study, the one-group pretest–posttest design, and the static-group comparison are three commonly used preexperimental designs.

Generally, studies that use one of the preexperimental designs are retrospective. The designs are frequently used in clinical sciences. The preexperimental designs often are justified on the basis of their practicality and clinical relevance. Studies that use these designs are typically considered to be exploratory. They can help identify potential causal relations. In clinical sciences, case studies and one-group pretest–posttest designs are useful in generating suggestions for studies involving more rigorous designs.

Because of their limitations, investigators using a preexperimental design must exercise caution in interpreting their results. The investigators should point out that any hint of causation is just that—only a hint that should be confirmed by more powerful designs. Readers of studies based on preexperimental designs should exercise similar caution in their evaluation of those studies. The readers should be especially careful not to accept an author's conclusions when they seem to disregard the limitations of a preexperimental design.

TRUE EXPERIMENTAL DESIGNS

As noted in Chapter 7, an experimental design should help establish a functional relation between an independent and a dependent variable. Among group designs, true experimental designs can do this by ruling out many of the potential extraneous variables. Therefore, true experimental designs are those that reveal a reasonably clear cause–effect relation between the manipulated independent variable and the measured dependent variable. Therefore, the designs have internal validity.

Most investigators who do not consider alternatives to the group design strategy claim that a single study with a true experimental group design can have external validity as well. As discussed in Chapter 4, such a claim is questionable because of the nature of generality and the limits of the probability theory.

As noted in Chapter 4, true experimental designs within the group strategy rule out the influence of extraneous variables, mainly through the use of experimental and control groups. The two groups are formed on the basis of the preferred randomization or its alternative, matching. See Chapter 4 for details on the conceptual background, methods, and potential problems.

I shall describe several true experimental designs. Some of the true experimental designs involve a single treatment (independent) variable, whereas others involve multiple treatment variables. The pretest–posttest control group design, the posttest-only control group design, and the Solomon four-group design (Solomon, 1949) involve a single treatment variable. On the other hand, multigroup pretest–posttest design, multigroup posttest-only design, and the several types of factorial designs make it possible to evaluate the effects of multiple independent variables. Because all true experimental designs are expected to use randomization to achieve sampling equivalence between groups, the diagrams of each design shows R for randomization, but it may be substituted with M for matching.

Pretest–Posttest Control Group Design

The pretest–posttest control group design is prototypical of the true experimental group designs. It also is the simplest. This design elegantly illustrates the logic and the strategy of the group designs. It requires two groups: an experimental group, which receives treatment, and a control group, which does not.

The design is based on the logic that to assess the effects of an independent variable, the only difference between the groups shall be that variable. Therefore, the investigator should start with two groups that are very similar if not identical. If the groups are different on some known or unknown variables other than the treatment, then the effect of that treatment variable cannot be experimentally isolated. In essence, achieving the equivalence of the experimental and control groups is the most critical task in forming the groups for this design. This task may be accomplished with randomization or matching.

The pretest–posttest control group design is illustrated in Figure 8.4. The diagram shows that the participants were randomly selected (R) from a population and were randomly assigned to the two groups. The experimental group (E) is exposed to the treatment variable (X), whereas the control group (C) is not. The dependent variable is measured (O) twice in each group, once before and once after the experimental group has received the treatment. This basic arrangement permits a relatively unambiguous evaluation of the effects of most independent variables.

The typical pretest–posttest control group design has only one treatment variable and a true control group that does not receive treatment. However, randomized clinical trials in medicine use variations of this de-

E	R	O_1	X	O_2
C	R	O_1		O_2

Figure 8.4. The pretest–posttest control group design. Note that this is the prototype of group experimental designs, with randomly selected and assigned groups.

sign. In one such variation, both the groups receive treatment, but the treatments are different. One of the two treatments is a new one, and the other is an older, well-established, and already evaluated treatment. Investigators in this case evaluate a new treatment against an older treatment; the research question is whether the new treatment is at least as good as the older treatment.

In yet another variation of the basic pretest–posttest control group design, the investigator may have three groups. One may receive the new treatment being evaluated, the other may receive a placebo (see Chapter 4 for details), and the third may receive a standard treatment. In all these variations, the main concern is to establish the effectiveness of the new treatment. The effects of the standard or common treatment are already known and not under investigation. Therefore, groups that receive a standard treatment may technically be called control groups (along with, of course, the placebo group).

In the analysis of the results of the basic version of the design, it is important to avoid some common mistakes. In one of the mistaken analyses, the pretest and posttest scores of the experimental group may be compared with one *t* test, and the scores of the two tests of the control group may be compared with a different *t* test. These two comparisons are based on the assumption that if the experimental group's posttest mean is significantly higher than the pretest mean, and the control group's pretest and posttest means are comparable, then the effect of the independent variable has been demonstrated. Actually, this analysis does not involve a direct comparison of the performance of the two groups. Sometimes investigators compare the two pretest scores with a *t* test and the two posttest scores with another *t* test. This also is an inappropriate analysis of the results because it does not adequately reflect changes in the dependent variable across the conditions of an experiment.

The correct method of analysis involves either a gain score procedure or an analysis of covariance. In the former, each participant's pretest scores are subtracted from the posttest scores to obtain the gain scores. The individual gain scores are then averaged to obtain two mean scores, one for each of the two groups. The two means are then compared with either the parametric independent samples *t* test or the nonparametric Mann-Whitney U test.

A median test may also be used to compare the two means. An analysis of covariance is a more complex and more efficient method of analysis and is preferred by many investigators.

The basic version of the design, which has a control group that does not receive treatment, is able to rule out extraneous factors relative to history and maturation. Events in the lives of the participants (history) or maturational changes that may affect the dependent variable are assumed to be common to the two groups. Therefore, significant changes in the dependent variable, if shown by the experimental group, cannot be attributed to history or maturation.

Regression to the mean can occur, but to the extent that the groups were equal to begin with, this phenomenon will be held constant across the two groups. For example, if stuttering rate returns to the mean level in the experimental group some time after the pretest, the same thing can be expected to happen in the control group also. Similarly ruled out is the factor of participant selection as long as the samples were drawn, or at least assigned, randomly. However, if participants are matched, then none of the sources of participant selection bias can be ruled out (D. T. Campbell & Stanley, 1966).

Testing as a factor of internal validity is controlled for in the design because both the groups were pretested; therefore, changes due to measurement of the dependent variable should be common across the two groups. When the same instruments are used in obtaining all measures of the variables in both the groups, the effects of the instrumentation also are not of concern.

Differential participant attrition can be a problem in the pretest–posttest control group design. The experimenter, however, would know whether attrition could have affected the results. Any dropout of participants from the experimental group is suggestive of this potential problem. It is difficult to determine the nature or extent of the effect of attrition when it is known to have occurred, however. Unfortunately, the effects of participant attrition are "commonly swept under the rug" (D. T. Campbell & Stanley, 1966, p. 15). The loss of participants during the course of the experiment may be reported but not handled in the data analysis. This mistake is easy to commit in a group design in which, despite some participant loss, the investigator seems to have some data to be analyzed.

The external validity of this, or in fact any design, is a different matter. Most textbooks tend to advise that as long as a random sample has been drawn from the population, the results should have generality. As noted in Chapter 4, clinical treatment studies—including randomized clinical trials—typically do not select participants randomly. Because of the requirement of informed consent, all participants in current treatment research are self-selected. In the absence of random selection, there is no generality without replication.

Another problem with the assumption of generality of pretest–posttest control group design is that it takes into consideration only inferential generality. There is no empirical basis to assume that other kinds of generality, which are equally if not more important, are assured by even the best random sample. For instance, generality across responses, settings, and experimenters is not known unless the experiment is repeated with different responses, under different settings, and by different investigators. The position advocated here, and expanded in Chapters 4 and 10, is that generality is a function of replication; therefore, a single study using even the best of the experimental designs of either the group or the single-subject strategy does not assure it.

Posttest-Only Control Group Design

In the posttest-only control group design, neither the experimental nor the control group participants are given a pretest. After randomly selecting and assigning participants to the two groups, the treatment variable is applied to the experimental group. At the completion of the experimental treatment, the two groups are given a posttest. The design is illustrated in Figure 8.5.

A pretest is considered indispensable by many investigators. Therefore, this design is not used very frequently. However, D. T. Campbell and Stanley (1966) suggested that pretests are not at all necessary when the participants are selected randomly. Therefore, they strongly recommend this design and consider it superior to the pretest–posttest control group design. It certainly avoids the pretest–posttest sensitization to treatment because there is no pretest. The design can also control for other sources that affect internal validity, except for differential participant attrition.

The justification for this design rests heavily on the adequacy of randomization. The argument is that when participants are selected and assigned randomly, the groups are equal at the beginning. The pretest is only a confirmation of this fact. However, if pretests are expected to create problems, or for some reason are not practical, then they can be avoided without loss of scientific rigor because the groups are comparable anyway. A statistically significant difference in the posttest scores of the two groups should be due to the experimental variable only. An analysis of such a difference usually involves a t test.

E	R	X	0
C	R		0

Figure 8.5. The posttest-only control group design. Note that the design lacks pretests and assumes that pretest scores would have been similar to the posttest scores of the control group.

If the probability theory and random procedures were as practical as they are elegant, there would be no problem with this design. However, in most clinical sciences that need to evaluate the effects of treatments in persons with various diseases and disorders, randomization is the least practical of the procedures of participant selection. In other designs, the pretest will at least let the investigator know that the groups are not equal. When there is no pretest, the experimenter has no way of checking sampling equivalence of the two groups. The design places too heavy a burden on the theory of random samples and too great a confidence in its practicality. Unfortunately, the probability theory promises much at the level of theory but delivers less at the level of clinical research.

Solomon Four-Group Design

The four-group design was originally proposed in 1949 by Solomon and quickly became one of the most prestigious of the group designs used in social and psychological research. Solomon was the first to formally recognize the interaction of pretest sensitization and treatment as a potential threat to external validity. However, this problem must have been implicitly acknowledged by previous investigators because the design without a pretest was already available. Solomon proposed a design that provided not only an opportunity for the interaction to take place but also a method to measure its magnitude.

The four-group design is considered the most appropriate strategy for investigation when the pretest sensitization is expected to interact with the independent variable (see Figure 8.6). It is clear from the diagram that the design is actually a combination of two previously described designs: the pretest–posttest control group and the posttest-only control group. The

E	R	O_1	X	O_2
C	R	O_1		O_2
E	R		X	O
C	R			O

Figure 8.6. The Solomon four-group design. Note that the design has two experimental groups and two control groups; one experimental group and one control group receive no pretests.

design has two experimental and two control groups. One of the experimental groups receives both the pretest and the posttest. The second experimental group is not pretested; it receives only the posttest. One of the two control groups receives both tests, whereas the second control group receives only the posttest.

The design controls for all the factors that affect internal validity. Therefore, the design can evaluate treatment effects. In addition, it also demonstrates the presence and the extent of pretest sensitization as a threat to external validity. A difference between the means of the pretested groups and an absence of such a difference between the means of groups not pretested reveals the effects of sensitization. Also, from a descriptive standpoint, if the pretest sensitizes the participants, the treatment effects are larger in the first experimental group than in the second. Because the first experimental group receives both tests whereas the second receives only the posttest, the performance of the second group is free of pretest sensitization. The two control groups also indicate any effects of the pretest on the dependent variable (a factor of internal validity). If the pretest has a direct effect on the dependent variable, the control group receiving both tests behaves differently than the one receiving only the posttest.

It has been recognized that analysis of the results of the Solomon design is difficult. A single statistical technique that can simultaneously analyze all the observations of the design is not available. Therefore, the pretest scores are ignored and a two-way analysis of variance is performed. This analysis is arranged in terms of the scores of participants who have been pretested/not pretested and treated/untreated.

The design, though considered ideal in many respects, is of limited practical and paradigmatic value. It presents the immense practical problem of finding a population from which four groups of participants can be drawn randomly. Because it is a combination of two designs, it is about twice as hard to implement as any of the basic group designs. Therefore, there are hardly any clinical treatment studies in which the four-group design was used. The design is simply not used often even in nonclinical social research where it is more practical.

It can also be argued, in an admittedly controversial manner, that the design offers a methodological solution for the problem of paradigm. Obviously, the design is needed only when pretest sensitization is a consideration. It is a consideration mostly in research that addresses reactive measures such as attitudes and opinions. In other words, the design is needed when the dependent variables are weak and at best offer indirect measures. For example, the attitude of a group of speech–language pathologists toward people who stutter in public schools can be measured, as several researchers have done. One would assume that this type of research is done to determine whether clinicians are unlikely to treat people who stutter because of their negative attitudes or whether, when they do treat people who stutter, the outcome may not be favorable, again because of negative attitudes. Or the researcher may wish to change the clinicians' negative attitudes with an informational package (the treatment variable). In this second instance, the researcher would need the four-group design. Incidentally, much of the research on attitudes in communicative disorders is done only to uncover negative attitudes; hardly anything is done about them. A conceptually different approach to the issue is to find out how many people who stutter are not receiving treatment in a given setting and then proceed to find out why.

The finding that some clinicians have a negative attitude toward stuttering is hardly illuminating. It is probably better to look into the clinicians' training and expertise in the treatment of stuttering deficiencies in which may have originated a side effect described by some as negative attitudes. In essence, a conceptual solution to the problem of reactive measures is to try to avoid such dependent variables in favor of those that are less reactive, more stable, and perhaps more meaningful. Obviously, those who think that attitudes and opinions are important variables would disagree with this suggestion.

DESIGNS TO EVALUATE MULTIPLE TREATMENTS

The previous text described group designs to evaluate the effects of a single treatment. In many cases, though, the effects of more than one treatment may be of interest. In clinical sciences, it often is necessary to determine whether one treatment is more effective than the other. This generally is the question of relative effects (as opposed to absolute or independent effects) of treatments.

Group design strategy offers some excellent options to study the relative effects of two or more treatments. I will describe two designs that are an extension of the designs presented earlier: multigroup pretest–posttest design and multigroup posttest-only design. I also will describe a separate class of designs, known as *factorial designs*, which help evaluate multiple treatment effects and their interactions.

Multigroup Pretest–Posttest Design

In the evaluation of two or more treatment techniques, the basic pretest–posttest control group design may be extended to include the needed number of additional groups. Theoretically, several treatment procedures can be studied in multiple groups within a single design. However, extensions are limited by the ease with which the groups can be formed; each treatment built into the study will need an additional group. Also, data analysis will become increasingly complex with the addition of groups. Even an extension of the basic design by a single additional treatment can introduce a considerable amount of complexity.

The multigroup pretest–posttest design can evaluate the relative effects of selected treatment techniques. In other words, the design can answer the question of whether one treatment is more effective than the other, and in the case of three or more treatments, the design can help evaluate their progressively increasing or decreasing effects.

It may be noted that the control group is placed within parentheses to suggest that it is an optional arrangement. In many cases, the researcher who designs studies on relative effects of treatments already has data that demonstrate their absolute effects. Each treatment will have been compared with a no-treatment control group. Therefore, when one asks questions of relative effects, it is not necessary to have a control group. In randomized clinical trials, questions of relative effects are often researched without having completed research on absolute effects (Hegde, 2002). An added control group in any case will help evaluate both the relative and the absolute effects of the treatment techniques and will improve the study's internal validity as well.

A multigroup design that can evaluate the relative effects of three treatments is illustrated in Figure 8.7. The design affords a chance to determine the most and the least effective of the three techniques. Research involving this kind of design is highly desirable in areas where multiple treatment techniques are recommended by different clinicians to treat the same disorder. Such therapeutic diversity exists in the treatment of most disorders of communication.

In medicine, randomized clinical trials often employ this design. In such trials, one of the experimental groups may receive a new drug whose effect is being evaluated for the first time. The other experimental groups may receive more established treatments to see which one produces greater benefits for the patients. More often, the control group will receive a placebo,

E	R	O_1	X_1	O_2
E	R	O_1	X_2	O_2
E	R	O_1	X_3	O_2
(C	R	O_1		O_2)

Figure 8.7. The multigroup pretest–posttest design. Note that the design can evaluate the relative effects of multiple treatments and may include an optional control group.

in which case, the study is called a placebo-controlled randomized clinical trial. Placebo controls are relatively uncommon in behavioral and educational research although a new method can always be compared against an established treatment or teaching method.

The results of the design can be analyzed with a variety of statistical techniques, including analysis of covariance, analysis of variance based on gain scores for each participant (see pretest–posttest control group design), or a Lindquist Type I repeated measures analysis of variance. Most of these techniques of analysis simply indicate whether there is a significant difference in the performances of the groups. Therefore, when a significant difference between the groups is evident, additional analysis involving pairwise group comparisons is necessary.

Multigroup Posttest-Only Design

The multigroup posttest-only design is an extension of the posttest-only control group design presented earlier. In this design, two or more treatments are evaluated for their relative effectiveness in the absence of pretests. A diagram of the design with three treatments is presented in Figure 8.8. As in the original design, the participants are selected and assigned to the groups randomly, resulting in equivalent groups that need to be retested. Each group is exposed to a different treatment. The diagram shows an optional control group.

The results of the multigroup posttest-only design can be analyzed with a one-way analysis of variance or with nonparametric statistics such as the Kruskal-Wallis and chi-square tests.

The design shares the same strengths and weaknesses as the posttest-only control group design. It is needed when pretest sensitization is ex-

E	R	X_1	0
E	R	X_2	0
E	R	X_3	0
(C	R		0)

Figure 8.8. The multigroup posttest-only design. Note that the design lacks pretest scores, which are assumed to be similar across groups because of randomly drawn and assigned samples.

pected to interact with the treatment variable. Unless the investigator is sure that the groups were equal to begin with, there is no assurance of internal validity. The design is as good as the random procedure in practice.

FACTORIAL DESIGNS

Factorial designs also are true experimental designs. They are an excellent example of research strategies based mostly on the method of analysis of variance that Fisher developed in his agricultural research. Most of the factorial designs, too, were originally described by Fisher (1925, 1942). Fisher discovered that instead of applying multiple treatments (e.g., different levels of fertilization or watering) to multiple agricultural plots in a systematic manner, applying treatments across randomly selected plots reduced errors of observation. This discovery has led to factorial designs which are now used in educational, medical, social, and behavioral research.

Analysis of variance is a collection of related techniques, the complex forms of which can be used in the simultaneous analysis of two or more variables and their interactions. In the terminology of factorial designs, a **factor** is the same as an independent variable (teaching or treatment).

Factorial designs have two or more independent variables. The independent variables may be either active, assigned, or a combination of the two. It may be recalled that active independent variables are manipulated by the experimenter, whereas assigned variables may affect the results but cannot be manipulated. Assigned variables are typically participant characteristics such as age, gender, education, intelligence, socioeconomic status, and the severity of various disorders (see Chapter 3 for details). A factorial design that includes only assigned variables is not an experimental study, but belongs to the ex post facto category. Therefore, that type of design will not be discussed here. An experimental factorial design will have at least one active independent variable. Many factorial designs have a combination of active and assigned variables.

An independent variable used in a factorial design has a minimum of two different levels. For this reason, certain factorial designs are referred to as **treatment-by-levels** designs. The levels of an active (manipulated) independent variable may be the presence or the absence of it (treatment versus no treatment). Two techniques of treatment can also be considered levels. Furthermore, a technique whose intensity is varied can create different levels. For instance, in randomized clinical trials in medicine, different dosages of the same medicine will create levels.

As a further example from special education, an investigator may wish to evaluate the manual and oral methods of teaching individuals who are hard of hearing. In this case, the treatment variable has two levels, which are actually two separate treatments. A third level can be created by having a control group that is not exposed to either of the two teaching methods. Another clinician may wish to test regular (twice a week) versus intensive (five times a week) scheduling of clients while using a single treatment procedure. The two schedules create two levels.

An assigned variable also typically has two or more levels. For example, individuals who are hard of hearing and deaf selected for a certain treatment evaluation may be grouped according to the degree of hearing loss: mild, moderate, and severe. These three categories are the three levels of the assigned variable. Most other assigned variables such as age, gender, socioeconomic class, and intelligence have two or more levels.

Within the group design strategy, factorial designs are the primary techniques of assessing the interaction of two or more variables. An **interaction** is an effect that emerges when two or more independent variables are combined to produce an effect that is different from the separate or independent effect of each variable combined. For instance, drug A may effect a 20% reduction in some symptoms whereas drug B may effect a 30% reduction. But when the two are administered in combination, a 90% reduction in symptoms (not merely the additive 50%) may be observed. The increased magnitude of the effect, which goes beyond the mere additive effect, is known as interaction.

Interaction may be positive or negative. The example just given illustrates positive interaction in which the combination of treatments enhance each other's effects. Negative interaction is the antagonistic effects of one treatment on the other in a combination of treatments. In negative interaction, one variable may suppress the positive effects of another variable or may even induce harmful effects as in certain drug combinations that produce toxicity.

It is believed that most phenomena studied are multiply determined in an interactive fashion. In other words, most events have several causes, which in various combinations produce the effects normally seen. The designs that manipulate single variables at a time actually simplify the phenomenon for the sake of clearer analysis. Designs that permit the manipulation of multiple variables are more powerful. They also better approximate reality.

The factorial design also is based on the random procedure. The participants should be selected and assigned to the groups randomly. Once the participants are selected randomly, however, only the active variables permit random assignment. In the previous example, the clinician may be able to assign participants to the treatment and control conditions but not to either mild, moderate, or severe categories of hearing loss. Each participant's hearing loss, not the power of randomization, determines whether he or she is assigned to one or the other category of severity.

There are several factorial designs; some are simpler than the others. The complexity of a factorial design is directly related to the number of independent variables (assigned and active) and the number of levels of each of those variables.

Randomized Blocks Design

A 1920s invention of Fisher (1942), a randomized blocks design has at least one active variable and one assigned variable. It can have more than two variables, but one of the variables should be assigned. If each variable has two levels, then it is the basic randomized design, which often is represented as the 2 × 2 (two-by-two) design. Such a design also may be referred to as a two-way factorial design. Teaching or treatment methods are examples of active variables. The clinician or the educator can directly manipulate those methods. The participants' level of intelligence or the severity of a disorder, when categorized into levels, creates nonmanipulable assigned variables.

A 2 × 2 randomized blocks design would have four cells or conditions; a 2 × 3 design would have six. A 2 × 3 randomized blocks design is illustrated in Figure 8.9. The design has two independent variables, one manipulated treatment variable with two levels (manual and oral teaching methods) and one assigned variable with three levels (mild, moderate, and severe hearing loss). To conduct such a study, a population of individuals who have mild, moderate, and severe hearing loss (defined in some operational manner) are first identified. Next, a certain number of individuals is randomly drawn from each level of hearing loss in what is known as a stratified random sample (see Chapter 4). The samples are then assigned to the teaching methods as shown in Figure 8.9.

Each level of the assigned variable is considered a block from which a random sample is drawn. The design can include a control group that does not receive treatment. The participants of the control group should also

	Levels of Hearing Loss		
Treatment	**Mild**	**Moderate**	**Severe**
Manual			
Oral			

Figure 8.9. A 2 × 3 randomized blocks design. Note that the design includes two active (treatment) variables and three levels of participant characteristics; each cell represents a certain number of participants with defined characteristics.

represent the levels of the assigned variable. Other research examples for which the randomized blocks design is appropriate include the effects of two aphasia treatment programs administered to persons who have had a stroke during the past month versus those who had a stroke 6 months ago (a 2×2 design). In medicine, the effects of two new drugs may be evaluated for their effects in women whose breast cancer was diagnosed early compared to those whose cancer was diagnosed late, defined in some operational manner.

Factorial designs can help determine the separate (independent) effects of the treatment methods as well as their interactions. The main effects in an analysis of variance of the results of a factorial design are the effects of the separate treatment variables. In our example, the oral and the manual methods of teaching produce two main effects in the study.

The other important effect the analysis can reveal is the interaction of treatment with participant characteristics. It is possible that the oral method of instruction is most effective with participants who have only a mild hearing loss and that the manual method is more effective for those with severe hearing loss. Individuals with a moderate level of hearing loss may benefit equally from the two procedures. This kind of relation is what is implied in an interaction. Obviously, discovery of such relations is important in offering effective services. When such interactions exist, simpler questions that address the effects of single variables in isolation do not reflect the complexity of the phenomenon under investigation. For example, the question of whether the oral or the manual method of teaching is more effective may not be answered unless the level of hearing loss is taken into consideration.

When the number of variables and their levels are increased, the complexity of the design increases. The need for participants is directly proportional to the number of variables and levels in a factorial study. In the design illustrated in Figure 8.9, there are six cells, and assuming that at least 15 participants to a cell are needed, the investigator will have to find 90 participants to complete the study. A control group, when used, creates a need for additional participants.

Completely Randomized Factorial Design

In the previous design, one of the two factors is active (treatment) and the other assigned (levels of hearing loss). It is possible to design a factorial study in which all the factors are active, however. Such a design is known as the completely randomized factorial design. No assigned variable is included in this type of design. Hence, there is no blocking in a completely randomized factorial design.

It is evident that complete randomization of participants is possible only when all the factors are active. An experimenter cannot assign participants randomly to the experimental conditions on the basis of their gender or intelligence. Participants can be assigned randomly only to treatment conditions that are under the experimenter's control. Another invention of

Fisher (1942), the completely randomized factorial designs use only active variables and do not address issues relative to potential interactions between treatment variables and participant characteristics.

A completely randomized factorial design is illustrated in Figure 8.10. It shows a 2 × 2 design in which two independent variables, both active, are studied. The research question of the example is whether the airflow or the syllable prolongation component of stuttering therapy is more effective and whether the effects depend upon the presence or absence of contingent feedback on participant performance during treatment sessions. Both the forms of treatment and feedback are active; the experimenter controls all of them. The participants are randomly assigned to the conditions of the study. In other words, who receives airflow or prolongation treatment and who receives either of these with or without contingent feedback are decided randomly.

The 2 × 2 design just described would probably need at least 60 participants who stutter, 15 to each condition (the four empty boxes in the diagram). A control group, when used, would require an additional 10 participants. The design can be extended to include other active independent variables. For example, in an educational research study, two methods of teaching mathematical skills to children may be implemented with and without the help of computers, creating a 2 × 2 factorial design.

In a randomized clinical trial in medicine, two drugs may be evaluated at two levels of dosage, creating a 2 × 2 design. In medicine, often a variation of this design involves a combination of two treatments: Group 1 (cell 1) receiving treatment *A*, Group 2 (cell 2) receiving treatment *B*, Group 3 (cell 3) receiving both *A* and *B*, and Group 4 (cell 4) receiving placebo (Byar & Piantadosi, 1985; Freedman & Green, 1990). Although useful in studying the effects of multiple drugs and their interactions, factorial designs are not appropriate when combinations of drugs produce increased

	Contingent Feedback	
	Present	**Absent**
Airflow		
Prolongation		

Figure 8.10. A 2 × 2 completely randomized factorial design. Note that the design includes only active treatment variables; each cell may contain 10 to 15 participants.

toxicity or negative interaction (Lee, Lieberman, Sloand, Piantadosi, & Lipman, 2001).

Factorial designs are among the most powerful of the group designs. They can help answer complex and clinically significant questions. It is a common clinical observation that most treatment procedures do not seem to work equally effectively with all types of participants. Clinicians suspect that to a certain extent the effects of treatment procedures depend upon several participant characteristics, which often reflect other variables. Some of those variables may be related to the client's learning history, the precise nature of the disorder, unsuccessful treatment in the past, and so on. Even such characteristics as gender and socioeconomic class may be a mixture of variables, some of which are external factors in the life of the individual. It is important to know how different variables, including those the clinician calls "treatment," come together to produce the final, desirable effect in different clients. Factorial designs can help answer such important clinical questions.

The problems with factorial designs are mostly practical. Randomization, which is required at some or all levels, creates problems that have been discussed before. Although a factorial design can theoretically handle several variables, the complexity and the need for participants increase in proportion to the number of variables. Finding persons who stutter or have aphasia and are willing to participate in an experimental study in enough numbers to permit random assignment to the various cells of a factorial design is difficult. Clinical conditions that are relatively rare present the same problem with a much greater magnitude. The analysis of results also becomes more and more difficult with increases in the number of variables or their levels. As a result, firm and clear conclusions regarding the interaction between several variables and levels are difficult to offer.

Summary and Summative Evaluation of True Experimental Designs

True experimental designs have a minimum of two groups. The groups are formed on the basis of either randomization or matching. Randomization is preferred because it assures sampling equivalence of the groups on known and unknown variables. In most cases, one group receives the treatment and the other does not. However, it is possible to expose both of the groups to one of two treatments when the purpose is to evaluate the relative effects of those two treatments. Even then, an optional control group that does not receive treatment may be included.

The pretest–posttest control group design is the most prototypical of the true experimental designs. The posttest-only control group design and the Solomon four-group design are the two other true experimental designs that help establish the effects of a single treatment variable. The multigroup pretest–posttest design and the multigroup posttest-only design may be used to evaluate the effects of two or more independent variables. The factorial designs can be used to determine the independent and interactive effects of multiple treatment variables. Factorial designs may have some independent variables that cannot be manipulated, or they may have all manipulable independent variables.

Most true experimental designs have a pretest and a posttest. However, when participants are randomly selected and assigned to the groups of a study, the pretest may not be necessary, as in a multigroup posttest-only design.

True experimental designs, especially the factorial designs, are the most powerful of the group design strategies. When properly implemented, these designs assure internal validity. Through direct and systematic replications, they may also achieve external validity.

From a clinical standpoint, a major limitation of true experimental designs is that it is not always possible to randomly draw participants from particular clinical populations. Also, because of the informed consent requirement, randomly assigned participants may or may not continue in the group to which they are assigned. Therefore, self-selection of participants is the reality of randomized human experiments. Sampling equivalence, therefore, is difficult to achieve in clinical research that uses true experimental group designs. Besides, the group design studies may not allow an extension of results to individual clients. These and other issues have been discussed in Chapter 4 and are addressed again in a later section on group designs in clinical research.

QUASI-EXPERIMENTAL DESIGNS

Quasi-experimental designs are those in which the investigator is not able to exert full control over all the relevant variables and operations. Originally, they were suggested as a means of conducting experiments in natural settings rather than in well-controlled laboratories (D. T. Campbell & Stanley, 1966). In practice, quasi-experimental designs are used whenever practical considerations prevent the use of better (more controlled) designs of research.

Quasi-experimental designs are weaker than true experimental designs because certain control procedures are not used. When studies are conducted in natural settings, it is not always possible to use some of the control procedures, and yet the opportunity for limited experimentation may exist. For example, it may not be possible to draw a random sample of pupils in conducting an experiment on improving teaching methods in an elementary school. Similarly, when a new program of diet or physical exercise for the elderly is initiated in a nursing home, the investigator may not have a chance to select or assign participants randomly. Experimental evaluation of programs in various institutions necessarily uses existing participants and living arrangements. Therefore, some of the quasi-experimental designs do not have groups that are formed especially for the purposes of research. In such cases, the investigators often use already existing natural groups, called *intact groups,* of participants.

Those studies known as field studies are the same as, or very similar to, studies that use quasi-experimental designs. **Field studies** are those done in natural conditions or in less artificial conditions than laboratory studies. They also tend to use natural or intact groups. For this reason, they lack randomization and, as a consequence, lose control over some of the factors that affect internal validity.

Two specific quasi-experimental designs described here are the non-equivalent control group design and the separate-sample pretest–posttest design. In addition a separate class of quasi-experimental designs known as time-series designs is described.

Nonequivalent Control Group Design

The nonequivalent control group design is similar to the pretest–posttest control group design. It has two groups: one experimental and one control. Both are pretested. The experimental group receives the treatment. The posttests of the two groups follow. The nonequivalent control group design differs from the pretest–posttest control group design in only one respect: There is no random selection or assignment in the nonequivalent control group design. The design is presented in Figure 8.11. In the diagram, note the absence of R for randomization. A line of dashes separates the two groups to suggest that there is no assurance of equivalence based on the random sampling procedure.

The design can have more than two groups. Also, both the groups in a two-group nonequivalent design can receive treatment when the purpose is to evaluate the relative effects of two treatments.

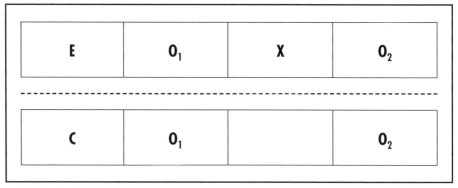

Figure 8.11. The nonequivalent control group design. Note that the design lacks random selection and assignment of participants, indicated by the dashed line.

The design often is necessary in settings such as schools, general and mental hospitals, nursing and extended care homes, and institutions for people with mental retardation. The same-grade children in different sections, groups of patients, or residents in different wards or housing units may serve as the different groups of the study. For example, all persons on the first floor of a residential facility may serve as the experimental group, while those on the second floor may serve as the control group. This results in intact experimental and control groups. Which group receives treatment and which serves as the control is determined randomly.

Some nonequivalent control group designs may have participants who volunteer for the study. In this case, the sample is self-selected. The investigator then has a self-selected experimental group. A control group may be created from those who do not volunteer for the study.

Intact experimental and control groups are better than self-selected experimental groups. Possibly, those who volunteer for a study are quite different from those who do not. When the investigator forms a control group, he or she may have no knowledge about the differences between those who wish to participate and those who do not. As a result, the experimenter is likely to have two groups that are so different as to make them unacceptable even within a quasi-experimental design.

It is important to realize that the design does not recommend dispensing with the notion of preexperimental equivalence of groups. It permits an experiment under conditions of no assurance of equivalence based on randomization. The investigator is still expected to take every feasible step to make the groups as similar as possible. For example, an investigator may be interested in the evaluation of a treatment program designed to increase verbal behaviors in institutionalized autistic children. It is possible that the residents of one ward are more verbal than the residents of another ward. In this case, the investigator should not select the ward with more verbal autistic children for the experimental group and the ward with less verbal children for the control group. The investigator cannot use these two intact groups.

The same statistical techniques used in the analysis of the results of pretest–posttest control group design are applicable to the nonequivalent control group design. However, the use of analysis of covariance, which is based on a strong assumption of preexperimental sampling equivalence of groups, is questionable.

The most critical problem with the nonequivalent control group design is the selection biases that threaten internal validity. Other threats include statistical regression and differential participant attrition. The participants (either selected or volunteered) may have had unusually high pretest scores to begin with that might regress to the mean during the course of an experiment. This may lead to an erroneous conclusion that the independent variable was responsible for the change. For example, in a study designed to evaluate a new exercise program for senior citizens, residents who are not making progress under the treatment program may withdraw from the study, leaving only those participants who do show improvement.

The design was originally recommended for experiments in natural settings where a better design is not suitable. However, in practice, many investigators in social and psychological research have used the design in laboratory-oriented research, partly because the requirement of randomization poses significant practical problems for all kinds of research, not just for field experiments. Nevertheless, when one of the true experimental designs can be used, the nonequivalent control group design is a poor choice.

Separate-Sample Pretest–Posttest Design

Sometimes investigators wish to study certain behaviors or practices of very large natural groups such as workers in a factory, children in large schools, people living in various parts of a city, or speech–language clinicians in a large school district. In such cases, it often is not possible to randomly select individual participants to form experimental and control groups. However, the investigators usually can randomly select groups of people who will be observed before and after treatment. The separate-sample pretest–posttest design is applicable in situations such as these.

This design is represented in Figure 8.12. Note that, unlike the non-equivalent control group design, this design uses the random procedure in selecting groups (not individuals). The two groups, therefore, are assumed to have sampling equivalence, although this might often be a questionable assumption because the individuals are not randomly selected. Only one sample is pretested, and then this sample is presented with a treatment variable not relevant to the study: the *X* in parenthesis. It is the second group, those participants not receiving the pretest, that is the true experimental group in the design. The treatment variable is applied to this group, and a posttest follows.

The design can be illustrated with a hypothetical example. Suppose a coordinator of speech–language services in a large school district wishes to find out the most frequently used articulation therapy technique before a

C	R	O	(X)	
E	R		X	O

Figure 8.12. The separate-sample pretest–posttest design. Note that the groups, not individuals, are randomly selected; the effects of one of the two treatments—the *X* in parenthesis—is ignored.

new technique is presented to the clinicians in a workshop. The coordinator also wishes to find out if the clinicians would be likely to change their techniques after the presentation. However, he or she needs to avoid the problem of pretest sensitization to treatment, a problem of external validity. Therefore, the investigator randomly selects two subgroups of clinicians in the district and randomly assigns the groups to the experimental and control conditions. A subgroup may consist of all clinicians in a certain number of schools in the district. One of the groups is pretested about the techniques of articulation therapy they use. Then they receive a presentation on the new articulation therapy whose effects are ignored. The other group, in the absence of the pretest, receives the same information. The posttest evaluates the effects of the presentation in terms of any change in the clinicians' inclination to use the new technique.

The results of a separate-sample pretest–posttest design can be analyzed with the parametric independent sample t test or nonparametric Mann-Whitney U or median test.

The separate-sample pretest–posttest design is one of the weaker group designs because it does not control for the effects of history, maturation, and differential participant attrition. Like all of the quasi-experimental designs, it is used when a more appropriate design is not feasible.

Time-Series Designs

The designs described so far, including the true experimental designs, involve at the most only two measures of the dependent variable: one taken before the introduction of the independent variable and one after the introduction. The typical pretreatment and posttreatment measures of the dependent variable may be sufficient to demonstrate the effect of the independent variable from a statistical standpoint. However, those measures do not give a total picture of the initial stability of the phenomenon and the subsequent systematic changes the dependent variables cause. An alternative strategy that tracks the dependent variable more often than the pretest–posttest designs is that of time-series designs. These designs are considered quasi-experimental.

Time-series designs are those in which the dependent variable is observed on several occasions both before and after the introduction of the independent variable. The time-series designs are a group of flexible designs that can be used with single participants or groups of participants and with one or more independent variables. They can be used with independent variables that have relatively temporary or permanent effects. They are especially suited for studying changes in social behaviors that are a result of new social or legal policies.

There are many time-series designs, and it is not possible to review them all here. Interested readers should consult other sources (Cook &

Campbell, 1979; Glass, Wilson, & Gottman, 1974). A few of the typical time-series designs are presented here.

Single-Group Time-Series Designs

In the basic single-group time-series design, one group of participants is observed several times before and after the introduction of an independent variable. The design has several variations. In the simplest form of the design, there is a single temporary treatment before and after which the dependent variable is measured several times.

The design is illustrated in Figure 8.13. The diagram shows that the treatment was applied once to a single group of participants. The dependent variable was measured four times before and four times after the introduction of the treatment. This design also is called a simple interrupted time-series design (Cook & Campbell, 1979). The multiple measures before the treatment provide a better picture of the variability, if any, in the dependent variable before the application of treatment. Repeated observations after the treatment can help evaluate the maintenance of the treated behaviors over time.

A temporary treatment of the kind suggested in the design is used frequently in clinical sciences. A group of patients with aphasia may be observed repeatedly by obtaining several conversational language samples before introducing a treatment program. The treatment may be continued for several days before it is terminated. Then the language samples may be resumed for the next several days or weeks in an effort to monitor the maintenance of the treatment effect.

The basic time-series design shown in Figure 8.13 has several variations. The first involves the continuation of treatment during some of the posttreatment measures of the dependent variable. This design is illustrated in Figure 8.14, which shows that the first four measures were taken before treatment and only the last two were truly the posttreatment measures. Measures 5 and 6 were made while the participants were still receiving the treatment, suggested by the dashed lines under X and the respective O measures. In the earlier example of research on the treatment of aphasia, the treatment may be continued until two measures of the dependent variable have been recorded before it is withdrawn.

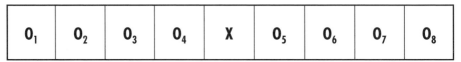

Figure 8.13. A single-group time-series design with temporary single treatment. Note that the dependent variable is measured four times before and four times after the introduction of treatment.

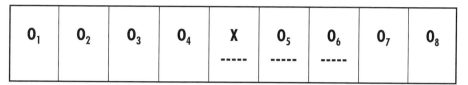

Figure 8.14. A single-group time-series design with continuous treatment and withdrawal. Note that the treatment is continued during observations 5 and 6.

In a second variation of the single-group time-series design, treatment is continued while the dependent variable is measured. This design is illustrated in Figure 8.15. The measurement of the dependent variable is continuous in the design as suggested by the dashed lines under X and all of the subsequent measures of the dependent variable.

The design is better able to track the effects of the treatment because it measures the dependent variable during the course of the treatment. In an institution for people with mental retardation, for example, a group language treatment program may be instituted after several measures of the clients' language have been taken. The periodic language sampling is then continued throughout the course of the treatment. In contrast, the traditional pretests and posttests are inadequate for the purposes of documenting the course of therapeutic changes that take place over an extended period of time.

The design often is used in social research. In many cases, the repeated measures of a dependent variable before treatment may have already been recorded simply as a matter of routine organizational policy. For example, a state department of motor vehicles may keep the records of bodily injuries sustained by people in traffic accidents. An investigator may gain access to such information recorded over a period of time. Incidentally, information of this kind often is called archival data. Such archival data can be used as the repeated pretreatment measures. Then the state legislature may pass a mandatory seat-belt law that requires all drivers and passengers to wear seat belts. The frequency of accidents involving bodily injury will continue to be recorded, providing the necessary repeated posttests. The treatment (the new law) continues to be applied while the dependent variable is measured. A significant reduction in the frequency of injury reports in the absence of a significant change in the accident rates may be interpreted as a favorable effect of the seat-belt law.

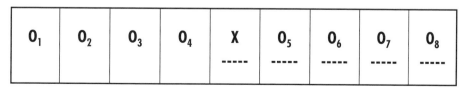

Figure 8.15. A single-group time-series design with single continuous treatment. Note that once initiated, the treatment is continued during all periods of observation.

In the example just given, it should be noted that the repeated measurements of the dependent variable do not necessarily involve the same group of participants. The persons who had accidents before the seat-belt law went into effect may not be the same as those who had them after the law went into effect. In other words, people who get into accidents do not constitute a single static group, although some individuals may have a longer membership in that group. In all probability, it is a group whose membership keeps changing. Therefore, in such situations, the measurements of the dependent variable are taken on **replicated groups,** which are groups with changing membership but a defined characteristic (such as those who have accidents). A replicated group contrasts with a **repeated group,** which is a group whose membership is constant. In this latter case, participants in the same group are measured repeatedly. In a majority of time-series designs, measures are taken on repeated groups.

A third variation of the single-group time-series design consists of repeated measures and two or more treatments. The design is illustrated in Figure 8.16. The diagram shows that after obtaining three measures of the dependent variable, the first treatment (X_1) was introduced. After the treatment was terminated, three more measures were obtained. Then, a second treatment was introduced (X_2), followed by three more observations of the dependent variable. The design can be extended to include additional treatments.

This design may be used in the evaluation of the temporary effects of two or more treatments on the same behavior. A program to teach language to a group of children with autism may contain two different treatment procedures. A language stimulation program that does not target specific language structures for treatment (X_1) may be evaluated against a program in which selected grammatic features are taught (X_2). The treatments are interrupted by a series of measurements of the dependent variable. In implementing a study such as this, it is necessary to have measures of dependent variables that are independent of each other. Also, the selected target behaviors should be equally easy or hard to learn.

The single-group time-series design with multiple treatments can be implemented with continuous treatment. After the initial set of observations, the first treatment is initiated and the measurement of the effects is continued until the treatment is terminated. The second treatment is then introduced and the measurement continued until the conclusion of the experiment.

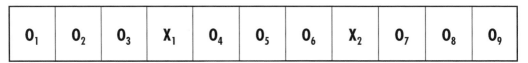

Figure 8.16. A single-group time-series design with multiple temporary treatments. Note that there are two treatments that are separated by observations without treatment.

All the single-group time-series designs described so far may be used with single participants as well. In fact, multiple observations before, during, and after treatment are one of the most important characteristics of single-subject designs. There are, however, some important differences between the single-subject and the time-series designs. In single-subject designs, the pretreatment observations are continued until the dependent variable shows an operational degree of stability. There is no such requirement in the time-series designs. Therefore, the pretreatment measurements are made a certain number of predetermined times. Furthermore, single-subject designs typically do not use archival data unless supported by independent observations. More importantly, single-subject designs differ in terms of how control is achieved. For instance, after a treatment is withdrawn, it is rarely reintroduced in a time-series design, but such reintroductions of treatment are typical of many single-subject designs (see Chapter 9 for details).

The analysis of the time-series designs involves complex statistical procedures, most of them designed especially for the kind of data generated by the strategy. The techniques are unique and involved. A set of statistical techniques often employed uses an **integrated moving-average model,** which takes into account the change in the level of the repeated measures and change in the slope. Whether or not there was a slope also may be considered in the analysis.

A serious limitation of single-group time-series designs is the lack of control over extraneous variables, especially those included in the history. The changes recorded at the time the independent variable was introduced into a time series may have been due to some other variables in the lives of the participants. The design is not able to rule out directly the influence of extraneous variables. However, when the repeated measures are reasonably stable before the introduction of the treatment and an abrupt and dramatic change is recorded soon after the introduction, the data may strongly suggest a relation that can be confirmed with additional research using designs that permit greater control.

The investigator has less confidence in the results of a single-group time-series design if the changes are small and gradual or highly variable or when a clear trend in the data was evident in the predicted direction from the very beginning of the study. With regard to this last point, the pretreatment measures of language in a language-treatment research project may show an increasing trend from the beginning of observation. When this trend continues with the introduction of treatment, the results cannot be interpreted to mean that the treatment was effective. The researcher cannot be sure that language measures would have continued to increase without treatment. One also could suspect an interaction between treatment and other unidentified variables that created the increasing trend in the first place. But the nature and extent of this interaction will not be clear.

Multiple-Group Time-Series Designs

The single-group time-series designs can be extended to include two or more groups. However, the groups in a time-series design are not randomly drawn from a population, and therefore they do not have sampling equivalence. Usually, intact groups are used in these designs.

There are several variations of the multiple-group time-series design, and it is not possible to describe them all here. A basic multiple-group time-series design has two nonequivalent groups, one of which is exposed to the treatment variable. Both the groups are repeatedly measured for the dependent variable before and after the experimental manipulation in one of the groups. This design is illustrated in Figure 8.17. The figure separates the two groups with dashed lines to suggest lack of sampling equivalence. It also shows four measures before and four measures after the introduction of the independent variable in the experimental group. The dependent variable in the control group also is measured to the same extent.

The design is similar to the nonequivalent control group design (see Figure 8.11) except that the dependent variable is measured repeatedly. The suggestions offered earlier on how to form the two nonequivalent groups are relevant here also.

Compared with the single-group design, the two-group design—even without sampling equivalence—is better because the investigator has a chance to compare treatment with a no-treatment control group. If the repeated measures of the dependent variable do not show significant change although such a change was evident soon after the independent variable was introduced into the experimental group, the possibility of a cause–effect relation is increased.

All the designs illustrated in Figures 8.13 through 8.16 can be modified into two-group or multiple-group time-series designs by adding one or more groups. An added group can receive treatment when the purpose is to evaluate the relative effects of two treatments. When people in institutions

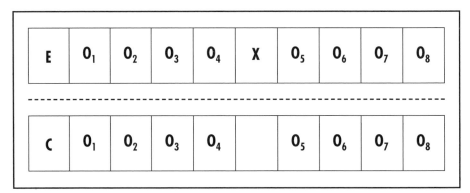

Figure 8.17. A nonequivalent two-group time-series design. Note that the dashed line suggests nonrandom formation of the groups.

or cities serve as experimental groups, people in other comparable institutions or cities may serve as the control groups.

An interesting multiple-group time-series design involves two staggered treatments. The design, illustrated in Figure 8.18, shows two groups that each receive a different treatment but in a staggered sequence. Possibly, treating both the groups simultaneously may be impractical for reasons of money or personnel. In such cases, one group is treated first and the second group next. In clinical research, one group of clients may be treated first and clients on the waiting list treated next. When measures are repeated before and after the treatment (or during it), a staggered multigroup time-series design is in effect.

Summary and Summative Evaluation of Quasi-Experimental Designs

Quasi-experimental designs are eminently practical because they do not insist upon the random selection and assignment of participants to groups of a study. For the same reason, they are considered weaker than true experimental designs. There is usually no assurance of sampling equivalence within most of the quasi-experimental designs.

Quasi-experimental designs are appropriate for naturalistic studies conducted in nonlaboratory situations. The nonequivalent control group design and the separate-sample pretest–posttest design are two of the basic quasi-experimental designs. The nonequivalent control group design is similar to the pretest–posttest control group design except that there is no assurance of sampling equivalence. In the separate-sample pretest–posttest design, the random procedure is used to assign participants to the two groups of a study, but they may or may not be randomly drawn from a population. An interesting feature of this design is the presentation of an irrelevant independent variable to the control group.

Of the quasi-experimental designs, the time-series designs are probably more useful. In time-series designs, dependent variables are measured repeatedly both before and after the introduction of treatment. There are both controlled and uncontrolled varieties of the time-series designs.

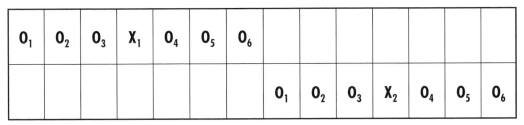

Figure 8.18. A two-group time-series design with two staggered treatments. Note that the second group's observation and treatment begins only after the first group's observation is completed.

Despite their lack of sampling equivalence, time-series designs are useful in showing systematic changes in the dependent variable over a period of time. The multiple measures taken before and after the treatment can demonstrate the reliability of the measures better than the single measures that are typical of the other group designs. Time-series designs are more flexible than other group designs. In terms of this flexibility and multiple measures of the dependent variables, time-series designs are similar to single-subject designs.

COUNTERBALANCED WITHIN-SUBJECTS DESIGNS

The common method of establishing cause–effect relations within the group design strategy involves two or more groups, but each group is exposed to at least one different condition of the design. In other words, the same participants do not experience all conditions of the experiment. While measurement of the dependent variable is common to the groups, experimental manipulation is not. One group receives treatment while the other does not. Or two groups each experience a different form of treatment. As a result, the basic strategy of analysis involves a comparison of different participants performing under different conditions. For this reason, the group designs discussed so far also are appropriately called the between-groups strategy.

There are, however, designs within the group strategy that do not compare the performance of different groups exposed to different conditions of an experiment. Such designs, known as **within-subjects designs** or **counterbalanced designs,** expose participants of all the groups to all the conditions of an experiment. Other names for these designs include *rotation experiments, crossover designs,* and *switchover designs.* Of these, the term *crossover design* also refers to a particular type of counterbalanced within-subjects design.

In recent years, the term within-subjects design has been occasionally used to refer to single-subject designs. This usage is avoided here. For a long time, the term within-subjects design has been a part of the group design terminology, and some of the group within-subjects designs have been known since the early 1920s (Edwards, 1960; McCall, 1923). Therefore, in this book, the within-subjects design refers only to a variety of group designs with counterbalancing as their major feature.

There are some similarities between counterbalanced within-subjects designs and single-subject designs, however. In either strategy, there is no control group that does not receive treatment. Also, in both the strategies, each participant is said to serve as his or her own control. When a controlled condition is a part of an experiment, all participants are assigned to it. Each participant experiences all the experimental conditions in both the strategies. These may be the reasons why some refer to single-subject designs as within-subjects designs. Nevertheless, there are important philosophical and methodological differences between the two approaches. Counterbalanced within-subjects designs are a part of the group design approach. The strategy typically uses two or more groups of participants. It uses the random procedure in participant selection and the assignment process. The results of counterbalanced within-subjects designs are analyzed through inferential statistics. Most single-subject designs do not share these characteristics. Therefore, single-subject designs are not within-subjects designs.

One-Group Single-Treatment Counterbalanced Design

The simplest form of a counterbalanced within-subjects design evaluates a single treatment. This is the one-group single-treatment counterbalanced design in which an investigator has only one group of participants who are all exposed to all conditions of an experiment. The design is sometimes described as *ABBA* counterbalanced design, which should not be confused with the single-subject *ABAB* design.

The one-group single-treatment counterbalanced design has two conditions that are exposed to all of the participants in the group: a no-treatment and a treatment condition. (In the *ABBA* terminology, the two conditions are designated *A* and *B*.) In exposing the participants to the two conditions of the study, the investigator can follow one of three sequences: (a) all participants first go through the control condition and then the experimental condition; (b) all participants first go through the experimental and then the control condition; or (c) the participants are divided into two subgroups: one of the subgroups goes through the first sequence, and the other goes through the second. The first two conditions do not involve counterbalancing. Therefore, those two sequences are not used.

The third sequence is the simplest form of counterbalancing, and therefore, one-group single-treatment counterbalanced design uses it. Note that the two subgroups do not make it a two-group design. There is only one treatment, and the formation of two subgroups is a means of counterbalancing the experimental and control conditions.

Suppose an investigator wishes to study the temporary effects of masking noise on stuttering with a single group of people who stutter. After having selected the participants, preferably on a random basis, the investigator randomly forms two subgroups with an equal number of participants. When the number of participants is small, and typically it is in a counterbalanced design, the random procedure accomplishes very little. In any case, the two subgroups are then exposed to the noise and no-noise conditions in the counterbalanced order. One possible sequence of the design is represented in Figure 8.19. Of course, the sequence shown can be switched across the groups.

	Sequence of Conditions	
	First Condition	**Second Condition**
Subgroup 1	Treatment ➡	No Treatment
Subgroup 2	No Treatment ➡	Treatment

Figure 8.19. One-group single-treatment counterbalanced design. Note that the treatment and no-treatment conditions are counterbalanced across the subgroups.

Whether the first subgroup should go through the noise and no-noise sequence or vice versa may also be determined randomly. A toss of a coin may determine the initial sequence. If it is determined that the first subgroup will experience the treatment condition (noise) first and the control condition (no noise) next, the second subgroup will automatically follow the opposite sequence. Thus, each half of the participants will have been exposed to one of the two possible sequences.

The results of each of the conditions are pooled and averaged from the two groups. That is, the mean number of stutterings exhibited by all the participants in the control condition is compared with the mean number of stutterings in the treatment condition. (This is yet another reason why the design is considered to have only one group.) A significant difference between the two means as evaluated by a statistical test of significance suggests the possibility of an effect of the treatment variable.

Counterbalancing is a method to eliminate the order as a factor that influences treatment effects. It is possible that when all the participants experience the noise condition first and then the control condition, their stuttering in the second condition may be higher or lower simply because of the previous condition. Counterbalancing—by having half the participants experience one condition first and the other half experience the other condition first—seeks to balance the effects of order across the groups. In this sense, counterbalancing can be seen as a method of equating the order and sequence effects in the groups.

Counterbalancing also can be done on an individual basis. Using the random procedure, the sequence with which each participant experiences the two experimental conditions may be determined. In this method of **intrasubject counterbalancing,** the first participant may go through the control–treatment sequence and the second participant may go through the treatment–control sequence. Care must be taken to ensure that there are equal numbers of participants in both the sequences. The more typical counterbalancing of subgroups, shown in Figure 8.19, is called **intragroup counterbalancing.**

The one-group single-treatment counterbalanced design does not control for extraneous variables of history, maturation, testing, differential participant attrition, and so on. Though it includes a control condition, it does not fully control all or even most of the factors that affect internal validity. The control over the extraneous factors is increased if the same participants, after having experienced no-treatment and treatment conditions, again experience a no-treatment condition. The investigator can then show that changes in the dependent variables follow both the introduction and the removal of an independent variable. Such designs are typical within the single-subject strategy.

Crossover Design

Another counterbalanced within-subjects design is known as the crossover design in which two treatments are evaluated with two groups, both of which are exposed to the two treatments in a crossover fashion. That is, halfway through an experiment, the participants switch over to another treatment. The design is represented in Figure 8.20. The diagram shows that the groups are formed on a random basis and both the groups receive the two treatments selected for evaluation. Therefore, there is no control group that does not receive treatment.

A hypothetical example can clarify the design arrangement. Suppose a clinician wishes to evaluate the effects of two treatment approaches to the remediation of articulation disorders in school-age children. The clinician selects a random sample of children with multiple articulation problems and divides the sample into two randomly formed groups. The children who have specific speech-sound errors may be selected, which would necessitate an access to a large number of children with those specific speech-sound errors. The participants are pretested (O_1), for example, by standardized tests

R	E	O_1	X_1	O_2	X_2	O_3
R	E	O_1	X_2	O_2	X_1	O_3

Figure 8.20. A crossover design with two treatments and two groups. Note that each group receives both the treatments in a counterbalanced order.

and conversational speech samples, to determine the specific speech sounds misarticulated by the children. Next, the order in which the groups will receive treatment is determined randomly. Each group then receives the two articulation treatments in a different order. The design requires an assessment in the middle of the study when the participants are crossed over to the other treatment. A final assessment at the end of the study also is required of both the groups.

Complex Counterbalanced Designs

When only one or two treatment variables are evaluated, the counterbalanced designs are somewhat simple. Without much difficulty, the investigator can make sure that each treatment appears in the first and the second position in the sequence. However, experiments involving three or more treatments require complex counterbalanced arrangements. The basic requirement of counterbalancing is that each treatment appear at least once in each of all possible positions. To achieve this, the investigator should initially identify all possible sequences of the selected number of treatments.

A counterbalanced design involving only three treatments is already fairly complex. The three treatments *A*, *B*, and *C* combine into six sequences: *ABC, ACB, BAC, BCA, CAB,* and *CBA.* In this arrangement, each treatment appears twice in each of the initial, medial, and final positions. If the investigator were to use intrasubject counterbalancing, each participant would be randomly assigned to one of the six sequences. However, one should make sure that each order has a comparable number of participants. This often results in ad hoc modifications in the random procedure. In intragroup counterbalancing, six comparable groups are initially formed, and each group is randomly assigned to one of the sequences.

A counterbalanced design with four treatments would have 24 sequences ($1 \times 2 \times 3 \times 4 = 24$). However, when the number of treatments is increased by just one to a total of five, the number of sequences increases to a formidable 120 ($1 \times 2 \times 3 \times 4 \times 5 = 120$). Obviously, arithmetic increases in the number of treatments result in factorial increases in the number of sequences that need to be counterbalanced. As a result, the need for participants, the number of groups, or both increases dramatically. This can be a serious problem in clinical research where the required number of comparable clients with specific disorders may not be found. For these reasons, completely counterbalanced designs are generally limited to fewer than four treatment variables. Even then, the designs are used infrequently in clinical treatment research.

The practical difficulties involved in achieving complete counterbalancing of multiple treatment variables have led to a compromised procedure of incomplete counterbalancing. Some of the designs that use incomplete counterbalancing also are known as Latin square designs. In a **Latin square design,** each treatment in each position appears only once in each group.

Therefore, conditions do not precede or follow each other in all sequences or in equal numbers. Therefore, not all combinations of multiple treatment variables are implemented in a Latin square design.

A Latin square arrangement is represented in Table 8.1. The numbers of groups, treatments, and positions (sequences) are all equal when a Latin square design is represented in the form of a table. Such a table has the same number of rows, columns, and cells in relation to any one group. The same four treatments (*ABCD* in the table shown) permit other combinations. A given set of treatments can be represented by different Latin squares. It must be emphasized that the arrangements of treatment sequences in a Latin square are limited. As noted before, complete counterbalancing of the four treatments shown in Table 8.1 would have required not 4 but 24 groups.

Limitations of Counterbalanced Within-Subjects Designs

When several treatments are administered to the same individual or the same group of participants, several potential problems may make it difficult to interpret the results. One should take these limitations into consideration in designing and interpreting the studies of counterbalanced within-subjects designs. Some of these problems can be seen in a few single-subject designs as well.

Order Effects

The influence a particular sequence with which multiple treatments are offered to the same individual is known as the **order effects.** In this case, some or all of the effects of two or more treatments can be explained on the basis of the specific order in which they were administered. Obviously, designs with multiple treatments that are administered to the same participants

TABLE 8.1
One of the Latin Square Arrangements of Four Treatments

| Groups | Order of Treatment | | | |
	1	2	3	4
I	A	B	C	D
II	B	A	D	C
III	C	D	A	B
IV	D	C	B	A

Note. This counterbalanced design requires four groups (I–IV). Note that each group receives the four treatments in a different order.

necessarily have an order. Therefore, order as a factor cannot be ruled out on a priori grounds.

The problem of the order effect can be understood clearly when two treatments are administered in a single, fixed order to all participants. Suppose that an investigator wished to evaluate the relative (and interactive) effects of a new and an established articulation therapy. If the investigator were first to apply the traditional articulation therapy to all the clients and then to follow it with the new therapy, the results—especially of the new therapy—would be mostly uninterpretable. The effects observed during the administration of the new therapy may be due to the order in which it was administered. The investigator would not know whether the same results would be obtained if the treatments were to be administered in a different order.

The order effect is sometimes described as *practice effect*. The second treatment may be more effective simply because of the increased familiarity with the experimental tasks, arrangements, and repeated practice of some of the response skills measured in the sessions. In other words, the treatment itself may not have contributed much to the changes observed in the dependent variable under treatment.

Theoretically, order effects are neutralized in a completely counterbalanced design, which provides for all possible orders in which the selected set of multiple treatments can be administered. However, when the orders included in a study do not exhaust all possible positions for all treatments, then the order effects cannot be ruled out. Generally, the greater the number of treatments, the harder it is to present each of them in every possible order and the higher the chances of order effects.

Carryover Effects

The second problem associated with the administration of multiple treatments to the same participants or group of participants is known as *multiple-treatment interference* or *carryover effects*, also referred to as *sequential confounding* or *sequential effects*. While the order effect is due simply to the position in which a given treatment appears, the **carryover effect** is due to the influence of the previous treatment on the succeeding treatment. The prior treatment may have a positive or a negative effect on the succeeding treatment.

When the carryover effect is positive, the second treatment will appear stronger than it really is, and when the carryover effect is negative, the second treatment will appear weaker than it is. When administered alone, they may produce effects that are different from those observed in a sequential arrangement. The carryover effects may be cumulative over repeated phases, or they may be limited to adjacent phases. Cumulative carryover effects show increasingly larger magnitude across experimental conditions.

Whether the carryover effects have occurred or not can be assessed in a completely counterbalanced design in which each treatment precedes and follows every other treatment more than once. The presence of a positive carryover effect is suggested when the effect of a treatment is typically larger when it follows a given treatment and smaller when it precedes the same given treatment. This relationship between two treatments is illustrated in Figure 8.21. A negative carryover effect is suggested when the effect of a treatment is typically smaller when it follows a given treatment and larger when it precedes the same treatment. This relationship is illustrated in Figure 8.22.

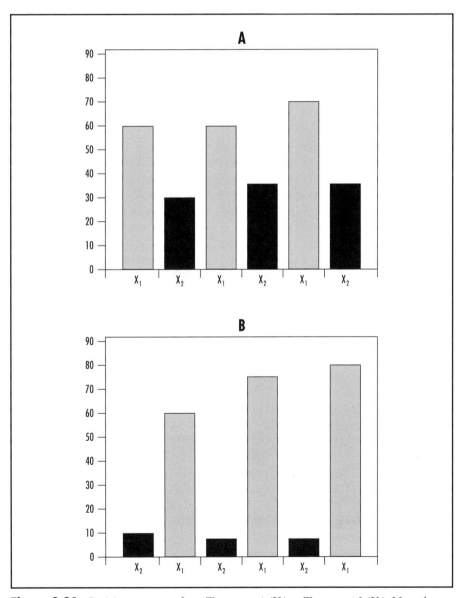

Figure 8.21. Positive carryover from Treatment 1 (X_1) to Treatment 2 (X_2). Note that Treatment 2 had a larger effect when it followed Treatment 1 (A) than when it preceded Treatment 1 (B).

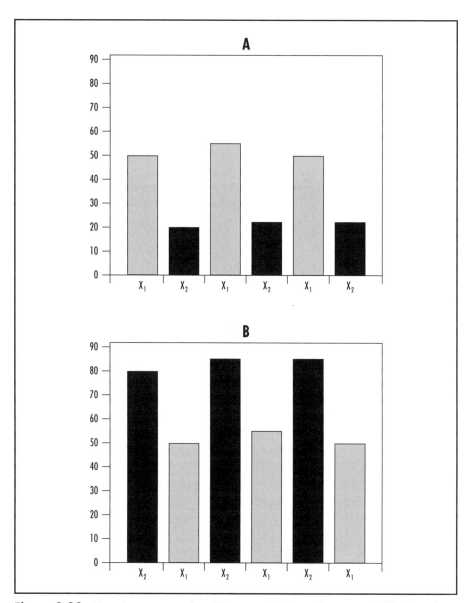

Figure 8.22. Negative carryover from Treatment 1 (X_1) to Treatment 2 (X_2). Note that Treatment 2 had a smaller effect when it followed Treatment 1 (A) than when it preceded Treatment 1 (B).

Ceiling and Floor Effects

Two other problems associated with counterbalanced multiple-treatment designs are the ceiling and floor effects. The **ceiling effect** refers to the maximum extent of change produced by a prior treatment, leaving the next treatment no room to show its effect. In a study done to evaluate the effects of two treatments on stuttering, the first method may reduce stuttering to a very low level, perhaps less than 1%. When the second treatment is applied, only a minimal reduction in stuttering may be evident. This small change associated with the second treatment may be due to the ceiling effect created by the first treatment.

As long as the first treatment has any effect at all, the second treatment in a sequence starts with a different floor created by the first. The **floor effect,** or the base level of performance, may be high or low, depending upon the effect of the previous treatment. This can also limit the extent of change that a variable can produce. The floor effect is actually a counterpart of the ceiling effect.

The ceiling and floor effects are striking when one treatment is stronger than the other. However, the effect can be seen when both are equally strong. In this case, the first treatment creates a ceiling effect on the second treatment, and the effect is mutual. Automatically, a new floor is created for the next treatment.

Most of the problems associated with counterbalanced designs discussed so far do not exist when all the treatments being evaluated are equally ineffective. Also, the problems are not serious when the treatments have only a temporary effect. That is, when the effects of a treatment disappear as soon as the treatment is stopped, the carryover, ceiling, or floor effects are not serious considerations. Therefore, the designs are more applicable to behaviors that take a relatively long time to change permanently but can show temporary but clear-cut changes in the short term.

Summary and Summative Evaluation of Counterbalanced Within-Subjects Designs

Counterbalanced within-subjects designs are those that expose all participants of a group to all the conditions of a study. There are no groups that do not receive treatment within a counterbalanced within-subjects design. However, within-subjects designs are still a variety of group design and, as such, should not be confused with single-subject designs.

The one-group single-treatment design and the crossover design are the simplest of the counterbalanced within-subjects designs. In the one-group single-treatment counterbalanced design, the participants are divided into two groups, and each group follows an opposite sequence of treatment and no-treatment conditions. In the crossover design, two randomly formed groups are used; initially, each receives one treatment and then crosses over to the other treatment.

Complex counterbalanced within-subjects designs are not very practical in clinical research because of the difficulty involved in counterbalancing all the sequences in which different treatments are presented. Ideally, when multiple treatments are evaluated, all combinations and sequences are used so that the order effects are neutralized. This then creates a need for many participants, who are divided into subgroups. However, complex counter-balanced designs do permit evaluations of multiple treatment variables. Problems involved in presenting all conditions of a study to all of the participants include the order effect, the carryover effect, and the ceiling and floor effects.

CORRELATIONAL ANALYSIS DESIGN

The final type of group research design to be considered is variously called *correlational analysis design, correlational design,* or *correlational studies.* Most of the designs considered so far permit some form of manipulation of an independent variable. In a **correlational analysis,** relation between events is studied, but there is no possibility of experimental manipulation of an independent variable. Therefore, the correlational analysis designs are not experimental designs. Many of the studies using correlational analysis are of the ex post facto variety described in Chapter 4. Therefore, the discussion of these designs will be brief.

A **correlation** is a statistical procedure that suggests that two events are somehow related. The relation may be positive or negative. Possibly, no relation may be revealed when a suspected relation is tested. A correlation is positive when the measured values of two variables are equally high or low; the variables seem to change in the same direction. When one increases, the other also increases and vice versa. The negative correlation is evident when one variable is high and the other is low and vice versa. A negative correlation suggests that when one event increases, the other decreases. Two events are not related (neutral) when their measured values do not correspond in any particular way.

Such measured values of two variables may be subjected to certain statistical analyses to derive a correlation coefficient that ranges between a perfect negative correlation of –1.00 to a perfect positive correlation of +1.00. Actual correlational coefficients rarely reach these perfect values. Even if the events are perfectly correlated, the measurements are not perfect, and therefore, the correlation will not reach either –1.00 or +1.00.

When an independent variable is not manipulable, one may look for natural events that seem to be related in some specific manner. Two selected variables may be measured once or repeatedly to determine if the measures reflect systematic changes in one or the other direction. A correlation coefficient is calculated for the measured values. Significant positive or negative correlations are interpreted to suggest a relation between the variables.

A correlation does not prove a cause–effect relation. Even if two events are causally related, the correlation itself does not specify which is the cause and which is the effect. Once a significant correlation is found, causes and effects are usually sorted out on the basis of prevailing theories and empirical knowledge. For example, when it is shown that academic performance and intelligence are highly (and positively) correlated, one concludes that the intelligence is the cause of better academic performance on the basis of available knowledge about these two variables. Such conclusions are not firm statements regarding functional relations between variables that are correlated. In many cases, causal relation inferred from correlation may be totally erroneous: Two variables may be correlated because they are both an effect of a third variable not observed by the investigator at all.

Once significant correlations between certain events have been found, experiments may be designed to manipulate one of the variables to see what effects follow. Unless this kind of experimental research is performed and the extraneous variables ruled out, it is not possible to draw firm conclusions regarding the meaning of correlations.

It is obvious that correlation is a statistical method of data analysis, not an experimental design in which variables are manipulated, controlled, and measured. As a statistical procedure, it is seen most frequently in the ex post facto type of research.

GROUP DESIGNS IN CLINICAL RESEARCH

The group design strategy described in this chapter has evolved over many years of research in several disciplines. The most significant impetus to this design strategy has come from the development of mathematical, psychological, medical, and agricultural statistics. Research needs in agriculture, psychology, many social sciences, medicine, and biological sciences have shaped the research methods, terms, and strategies used in the group approach. The statistical theory of probability, random selection and assignment of participants, inferential statistical analyses of differences in the mean performance measures of groups, evaluation of the effects of independent variables against a background of chance variability, and extension of the conclusions to the population from which the sample was drawn are all distinguishing characteristics of the group design strategy.

The group design strategy, like any other strategy, has its strengths and weaknesses. It works better with certain kinds of research problems investigated in certain settings. It does not work as well with certain other kinds of problems faced in other settings. From a theoretical standpoint, the group design approach offers an attractive and efficient strategy for investigating research questions. Various designs make it possible to isolate a cause–effect relation between events. The object of all scientific inquiry is to develop evidence of generality, though special cases also are of scientific interest. Nevertheless, most events cannot be studied in the population as a whole, and therefore, sampling techniques are needed. Statisticians have shown that a randomly selected representative sample can help extend the conclusions of the sample to the population.

Significant problems arise when the same strategy that has worked well in large-scale social, agricultural, and certain kinds of psychological research is applied to clinical problems of treatment evaluation. To be sure, the clinician also is interested in drawing conclusions that apply to the clinical populations, not just to one or two clients that he or she may conduct research on. However, the nature of the everyday clinical business and the feasible strategies of clinical research make the widespread application of the statistical approach impractical.

Medicine has been more successful than other clinical disciplines in using the group approach in evaluating treatment effects. However, as noted in Chapter 4, randomized clinical trials have made significant methodologic compromises in using the group design strategy. Many of these compromises have been forced by the nature of clinical populations and the nature of medical and nonmedical treatments. The biggest problem a clinician faces is to achieve sampling equivalence of groups through random procedures to investigate questions of treatment effectiveness. Clinical populations are generally not accessible for random sampling. Populations with language, articulation, fluency, and voice problems are not readily available for random sampling in which every patient or client has an equal chance of being selected for the study.

Self-selection of participants is a more serious problem than lack of accessibility to clinical populations for random selection. Available participants who are selected for the study may refuse participation because of the legal rights afforded to clinical populations under the National Research Act of 1974 (P.L. 93-348). When potential participants are informed about the purpose of a clinical experiment, nature of the treatment to be evaluated, and the alternative treatments available to them, many patients refuse to be randomized. As discussed in Chapter 4, such refusal results in self-selected participants. It means that those who eventually participate in a randomized clinical trial are not randomly selected, but self-selected. Consequently, the results of a group treatment study cannot be generalized to the population of patients needing the same or similar treatment. Therefore, the claimed superiority of group designs in demonstrating statistical (inferential) generality of findings of a treatment evaluation study is not realized.

Implementation of group design studies in speech–language pathology presents additional problems. In medicine, a new treatment (e.g., a new drug) may be relatively easily administered to large number of patients in multiple centers. To the contrary, the behavioral treatment techniques used in speech–language pathology and special education are difficult to apply to a large number of participants. Much clinical work in speech–language pathology and education is specific to the individual. In nonclinical research the independent variables can be presented in groups. A film on attitudes or sensitivity, a set of slides that are supposed to change participants' rated moods, a training program designed to enhance sales clerks' skills, and so on can be easily presented in groups. However, in a treatment method with various steps in which individual clients' behaviors have to be changed to a substantial degree, group presentation of the independent variable is inefficient at best and useless at worst. Whenever it is tried, the worst case is realized more often than the best case.

Within the group strategy, the changes produced by the independent variables can be small but the study can be considered a success. Because there are statistical techniques to identify changes that are not clear when visually inspected, small changes in clients' behaviors under treatment can be considered successful. Such small changes may certainly have theoretical significance and clinical potential, but they are not of immediate clinical significance. However, in clinical sciences, the changes in stuttering or language disorders induced by experimental or routine therapies should be large enough to make a difference in the lives of the clients. A statistical difference at the .001 level may or may not correspond to the magnitude of change required by real-life conditions. Therefore, the clinician painstakingly shapes and changes individual behaviors to a point where even a layperson can recognize those changes. Once this is done, the use of statistical techniques that are especially designed to detect small changes seems unnecessary as well as unimaginative. When one can talk about individuals in a meaningful manner, the statistical average is as irrelevant as it is mythical.

The relevance of inferential generality to clinical work is typically overestimated. When a clinician reads a report on a new treatment technique in a professional journal, he or she is not especially worried about the population of clients to which the conclusions may be applied. Such a concern about the behavior of the population is real to a politician seeking a majority vote, but the clinician faces a different kind of problem. The clinician's immediate concern is whether the treatment is applicable to a few individual clients he or she may be working with. This means that the clinician's immediate concern is logical, not inferential, generality. Group designs do not offer much help in this regard.

Group strategy is more effectively used in such nonexperimental research as sample surveys, ex post facto studies, normative research, and standard-group comparisons. Experimental research in which cause–effect relations are analyzed with randomly drawn and assigned experimental and control groups are few and far between. In medicine, where randomized clinical trials are common, the random selection of participants is not possible, but an initial random assignment may be attempted and adhered to as much as possible. Therefore, the results have neither inferential nor logical generality. In communicative disorders, difficulties involved in forming large enough clinical groups representative of the populations necessary to conduct experimental treatment evaluations have resulted in sparse experimental data.

I shall not attempt a more complete evaluation of the group research strategy here, as that will be done in Chapter 11. Because the advantages and disadvantages of a given approach are better understood in a comparative context, both group and single-subject design strategies will be evaluated after the latter has been considered in the next chapter.

SUMMARY _____

Group designs were originally developed in agricultural and social research. They are based on the theory of probability. The group design approach requires the formation of two or more groups for the purposes of experimentation. The groups may be formed on the basis of either random selection of participants from a defined population or by matching participants of similar characteristics. The basic method of group designs is to initially have two or more comparable groups that represent the population from which they were drawn (especially when the random procedure is used). At the least, one of the groups receives a treatment variable and another group does not. Table 8.2 offers a summary of major group designs and the kinds of questions they can address (i.e., their applications).

Typically, the performance of the two groups is measured before and after the presentation of an independent variable to the experimental group. The performance of the groups is expressed in terms of the statistical mean,

TABLE 8.2
Summary of Major Group Designs and Their Applications

Design	Research Questions	Strengths and Limitations
One-shot case study	Does the history suggest a cause?	Clinically useful; results are only suggestive
One-group pretest–posttest design	Is there an apparent change due to treatment?	Clinically useful; lacks control; cannot isolate cause–effect relations
Static-group comparisons	Does a treated group differ from an untreated group?	Uses existing treated and untreated groups; lacks pretests
Pretest–posttest control group design	Is a treatment effective? Is there a cause–effect relation?	True experimental design; well controlled; can isolate cause–effect relations; often clinically impractical
Posttest-only control group design	Is a treatment effective? Is there a cause–effect relation?	Well controlled when randomization is used; clinically impractical
Solomon four-group design	Is there an interaction between pretest and treatment? If so, what is its extent?	Useful in studies on reactive variables; impractical in clinical research
Multigroup pretest–posttest design	Is one treatment more effective than the other? What are the relative effects of treatment?	Well controlled; useful to the extent practical; clinically important
Multigroup posttest-only design	Is one treatment more effective than the other? What are the relative effects of treatment?	Well controlled; useful to the extent practical; lacks pretests

(continues)

TABLE 8.2 *Continued.*

Design	Research Questions	Strengths and Limitations
Factorial designs; randomized blocks design; completely randomized factorial design	What are the effects of two or more treatments? Is there an interaction between treatments or between treatments and client characteristics?	Excellent designs to study interaction; the most effective strategy to study interaction between participant characteristics and treatment; difficult to find enough participants in clinical research
Single-group time-series design	Is there a change following treatment? Do multiple treatments seem to produce change?	Multiple measures help demonstrate changes in dependent variables; relative effects of treatment can be evaluated; lack of control
Multiple-group time-series design	Is a treatment effective? What are the relative effects of two or more treatments?	Multiple groups ensure some control; multiple measures help demonstrate reliability; no sampling equivalence
One-group single-treatment counter-balanced design	Do treatment and no-treatment conditions differ significantly?	Has a control condition instead of a group; clinically useful
Crossover design	Do the same participants react differently to two different treatments?	Useful when two treatments should be exposed to the same participants; somewhat weak control
Correlational analysis	Do the selected variables covary?	Can show covariation, not causation

which is used in evaluating the effects of the independent variable. Such an evaluation usually consists of various statistical analyses of data to determine if the differences in the mean posttest scores of the groups are due to the experimental variable.

True experimental designs make it possible to evaluate the effects of various independent variables. There are many designs within the group strategy, but the basic pretest–posttest control group design is the prototype of this strategy. However, when complete randomization of participant selection is assured, the posttest may be avoided. This results in the posttest-only control group design. An extended design with four groups, known as the Solomon four-group design, may be used when the pretest sensitization is expected to interact with the treatment variable.

Group designs that permit the evaluation of multiple treatments include the multigroup pretest–posttest design, the multigroup posttest-only design, and the factorial designs. In the former two designs, different groups of participants experience different treatment variables. Factorial designs help assess not only the effects of multiple treatments but also any interactions between those treatments. Besides, they can help determine an interaction between treatment variables and participant characteristics (assigned variables).

Quasi-experimental designs are those that do not have full control of extraneous variables. Nevertheless, they are useful in identifying potential causal relations, which may be further verified through one of the true experimental designs. Of the many quasi-experimental designs, time-series designs are especially useful in clinical research. In the time-series designs, the dependent variable is measured on several occasions both before and after treatment. Therefore, the dependent variable measures may be more reliable than the single pretest and posttest measures. Time-series designs also are highly flexible. The dependent variables may be measured as often as necessary. Measures may be repeated during the treatment as well. Also, one or more groups may be used in evaluating the effects of single or multiple treatments.

Counterbalanced within-subjects designs are a variation of group designs. In these designs, all the participants of a study are exposed to all the experimental conditions. Each participant experiences a control condition and an experimental condition. If multiple treatments are evaluated, different combinations of treatment are presented in a counterbalanced manner. Counterbalanced designs are capable of evaluating multiple treatments although such designs tend to be complex and impractical. The limitations of counterbalanced designs include the order effect, the carryover effect, and the ceiling and floor effects. Most of these problems arise when the counterbalancing is not complete and treatments produce strong, relatively permanent effects.

Finally, the group design strategy offers correlational analysis designs based on statistical methods of correlation. These are not experimental designs because correlational studies do not involve manipulation of independent variables. The studies seek to find out if two events are related and, if so, whether the relation is positive or negative. Possibly, one may find that the two events are not related. Correlational designs do not permit statements on causation, but a relation found within these designs may be verified by one of the experimental designs.

Group designs are powerful tools when the requirements of the sampling equivalence based on the random procedure can be fulfilled. In clinical research, this often is not possible. Well-done group design studies are able to demonstrate internal validity, but external validity requires replication. Group designs that randomly draw a representative sample may permit inferential generality, but this type of generality is not useful in predicting the performance of individual clients.

STUDY GUIDE _____

1. Distinguish between statistics and research designs. Specify why statistics should not be equated with research designs.

2. Whose work specifies an entirely statistical approach to research?

3. What is sampling equivalence? How is it achieved in the group strategy?

4. How frequently are the dependent variables measured in most of the group designs?

5. Can a control group ever receive treatment?

6. What do *X, Y, O*, and *R* stand for in a diagram showing experimental designs?

7. What are preexperimental designs?

8. What is the greatest weakness of a one-shot case study?

9. What statistical tests may be used in the analysis of results of a one-group pretest–posttest design?

10. Describe how a one-group pretest–posttest control group design would not be able to demonstrate internal validity of its results.

11. Give a hypothetical example of the static-group design. Use a clinical problem for illustration.

12. What are the limitations of preexperimental designs?

13. What is the main mechanism through which true experimental designs rule out the influence of extraneous variables?

14. Describe two methods of drawing a random sample from a population.

15. Why is randomization considered the best method of achieving sampling equivalence?

16. Distinguish between random selection and random assignment of participants. What different functions do they serve?

17. Describe two methods of matching participants. What are the limitations of matching?

18. Draw a diagram of the pretest–posttest control group design.

19. A clinician wishes to evaluate the effects of a language treatment procedure with the help of the pretest–posttest control group design. The participants are school-age children. Design this study and justify its procedure.

20. Specify one incorrect and one correct method of analyzing the results of the pretest–posttest control group design.

21. Describe the factors of internal invalidity the pretest–posttest control group design does and does not control for.

22. Are pretests absolutely necessary in a true experimental design? Why or why not?

23. What specific problem is the Solomon four-group design thought to avoid?

24. What are the limitations of the Solomon four-group design? What is your alternative to using that design?

25. Suppose you wish to evaluate the effects of three treatment techniques used in the management of stuttering. What would be your experimental design? Draw a diagram of the design.

26. What are factorial designs? What purposes do they serve?

27. Describe a randomized blocks design. Give an example, complete with all the variables involved.

28. How many conditions or cells does a 2 × 3 factorial design have?

29. Define a block and a level in a factorial design.

30. Describe a completely randomized factorial design. Identify all the levels, variables, and cells. How many participants do you need? How do you plan to get them?

31. What are quasi-experimental designs? When do you use them?

32. In what respect does the nonequivalent control group design differ from the pretest–posttest control group design?

33. What is meant by intact experimental and control groups? Give examples.

34. Illustrate the use of a separate-sample pretest–posttest design with an example of your own.

35. What is the most important characteristic of time-series designs?

36. A clinician evaluated a certain treatment procedure used in the management of language disorders. The clinician measured the language performance of the clients four times before starting treatment. The treatment was then applied for 3 months. Finally, the clinician took four more measures of language behaviors in the absence of treatment. What kind of design did the clinician use? What kinds of conclusions were possible?

37. Draw a diagram of a single-group time-series design with continuous treatment and withdrawal.

38. In a time-series design, can treatment be continued while the dependent variable is measured? If so, what is the name of the design?

39. Demonstrate how you can evaluate the effects of two or more treatments in a time-series design. Illustrate your answer.

40. Show how a control group can be built into a time-series design.

41. What are counterbalanced within-subjects designs?

42. As described in the text, are within-subjects designs the same as single-subject designs? Justify your answer.

43. Illustrate a one-group single-treatment counterbalanced design. Identify your variables, experimental conditions, and the sequences.

44. What is a crossover design? Do you evaluate a single treatment or multiple treatments in this design?

45. What is a Latin square design? What are its limitations?

46. Define order effects. How do you handle them in a counterbalanced within-subjects design?

47. Distinguish between positive and negative carryover effects. Give examples.

48. Distinguish between ceiling effects and floor effects. Under what conditions are they significant in a study?

49. What are the limitations of correlational analysis designs?

50. Evaluate the usefulness of group designs in clinical treatment research.

Chapter 9

◆◆◆◆◆◆◆◆◆◆◆◆◆◆◆◆◆◆◆◆◆◆◆◆◆◆◆◆◆◆

Single-Subject Designs

In the previous chapter, I described a research strategy in which the data represent the performance differences between groups of participants. In this chapter, I shall describe a different strategy of research in which the data represent differences in performance of the same participants under different conditions of an experiment. The research designs of this strategy are known as single-subject designs.

The single-subject design strategy is now well established, although the group strategy is still the most widely known and traditionally taught approach to experimental research. Single-subject approach is appropriate for establishing cause–effect relations in animal and human behavior. It is also as effective as the group design strategy in evaluating treatments in most disciplines, including medicine, physical therapy, counseling, social work, clinical psychology, and speech–language pathology. Its usefulness is proven in regular and special education and behavioral research. Single-subject designs are the preferred method of evaluating behavioral intervention techniques (Barlow, Hayes, & Nelson, 1984; Barlow & Hersen, 1984; Johnston & Pennypacker, 1993; Kazdin, 1982; Sidman, 1960), which include almost all of the treatment procedures used in communicative disorders.

HISTORICAL BACKGROUND OF SINGLE-SUBJECT DESIGNS

The single-subject approach, though fully developed by behavioral scientists in the 20th century, has a historical record that includes the work of early psychologists who studied psychophysics; physiologists and neurologists who studied individual differences in anatomy, physiology, and neurology; and psychiatrists and clinical psychologists who studied behavior disorders and their unique manifestations in individual clients.

Generally speaking, the work of these diverse scientists was concerned mostly with the individual, not groups of people. Scientifically, understanding patterns of individual behaviors and their experimentally manipulable causes, and clinically, understanding the uniqueness of individual symptoms and responses to treatment were the main concerns that led to the development of single-subject approach.

Study of the Individual

Studying the behavior of single individuals, as against the behavior of groups of individuals, has a long and productive history in both clinical and basic sciences. Whereas the statistical developments in the early 20th century established the study of groups and differences between groups, certain academic and clinical developments in late 19th century, and continuing into the present have helped establish a parallel trend of studying the individual.

Academic developments that led to systematic observations of individuals first took place in early psychology and physiology. First, a few major trends in early psychology, physiology, and clinical disciplines are reviewed, followed by a discussion of the experimental and applied behavior analysis that fully developed not only the study of individuals but experimental demonstration of certain cause–effect relations.

Psychological and Neurophysiological Study of the Individual

Much of the early descriptive and experimental psychology was concerned with single or a few individual participants. Group comparisons were uncommon in the first few decades of experimental psychology, and as noted in the next section, uncommon in the early development of most clinical sciences as well.

Experimental psychology began in the 1860s in the works of German mathematicians, philosophers, physiologists, and psychologists of the time. It was the works of Gustav Fechner (1801–1887) and Wilhelm Wundt (1832–1920) that gave birth to the basic science of psychophysics, which laid the foundation for experimental psychology in Germany (Boring, 1950). What is of interest to us is that the method used by early experimental psychologists was self-examination and examination of a few participants who experienced different kinds of sensation. Early psychophysics was a study of human experience in relation to precisely measured and presented sensory stimuli of various kinds. In psychophysical experiments, a few well-trained individuals would receive such stimulation and report their experiences (sensation and perception) in a method called *introspection.* The participants were trained in reporting their experiences in an objective and scientific language. In fact, Fechner is reported to have injured his eyes because he was his own single subject in experiments on visual after-images as he gazed at the sun through colored glasses (Boring, 1950).

The tradition of self-experimentation was continued in the works of Hermann Ebbinghaus (1850–1909), the inventor of the nonsense syllable, who did the earliest experiments on memory. He was his own single subject and learned various nonsense syllables and recalled them under varied conditions to find out the relationship between such variables as learning and the length of the material learned, frequency of repetition and the strength of recall, forgetting and the amount of time that lapses since learning, and so forth.

There are numerous examples of fundamental processes in sensory physiology and psychology that were discovered in experiments with few or single participants (Dukes, 1965). In learning and conditioning, most experiments have been conducted with few animal or human subjects. Pavlov's experiments on classical conditioning, for example, had only a few dogs as subjects. Nonetheless, the principles of conditioning that Pavlov formulated have been shown to have generality. Pavlov's experiments (and Skinner's as will be shown) produced data of such generality mainly because of the degree of experimental control achieved in his experiments and the precision with which the dependent and independent variables were measured. Similarly, Watson and Rayner's (1920) well-known experiment on conditioning of fear in a single child to white rats eventually demonstrated that data generated from single participants may have generality.

Early physiological and neurological research, too has been based on systematic observations of, and experimentation on, one or a few individuals. It is well known that Broca's discovery of the motor speech center in the third frontal convolution of the left cerebral hemisphere was based initially on a single case, and subsequently on just a handful of cases. By carefully examining a patient with aphasia, Broca kept detailed records of the patient's speech problems and ruled out any pathology of the larynx or paralysis of the speech muscles. When the patient died, Broca performed a brain autopsy and found a lesion in the third frontal convolution in the left cerebral hemisphere. Broca's speech area and Broca's aphasia are now generally accepted although not without some controversy. His careful observations of single patients affirmed the value of intensive study of a single or a few individuals in making valid contributions to scientific knowledge.

Other early neurophysiological discoveries also used single or few participants. For instance, the discovery of localization of motor functions in the brain by Fritsch and Hitzig in 1870 was based on human single-case observations and few animal experiments (Boring, 1950). Similarly, Wernicke's discoveries of a sensory speech area in the posterior portion of the left superior temporal gyrus and a type of aphasia associated with lesions in this area were based on single-case observation. Mapping of the brain functions has always been done only with small number of participants, often single participants, who had to undergo brain surgery for such diseases as epilepsy (Calvin & Ojemann, 1980).

Case Study Method

The case study method was born out of clinical case histories, which are a description of an individual's clinical problem, conditions that led to the problem, variables that are associated with the problem, and other personal details that help diagnose a disease and suggest treatment for that individual. Case studies, however, go beyond the case history in the sense that they are a more scientific method of studying a phenomenon by making systematic observations and measurement. Although often used in the context of diseases and disorders, the case study method has been found to be effective in studying clinical as well as nonclinical phenomena in most disciplines, including such diverse disciplines as psychiatry, history, anthropology, medicine, psychology, linguistics, speech–language pathology, and sociology (Bolgar, 1965; Dukes, 1965).

The distinguishing characteristic of the case history and case study method is the attention paid to the individual. It is the case study method that has provided careful and detailed description of diseases and disorders in individual patients. The knowledge that clinicians use in diagnosing and treating disorders could not have been possible without the case study method where an individual patient's symptoms and conditions were systematically observed and documented. In psychiatry, thorough observations of patients to describe their symptoms by such early German psychiatrists as Kraepelin (1856–1926) have been the beginnings of the case study method (Bolgar, 1965).

Freud's psychoanalysis was founded entirely on the basis of observations generated by the method of case study. His accumulated observations of individual patients led to the influential psychoanalytic school of psychology and psychiatry. Freud believed that based on his observations of individual patients, he could make generalizations that would apply to most human beings. He thought that the psychodynamic principles he discovered in the context of his patients were valid in both clinical and nonclinical populations (Freud, 1944).

Clinical psychology, which flourished after World War II, fully exploited and extended the potential of the clinical case study method. Clinical psychologists continued to use the case study method to systematically observe and record various symptoms and behaviors associated with mental and behavioral disorders. Speech–language pathology, a clinical discipline, also began to use the case study method to document various disorders of communication.

As noted before, usefulness of the case study method is not limited to clinical problems. The method has been widely used in the study of other issues in human and animal research. For instance, the study of language acquisition in children has been greatly advanced by the case study method involving longitudinal observations of one or a few children. Parents' systematic observation of their single child's language behaviors, recorded over an extended period of time, is a standard method of tracing language acquisition (McLaughlin, 1998). Brown's (1973) well-known research on language acquisition had only three young children as participants. Much of Piaget's (1952, 1959) famous work on intellectual development in children was based on extended observations of his three children.

Experimental Analysis of Behavior

Although systematic observations of individuals has been a well-established scientific method in several disciplines, such observations were often nonexperimental. For instance, most research on language acquisition in children is nonexperimental. Nonexperimental observations of individuals, while providing valuable insights and hunches, cannot establish a functional relation between the variables measured or recorded. In a systematic clinical case study, for instance, it is not possible to firmly establish the cause of the disorder. When a case study reports favorable results of a treatment, clinicians cannot be sure that the treatment actually caused those results. The typical case study is an ex post facto analysis of factors that may have been responsible for an effect, but it lacks experimental control. Case studies rely heavily on the method of correlation, not experimentation. Therefore, while systematic observations of single participants are a good start, such observations need to incorporate experimental manipulations.

Skinner (1953) was foremost among the scientists who used the single-subject approach to develop an experimental method to create a science of behavior. To understand the basic processes of human behavior, Skinner developed the method of intensely studying individual behaviors under different experimental conditions. He did not believe that studying the behavior of large samples of individuals randomly drawn from a population would yield strong experimental data to build a science of behavior. In his view, large samples force superficial observations under weak experimental controls, resulting in data that fail to throw light on basic behavioral processes. He thought that only intensive study of individuals under well-controlled experimental conditions would provide strong data on behavior. To this effect, he stated that "instead of studying a thousand rats for one hour each, or a hundred rats for ten hours each, the investigator is likely to study one rat for a thousand hours" (Skinner, 1966, p. 21).

Skinner's experimental analysis of behavior has clearly shown that to achieve generality, one does not need randomized samples of a large number of participants. Most of the operant conditioning principles, including positive and negative reinforcement schedules, extinction, generalization, discrimination, and punishment were established with a few rats and later extended to human participants through various replications. Skinner's research has made it clear that to achieve generality, one only needs replication of findings. Single-subject experimental designs can achieve generality of findings through replication and produce scientifically valid knowledge.

Applied Behavior Analysis

Most of the currently used single-subject experimental designs in treatment research were developed in the process of applied behavioral analysis, which is based on Skinner's experimental analysis of behavior. Several of the currently popular designs were developed in the course of applied behavioral research. For instance, multiple-baseline designs were developed specifically to evaluate clinical treatment techniques and educational teaching methods. Therefore, most of the specific designs to be described had their origins in clinical or applied research. The kinds of dependent and independent variables manipulated in these designs have been influenced to a great extent by behavioral philosophy. Nevertheless, the designs themselves are strategies of research, which can be used to answer questions that may or may not have come from behavioral philosophy.

Applied behavioral research has clearly demonstrated that clinical and educational problems of social and personal significance can be meaningfully analyzed with single-subject experimental methods. Unlike traditional case studies, applied behavioral analysis is typically experimental. Both the methods use a single or a few participants, but the applied behavioral analysis makes its observations under controlled conditions and induces systematic experimental manipulations. The approach arranges different conditions for an experiment and rules out the influence of extraneous variables through controlled conditions. Because of this emphasis on the use of experimental methods in evaluating treatments and teaching methods, applied behavior analysis has made significant contributions to clinical literature.

CHARACTERISTICS OF SINGLE-SUBJECT DESIGNS

The single-subject designs also are described as single-case designs, intrasubject replication designs, and designs of behavioral analysis. As noted in Chapter 8, occasionally they also are called within-subjects designs. However, there exists a variety of group designs that has historically been known as within-subjects designs. Therefore, this term should not be used to describe single-subject designs.

Several characteristics are common to single-subject designs that are currently used in treatment research.

Intensive Study of Small Number of Participants

Single-subject designs avoid large samples and concentrate on fewer individuals. As noted previously, the philosophy of single-subject designs places a heavy emphasis on understanding the behavior of individuals. Intensive study of individuals makes much clinical sense. Clinicians are much more interested in changing the health status or undesirable behaviors of their individual clients. Clinical work, even if it involves a large number of individuals, is essentially concerned with how individuals react to different diagnostic and treatment procedures. Therefore, single-subject designs use a small number of available participants who meet the selection criteria. Clinical treatment studies with just few participants generate a significant amount of data largely because of extended observations of individual behaviors under such changing experimental conditions as baserate, treatment, and treatment withdrawal.

One of the mistaken notions about single-subject or single-case designs is that only one participant can be used in a study. Though some reported studies may have had single participants, the designs themselves are not restricted in this manner. Typically, multiple participants, perhaps six to eight, are used in most single-subject designs. Obviously, the number of participants used in single-subject designs is much smaller than in a group design.

Importance of Individual Differences

The emphasis on the behavior of individuals also means that individual differences are of both scientific and clinical interest. From a statistical standpoint, individual differences are within-group variance (variability). Such variability is considered an error in the group design strategy, which is most interested in variance between the experimental and control group. To the contrary, single-subject designs do not treat variations in an individual's behavior or among a few individuals as errors. There is nothing erroneous about individual differences. Behavioral variability within and across individuals is worthy of experimental analysis. It is only such experimental analysis of individuals and their behavioral variability that will lead to a better understanding of individual differences and commonalities. Controlling experimental conditions tightly to see if the behavioral variability is reduced is a unique characteristic of single-subject designs. If the variability is not reduced even under strict experimental conditions, efforts to understand why may then be initiated.

Because of its interest in behaviors of individuals, the single-subject strategy does not involve group comparisons. Instead of comparing the mean performance of participants receiving treatment with the mean performance of participants not receiving treatment, the single-subject strategy compares the same individual's performance under treatment and no-treatment conditions. Therefore, when several participants are used in a study, the results are not averaged across individuals. Each participant's results are described separately.

Repeated Measurement
of the Dependent Variables

Single-subject designs require repeated measurement of the dependent variables. There are no pretests and posttests, as in the group design approach. Both the terminology and the practice of pretests and posttests are determined mostly by educational research methods. In the single-subject strategy, the dependent variables are not *tested* or assessed with some standardized instrument, but are *measured* continuously—before, during, and after treatment.

Before the treatment is introduced, the dependent variables (skills that are treatment targets) are measured repeatedly. The repeated measures made before the introduction of treatment are typically known as baselines or steady states. As noted in Chapter 4, these initial baselines are held to a criterion of stability and reliability. In some cases, baseline observations may be done over several days to stabilize the behaviors under controlled conditions. Treatment is introduced only when the behaviors, stabilized across observations (or in other ways), provide contrast to treatment effects.

In treatment sessions, too, the target behaviors are continuously measured. This may not be the case in group designs that depend on a posttest administered at the end of the study. Session-by-session measures of target behaviors give a better picture of the course of changes in the dependent variables than the two-point measures of pretests and posttests.

Another measure of the dependent variable taken throughout single-subject studies is known as probes. **Probes** are measures of target behaviors in the absence of treatment. They may be taken in the treatment room or in many cases, outside the room. Probes help assess the stability of treatment effects when the treatment is temporarily discontinued. They also help assess generalized production of target skills in the natural environment. Such generalized productions in everyday situations enhance the social validity of treatment procedures.

Selection of Available Participants

In the single-subject strategy, participants are not selected randomly. No attempt is made to draw a representative sample from a defined population. Available individuals are considered appropriate for experimental analysis. As in group design studies, not all available participants are selected; only those who meet certain selection criteria thought to be relevant for the research question are chosen for participation. For instance, such variables as age, gender, severity of the disorder, prior treatment, or prior exposure to a certain technique may lead to specific selection criteria.

As in group design studies including randomized clinical trials, participants apparently selected by the investigator for a single-subject study are essentially self-selected. Only those who consent to participate in a study do so. Selected participants may refuse to participate, terminate their participation during the course of the study, and demand a treatment that is other than the experimental treatment being evaluated.

Because no effort is made to have a representative sample of a population, the conclusions of a single-subject study are not extended to the population on the basis of a single study or a few studies. In other words, unreplicated single-subject research does not claim inferential (statistical) generality. The single-subject researchers do believe that generality should be established for all treatment procedures. They take a different route to generality of treatment effects, however. These researchers believe that generality, including inferential generality, is a matter of replication and that even the most representative sample is not likely to have all kinds of generalities. Single-subject researchers believe that replication of studies, not a large randomized sample, is the key to establishing generality of treatment findings.

Strong on Logical Generality

Although single-subjects designs do not claim statistical (inferential) generality, they do claim logical generality. **Logical generality** is the extension of the conclusions of a single-subject study to individuals who match the profiles of study participants. Because single-subject study reports give full details on individual participants, it is easier for practitioners to match their client profiles with those of study participants.

Because single-subject design studies describe each participant's data separately, the reader of such reports knows who improved, who did not, and who deteriorated under the experimental treatment. The reader can thus match a participant's personal characteristics with the results obtained. For instance, if only those with a more severe disorder improved under an experimental treatment, the practitioner can then apply the treatment to such clients only. Group designs, even if they do have statistical generality, lack logical generality because the studies do not give individual profiles nor individual data in sufficient detail to be useful to clinicians.

Visual Inspection of Data Versus Statistical Analysis

The results of single-subject designs generally are not analyzed with statistical techniques. There are two main reasons for this. The first is that the experimental effects produced in single-subject designs are large enough to support conclusions without statistical analyses. Most statistical techniques are designed to detect small changes in dependent variables against a background of poorly controlled natural variability. Single-subject designs depend upon empirical significance in differences in conditions, not statistical differences. When conditions of an experiment differ markedly, visual inspection of data will reveal the effects of experimental manipulations. Therefore, in reading and evaluating single-subject studies, visual inspection plays a major role.

Figure 9.1 shows the difference between the group and the single-subject data of a hypothetical study. If a certain treatment of stuttering is evaluated within a two-group study and also a single-subject study, the kinds of results that are depicted in Figure 9.1 are likely. The data from the single-subject design, shown in the upper part as bar graphs (A), make the effects of treatment visually obvious. There has been a systematic and clinically

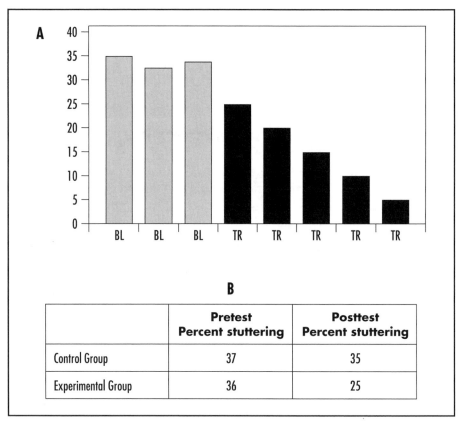

Figure 9.1. Differential visual effects of single-subject (A) and group design (B) studies of a hypothetical treatment effect on stuttering. Note that the single-subject data are presented for three baseline sessions (BL) and five treatment sessions (TR). The data for the group design study are the pretest and posttest means for the two groups.

impressive reduction in the frequency of stuttering. On the other hand, whether the difference in the mean frequency of stutterings of the two groups, shown in the lower portion (B) is due to the treatment or chance fluctuations is not so readily apparent. Therefore, the effects of treatment in group designs are better determined by statistical analysis.

The second reason for not using statistical procedures in the analysis of the results of single-subject designs is that a majority of statistical techniques are based on the random theory and require both random sampling and random assignment of participants. Such techniques may not be appropriate for evaluating data of individual participants. However, for those who prefer them, several special statistical techniques can be applied in the analysis of single-subject studies (Barlow & Hersen, 1984; Kazdin, 1982). A majority of single-subject investigators, though, do not use statistical techniques.

Mostly because of the characteristics just described, the single-subject strategy is highly suitable for clinical research. The need to work with a small number of clients, the problem of not being able to form large groups of clinical participants, the ethical implications of having to deny treatment to a control group that needs it, and the clinical requirement of having to produce large effects in individuals who receive treatment underscore the value of single-subject strategy for clinical professions.

EXPERIMENTAL CONTROL IN SINGLE-SUBJECT DESIGNS

Group and single-subject designs differ in the way they introduce experimental control to rule out the influence of extraneous variables to claim internal validity. Group designs rule out the influence of extraneous variables by the use of control groups that do not receive treatment and hence do not show significant change at the end of an experiment. Single-subject designs, on the other hand, rule out extraneous variables by a combination of control conditions. It was argued in Chapter 4 that control conditions and control groups are the primary and equally powerful methods of showing that a treatment, and no other variable, was responsible for the positive changes documented in an experiment. A variety of such control conditions have been described in Chapter 4. These include baselines, treatment withdrawal, treatment reversal, reinstatement of treatment, criterion-referenced change, rapid alternations, and simultaneous multibaselines.

The designs described in the subsequent sections of this chapter illustrate the use of multiple control mechanisms used in the single-subject approach. A mechanism common to most designs is the initial baselines. When the initial baseline data are contrasted with data recorded under treatment conditions, which are in turn contrasted with those obtained under treatment withdrawal, which are once again contrasted with those obtained under reinstatement of treatment, one can draw valid conclusions about the effects of a treatment. A main difference between the group designs and single-subject designs is that in the group designs, different individuals provide for control, whereas in the single-subject designs, the different response rates of the same individuals under different conditions of an experiment provide for control. The reader is referred to Chapter 4 for details and additional contrasts between the group and single-subject designs used in treatment research.

PREEXPERIMENTAL SINGLE-SUBJECT DESIGN

Preexperimental designs, as described in Chapter 8, do not have adequate control for the factors that affect the internal validity of an experiment. There is a single-subject design that parallels the group preexperimental one-shot case study. In the terminology of single-subject designs, this is known as the *AB* design.

The *AB* design is similar to traditional case studies. A case study is a rather detailed study of a single patient or client who undergoes a form of treatment. Such case studies are common in many clinical fields, including medicine, clinical psychology, psychiatry, and speech–language pathology.

In the *AB* design, a baseline of the target behavior is first established; the treatment is then applied and the dependent variable is measured continuously. When the treatment objective is achieved, a report is made on the recorded changes in the client behaviors. The design is illustrated in Figure 9.2.

It is obvious that the *AB* design lacks experimental control of extraneous variables. Therefore, it is not classified as an experimental design. It is similar to the traditional case study. The observed changes in the dependent variable may or may not be due to the influence of treatment. There is no assurance that in the absence of treatment, the behaviors would not have improved. Therefore, history and maturation, among other factors, may explain the results of case studies and *AB* studies.

The *AB* studies do not require control procedures that consume extra time and energy. Although they do not permit statements on cause–effect relations, *AB* studies are thought to suggest ideas for more controlled research while providing for a certain degree of confidence in the treatment procedure. If an *AB* study fails to show improvement, that is considered a significant finding because a treatment that does not produce an effect under uncontrolled conditions may not produce an effect under future controlled conditions either.

The matter of experimental control is not an either–or phenomenon because different designs have varying degrees of control. The *AB* designs

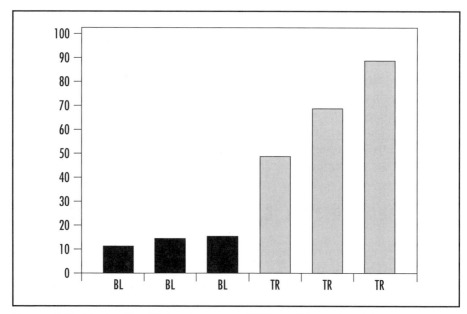

Figure 9.2. The baseline (BL) and treatment (TR) conditions of an *AB* (preexperimental) design.

can also vary in terms of the degree of confidence one can place in the results. Some of them can be more trustworthy than others. Multiple observations before, during, and after treatment with stable measures and good contrast can enhance the validity of *AB* studies. See Chapter 4 for other suggestions to improve the quality of evidence of case studies including *AB* studies.

EXPERIMENTAL DESIGNS FOR SINGLE-TREATMENT EVALUATION

Unlike the preexperimental *AB* design, **experimental single-subject designs** seek to rule out extraneous variables with appropriate control mechanisms. When adequate control mechanisms are used, the investigator may claim internal validity for the results.

Single-subject experimental designs are available to evaluate the effects of single or multiple treatments and interaction between two or more treatment procedures. This discussion first addresses designs that help evaluate the single treatments and moves on to more complex designs for evaluating relative and interactive effects of multiple treatments.

ABA and *ABAB* Designs

The basic experimental paradigm of the single-subject strategy is to establish baselines, introduce treatment, and then withdraw or reverse treatment. This is known as the *ABA* design and was developed in basic laboratory research. It is most appropriately used in demonstrating the control of variables that are not expected to produce lasting treatment effects. To demonstrate more permanent treatment effects, the *ABA* design can be extended to include the reinstatement of treatment resulting in the *ABAB* design. These two designs reveal the basic logic and the strategy of single-subject designs. Both have two versions: withdrawal and reversal.

ABA *Withdrawal Design*

The *ABA* withdrawal design, illustrated in Figure 9.3, is the original experimental design within the single-subject design strategy. In laboratory research involving animal behavior, subjects are typically run for an extended period of time to establish the operant level (baseline) of selected behaviors. It is not uncommon to run animal subjects for several weeks to achieve behavioral stability. Following a stable response rate, various kinds of stimulus and response-consequent contingencies are applied to assess the effects on behavior patterns.

Depending on the research question, the experimental contingencies also are applied over an extended time. A marked shift in the response rate

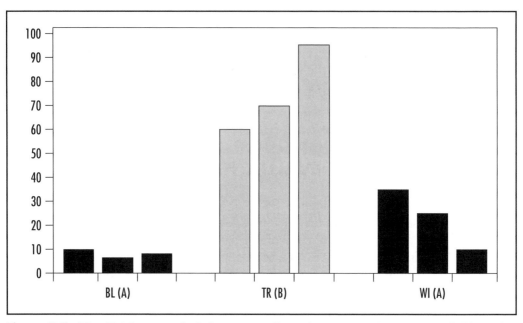

Figure 9.3. The *ABA* design in which the positive effects of a treatment (TR) are cancelled by withdrawal (WI).

creating a contrast between the baseline and the treatment conditions is sought by this prolonged experimental manipulation. After such a shift is observed, the independent variable is withdrawn, and the subjects or participants are allowed to respond. Normally, the response rate gradually decreases until it approximates the original baseline level. When the independent variable investigated is a reinforcer, the withdrawal condition also is known as the extinction condition.

In Figure 9.3, note that the first two conditions of the design show a comparable response rate. The response rate is higher under the treatment condition, which contrasts with the baseline and extinction conditions.

The *ABA* withdrawal design is a well-controlled design. When a stable response rate that is documented by baseline measures changes dramatically when the treatment is introduced but returns to the baseline level when the treatment is withdrawn, a convincing demonstration of the treatment effect will have occurred. The basic logic of the design is that when a variable is present, it produces an effect, but when the variable is absent, the effect disappears. When this happens, other factors cannot account for the presence and absence of the effect.

Much of the basic information about the principles of learning and conditioning including reinforcement, punishment, and the effects of various reinforcement schedules, has been generated by this *ABA* withdrawal strategy. It continues to be one of the most important experimental strategies of research in behavioral analysis.

It is clear that the final phase of the *ABA* withdrawal design does not involve treatment. When it is used in clinical settings, the improvement shown by the client in the treatment condition is neutralized in the final *A* condition. Therefore, it is not a clinical treatment design. However, the design has a place in clinical research. Its use in clinical research can be justified on certain discriminated grounds.

The design is not appropriate when a clinician expects to use a treatment procedure until the clinical goals of complete habilitation or rehabilitation are accomplished. However, the *ABA* design is appropriate when the effects of a new technique of treatment must be evaluated and there is no evidence yet that it will be the long-term treatment for the disorder under investigation.

There is a more important reason for using the *ABA* design. Whether a variable has any effect at all on a given behavior is an important research question. The effects may be temporary, in which case they may not lead to the development of a treatment effect. They may be relatively permanent, in which case the possibility of developing a new treatment technique exists. When the initial research question is whether a particular variable has any effect at all, the *ABA* withdrawal design is appropriate. For instance, it is reasonable to ask whether verbal or other kinds of stimuli have any effects at all on dysfluencies, misarticulations, vocal pitch breaks, or other kinds of speech–language problems.

If the answer produced by an *ABA* withdrawal design is positive, more clinically appropriate designs can be employed to develop treatment techniques. For example, much of the operant research on stuttering involving such aversive stimuli as shock, noise, and verbal stimuli was done with the *ABA* design. Hindsight would now justify the use of the *ABA* withdrawal strategy because stimuli such as shock and aversive noise have not led to routine clinical treatment procedures.

ABA *Reversal Design*

The reversal operation described as a control mechanism in Chapter 4 can be used in the *ABA* format. It is illustrated in Figure 9.4. In terms of the baseline and treatment, the design is the same as the *ABA* withdrawal design. However, during the second *A* condition, the experimental contingencies may be reversed. Instead of simply withdrawing the treatment from the target behavior (1), another, incompatible behavior (2) may be treated. As a result, it can be shown that the first behavior returns to the baseline and the second behavior shows new and systematic changes. This would help rule out extraneous variables.

For example, if the design is used in evaluating a treatment procedure for articulation disorders, the clinician first increases the correct production of selected phonemes and then reverses the contingencies to increase the original incorrect productions of the same phonemes. In the treatment of language disorders, participants' production of selected grammatical features may be first increased, and then the same treatment may be used to increase

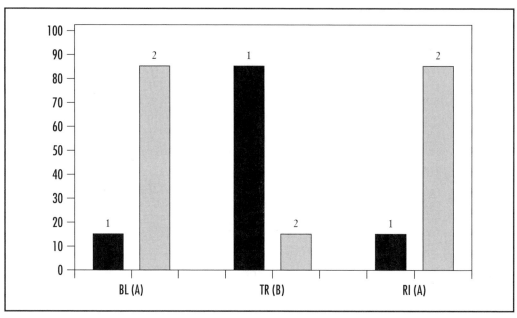

Figure 9.4. The *ABA* reversal design. Note the corresponding effects of treatment (TR) and reversal (RI) on a target (1) and its incompatible behavior (2).

the production of phrases or sentences without those grammatical features. For instance, if a child initially omits the auxiliary *is*, resulting in such responses as *boy running* and *girl writing*, the reversal involves a reinforcement of these responses.

It may appear that *ABA* reversal is clinically more problematic than the *ABA* withdrawal. An initial thought may be that in a withdrawal design the client is no better or no worse than his or her initial standing because at the end of the experiment his or her response rate will approximate the pretreatment baseline. The same client in a reversal design may appear to be worse off at the end of the experiment because the clinician reinforced the wrong response to increase it. These initial reactions may not be valid, however. Especially as the two designs are used in communicative disorders, clients in either case are in the same position: They are roughly at their baseline at the end of the experiment.

When a reversal is used, there is no need to increase the error response to a level that is higher than that observed at the baseline. When the baseline is at zero and the treatment increases the target behavior to 90% or higher, then the reversal need not be continued until the target behavior reaches zero. A reduction from 90% to 30% or 40% may be convincing. As such, reversal and withdrawal are both mechanisms either to recover the baselines or to force the target behaviors in that direction.

In withdrawal, the baseline is recovered rather slowly because the main mechanism is extinction of the treated behavior. It is known that extinction is a slow process. In reversal, the baseline may be recovered faster because reversal is a more active process. It increases an incompatible behavior, which indirectly decreases the treated target behavior. In this sense, reversal may be a more efficient control procedure.

As was suggested in the context of the withdrawal design, when there is no expectation of producing lasting effects, reversal may be just as appropriate as withdrawal. Questions of effects of various stimulus conditions on communicative behaviors and disorders may be researched within the reversal strategy because they have important theoretical implications. Whether a treatment procedure will eventually be developed out of this research may be an extraneous or a later consideration.

It must be noted that when either the withdrawal or the reversal strategy is used, the client participates in an experiment with no change in his or her problem situation. Taking appropriate human participant protection steps (see Chapter 12), the investigator can recruit clients for this kind of research. However, at the end of the experiment, it must be possible to offer those clients a treatment procedure that will remedy their specific clinical problem.

ABAB *Design*

To evaluate clinical treatment procedures, the *ABAB* design and its variations are considered better alternatives to the basic *ABA* design. It is a clinically more useful design because the treatment is the final condition of the experiment. Also, the treatment effects are replicated.

The *ABAB* design starts with the establishment of an acceptable baseline of the dependent variable (the first *A* condition). The treatment is then introduced in the first *B* condition and continued until the experimenter observes an unmistakable change in the dependent variable or concludes that a change is unlikely to take place. If found effective, the treatment is either withdrawn or reversed in the second *A* condition. The effects of this withdrawal or reversal are measured for an appropriate period of time. Finally, in the second *B* condition, the treatment is reintroduced to replicate and continue the treatment effects. The withdrawal version of the *ABAB* design is shown in Figure 9.5.

Assuming that the treatment is effective in changing the behavior when it is first introduced, a change in the opposite direction during the withdrawal or reversal (the second *A* condition) must be evident. When the treatment is reintroduced a second time, the response rate must change again in the opposite direction. If the treatment is expected to increase the rate of response, then the rate of response in the two treatment conditions should be higher than that in the two no-treatment conditions. If the treatment is expected to decrease a behavior, the rate of response should be lower in the two treatment conditions than in the two no-treatment conditions.

Let us suppose that a clinician wishes to assess the effects of verbal reinforcers on the production of selected grammatical features by a child with

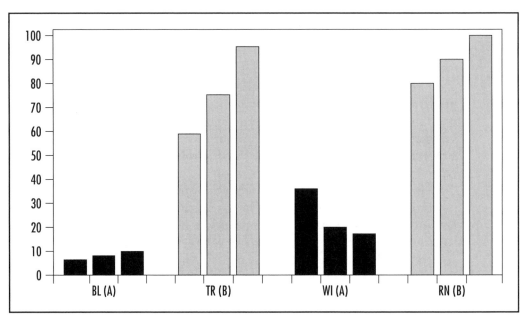

Figure 9.5. The baseline (A), treatment (B), withdrawal (A), and reinstatement (B) conditions of an *ABAB* design.

a language disorder who is producing those targets at a low rate. The clinician initially baserates the production of the selected morpheme by presenting it in the context of several sentences to be evoked by pictorial stimuli and an appropriate question. This is the first *A* condition, which may show that the morphemes are produced with 15% accuracy. Then the clinician shows selected pictures to evoke particular responses and reinforces the correct production of the target morpheme in sentences. This is the first treatment condition, *B*. During this condition, it may be observed that the production of the morpheme has increased to 86%. At this point, the clinician withdraws the verbal praise and continues to evoke the target responses on a series of trials. This is the second *A* condition, during which the response rate decreases to 21%. Finally, the clinician reintroduces the verbal praise for correct production of the morpheme, which may increase to 95% or better. This is the second *B* condition, in which the treatment is continued until the client has generalized and maintained the production of the morpheme in conversational speech evoked in naturalistic settings.

Introduction of additional treatment features such as generalization and maintenance during the latter part of the second *B* condition do not affect the conclusions that can be drawn from the study. The data needed to evaluate the effects of verbal praise on the production of the selected morpheme have been produced by the time such additional procedures are introduced. However, no firm conclusions regarding the effects of the additional procedures is permissible because those procedures have not been evaluated experimentally. For example, one cannot assume—because the child maintains the production of the morpheme after implementation of a maintenance program—that the program is indeed effective. The issue of evaluating maintenance programs will be addressed in a later section.

In the *ABAB* reversal version, the experiment just described involves reinforcement of productions that do not include the target morpheme but should. In other words, the contingency is placed on an incompatible behavior. In this case, the responses that do not include the morpheme would show an increase. In the final treatment condition, the reinforcer would be made contingent again on the correct production of the target morphemes.

A variation of the *ABAB* design is known as the *ABCB* design. In this design, the target behavior is baserated and a treatment applied, as in the *ABAB* design. However, the next condition involves neither withdrawal nor reversal. Therefore, this third condition is known as *C* instead of *A*. In this *C* condition, the reinforcer may be delivered on a noncontingent basis. In other words, the reinforcer does not follow correct production of the target behavior, but it may happen to follow any of the nontarget behaviors that happen to be produced. This may also result in a decrease in the target behavior, essentially showing the controlling function of the reinforcer. The amount of reinforcer delivered noncontingently is the same as that in the previous treatment condition.

The *ABAB* design permits the reinstatement and continuation of treatment until the clients are ready to be discharged. However, the design does require the use of either withdrawal or reversal of treatment to show that no other variable is responsible for the changes in the behavior. In this respect, it shares all problems associated with withdrawal and reversal. When the treatment is withdrawn, the rate of the target behavior may not show a decline. Reversal may take an unduly long period of time, raising questions of ethical justification concerning "teaching the wrong response."

Reversal or withdrawal may be totally undesirable when the behavior reduced during the treatment is either self-injurious or abusive of other persons. In such instances, reversal or withdrawal of successful treatment leads to injury to the self or to other persons. However, in many cases—especially in communicative disorders—withdrawal and reversal are achieved in a relatively short time so that the treatment is reinstated quickly without any negative effects on the client or other persons. When treatment is withdrawn, faulty articulation, dysfluencies, inappropriate vocal qualities, and inappropriate language responses show a relatively quick return to the near-baseline level, and reinstatement of treatment can result in equally quick recovery of the appropriate target responses. The *ABAB* design has been used extensively in modifying a variety of problem behaviors in clinical and educational settings.

In spite of its limitations, some clinical research questions require the *ABAB* strategy; for example, when one wishes to evaluate the effects that treating one behavior has on another behavior that is not treated, the *ABAB* is an excellent choice. This kind of research is able to identify behaviors that belong to distinct groups, called *response classes*. The clinician often faces the problem of not being able to identify target behaviors that are apparently different but are empirically the same. Conversely, the clinician may also face the problem of having a single category of responses that is actually a collection of different behaviors. The issue is important because a resolution of it often clarifies the number of clinical target behaviors in given treatment situations.

Take, for example, the question of subject noun phrase and object noun phrase. Are they separate clinical targets or are they one and the same? Are verbal auxiliary and copula one and the same or are they different clinical targets? In other words, what is the effect of training subject noun phrase on object noun phrase (and vice versa), and training verbal auxiliary on copula (and vice versa)? Questions such as these are appropriately answered by the *ABAB* design, in which one of the pairs in question is trained, the treatment is then withdrawn or reversed, and then it is reinstated while the production of both responses is measured. For example, the object noun phrase can be trained, reversed, and reinstated to see if the subject noun phrase also is produced, reversed, and reinstated without a direct application of the treatment variable. Such an outcome would suggest that the two are not separate clinical targets in spite of the structural distinctions between them. A study of this kind has suggested that subject and object noun phrases belong to the same response class (McReynolds & Engmann, 1974). Similarly, there is some evidence to suggest that the verbal auxiliary and copula belong to the same response class (Hegde, 1980b).

In the study of communication and its disorders, there are many structural categories such as semantic and pragmatic notions whose status as empirically valid responses is not clear. The *ABAB* design provides an excellent means of determining whether such structural categories are independent responses that can be clinically taught.

BAB *Design*

In the *BAB* design, which is a variation of the basic *ABA* format, the treatment is introduced in the first phase of an experiment. In this case, there is no initial baseline. The three conditions of the design, as shown in Figure 9.6 are the treatment *B*, baseline *A*, and treatment *B*. From a technical standpoint, it may be more appropriate to use the terms *withdrawal* or *reversal* for the second condition because it is unlike the original baseline, which precedes treatment.

One of the strengths of this design is that the experiment ends with treatment, and therefore, the design is more suitable than the *ABA* design for clinical evaluation of treatment techniques. Another strength is that the design involves intrasubject replication of treatment effects because the treatment is applied twice. However, the problem with this design is that there is no pretreatment baseline against which to compare the treatment effects. The treatment effects can be evaluated only in relation to the response rates under reversal or withdrawal of treatment. Nevertheless, the

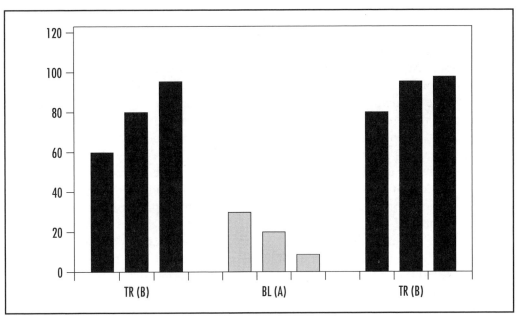

Figure 9.6. The *BAB* design with initial and final treatment conditions (TR) that increase a target behavior.

reversal or withdrawal in the second phase and the reintroduction of treatment in the third phase should provide a reasonable justification to evaluate the efficacy of the treatment variable. Treatment replication should enhance the internal validity of the experimental findings.

Multiple Baseline Designs

The multiple baseline designs are among the most desirable of the single-subject designs because they avoid the problems of withdrawal and reversal. The structure of the multiple baseline designs includes a series of baseline and treatment conditions across different behaviors, persons, settings, and some combinations of these. The design is essentially a multiple *AB* series. It is still able to control for the extraneous variables by arranging a series of simultaneous multibaselines in such a way that the dependent variables change *only* when they come under the influence of the treatment variable.

The multiple baseline design has three standard versions: multiple baseline design across behaviors, across subjects, and across settings. I shall discuss these standard versions as well as some variations.

Multiple Baseline Across Behaviors

Since its formal recognition in 1968 by Baer, Wolf, and Risley, the multiple baseline across behaviors has been used extensively in clinical research involving treatment evaluation. This design requires that the investigator have several dependent variables for experimental manipulation in a single participant or client. In most clinical situations, this is easily accomplished because clients usually need treatment for several target behaviors. For example, clients with articulation disorders typically need treatment for multiple phonemes, and clients with language disorders typically need treatment for multiple grammatical, semantic, pragmatic, or response class targets. Also, in most clinical situations, the clinician is not able to treat all target behaviors simultaneously. Single behaviors or just a few behaviors may be targeted for treatment at any one time. When the training is accomplished on certain behaviors, other behaviors are targeted for further training. This typical clinical situation is well suited for multiple baseline evaluation of treatment.

In the evaluation of a given treatment procedure with multiple baseline across behaviors, the clinician selects a client who needs treatment on several behaviors. To begin with, all of the target behaviors are baserated. When a stable response rate is established for at least one of the target behaviors, the treatment is applied to that behavior. The treatment is withheld from other behaviors that are still at baseline. The first behavior is trained to a specified criterion, say 90% accuracy on probe trials that do not involve treatment (no reinforcement, for example). Then the remaining behaviors are once again baserated to make sure that the behaviors not trained did not change relative to the original baseline. The second behavior is then trained to the selected criterion. The other target behaviors remain in baseline, which is reestablished before the third behavior is trained. After obtaining another baseline of untrained behaviors, the fourth behavior is trained. In this manner, every time a behavior is trained, the untrained behaviors are baserated to demonstrate their lack of change in the absence of treatment. The typical results of a multiple baseline design involving four target behaviors are illustrated in Figure 9.7.

There are two important considerations in the use of the multiple baseline design across behaviors. The first consideration is the number of target behaviors that are sequentially treated and the second is the independence of those behaviors. Both considerations have a potential for creating problems for interpreting data generated by the design.

It is generally thought that to demonstrate the controlling effects of the experimental manipulation, a minimum of three to four behaviors must be included in the design (Barlow & Hersen, 1984). Three to four behaviors give an adequate chance to show that the behaviors change only when treated and not when in baseline. In this case, the experimenter can establish a clear trend in the data that demonstrate the effect of an independent variable.

The second question—the independence of the behaviors selected for experimental manipulation—is more difficult for a priori judgments. The problem is that when two behaviors in a multiple baseline design are not independent of each other, then the treatment applied to one behavior may

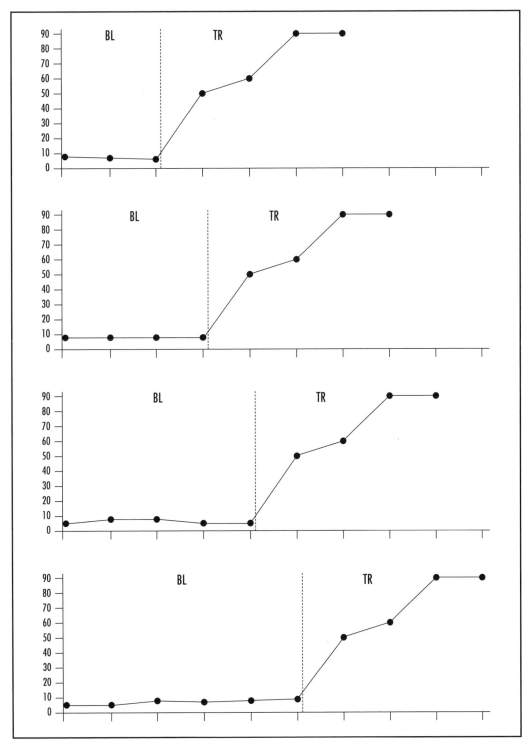

Figure 9.7. The multiple baseline design involving four target behaviors. Note the progressively increasing number of baseline observations (BL) for the second and subsequent targets. Each behavior increases only when brought under the influence of treatment (TR). Data from multiple baselines across participants and settings may be similarly charted.

affect the other, which is supposedly still in the baseline. Changes in untreated behaviors may be due to either uncontrolled independent variables or a dependence between the treated and changed, though untreated, behaviors.

The independence of behaviors selected for a multiple baseline design often is judged on the basis of theory, clinical experience, or empirical evidence. In given cases, these bases may or may not be valid. In this respect, untested theoretical grounds and unverified experience are risky. The best empirical basis is provided by past evidence. In speech–language pathology, the independence of behaviors is one of the most troublesome issues for clinical researchers because speech and language behaviors often are distinguished on the basis of response topography only. Behaviors are independent when they have different independent variables. However, distinctions among behaviors that are insensitive to the independent variables may prove misleading under conditions of experimental manipulations.

The misleading nature of behavioral distinctions based on untested theoretical grounds is evident in research on language treatment. The grammatical, semantic, and pragmatic theories of language have identified an endless variety of response categories that are based solely on the basis of *form* of responses. Distinctions between various grammatical categories, semantic notions, and pragmatic rules are based on structural theories with very little evidence regarding their empirical validity.

My associates and I had an opportunity to find out the hard way that some grammatical categories may not be real. An experiment on language training was designed to discover certain forms of contextual generalization (Hegde, Noll, & Pecora, 1978). A multiple baseline design across behaviors was selected to demonstrate the effectiveness of the treatment variable. The selected multiple target behaviors included contractible auxiliary (*he's* riding), contractible copula (*she's* happy), uncontractible auxiliary (*he was* painting), and possessive morpheme *s* (*lady's* hat). Initially, the four behaviors were baserated in a child with a language disability and mental retardation, 3 years and 9 months old. The correct production of the behaviors on the initial baseline was 0%. The contractible auxiliary was trained first, and a second set of baselines were then obtained on the remaining three target behaviors. During this baseline, the correct production of the second target morpheme, contractible copula, was produced with 100% accuracy. This raised the possibility that either contractible auxiliary and copula were not independent of each other or some extraneous variable was responsible for changes in the first target behavior.

Fortunately, two other baselines did not show any change when measured a second time (uncontractible auxiliary and the possessive morpheme). This supported the possibility that the contractible copula changed not because of an extraneous treatment but because it is not independent of contractible auxiliary. However, we could not be sure because within a multiple baseline design, change in an untreated behavior *must* be considered to represent weakened experimental control. We decided to see if we would get similar results by first treating contractible copula and then testing con-tractible auxiliary in a multiple baseline design applied to another client. This client was a 4-year-old boy who did not produce contractible copula, contractible auxiliary, uncontractible auxiliary, uncontractible copula, or the possessive *s* morpheme. In this case, there were five baselines.

After establishing the initial baselines on all five morphemes, we first trained the contractible copula and found that the production of the con-tractible auxiliary also increased to 100% on the second baseline. However, the three remaining untrained behaviors showed no change, and they contin-ued to show no change until each of them was brought under the influence of the treatment contingency. This once again suggested that the contractible auxiliary and copula probably belong to the same response class and hence are not independent behaviors. However, switching the sequence of the two morphemes across two participants was not considered a crucial test of the independence of the auxiliary and copula because a multiple baseline design could not provide such a test. An altered sequence was applied to another par-ticipant in the hope that some additional suggestive evidence might emerge. And it did. Eventually, an appropriate test of the independence of the two behaviors was made within the *ABAB* reversal design (Hegde, 1980b).

When the design includes four or more baselines (target behaviors), a potential interdependence between two of them may not be very damaging. The other baselines that do not show changes until treatment is applied to them will continue to serve the control function within the design.

Obviously, that lack of independence between behaviors, though trou-blesome, can provide interesting hints on responses that belong to the same class. When such hints are taken up for experimental analysis, a more spe-cific information on clinical target behaviors is likely to emerge. In this sense, interdependence of behaviors shown by a multiple baseline design, when confirmed, can be considered worthwhile accidents in research.

Multiple Baseline Across Subjects

When a given target behavior is baserated across individuals rather than across different behaviors of the same individual, the design is called multiple baseline across subjects. Thus, a speech–language clinician may baserate a single grammatical morpheme such as the plural *s* across four individuals. Then the language treatment to be evaluated may be given to the first indi-vidual while the other individuals remain in baseline. When the first par-ticipant's production of the plural morpheme reaches the training criterion, the baselines are repeated on the remaining participants. Assuming that the untreated participants are still not able to produce the morpheme, the clini-cian applies treatment to the second participant. The third and the fourth participants remain untreated until the second one is treated. After another set of baseline measures, the third participant receives treatment, and the fourth participant is baserated for the last time and then receives treatment.

Typically, the same behavior is baserated across different individuals. This practice is considered a standard, and perhaps safe, strategy. However, the basic logic of the design permits baserating different behaviors across different individuals (Barlow, Hayes, & Nelson, 1984). For example, four different morphemes such as the plural *z*, present progressive *-ing*, regular past tense *-ed*, and possessive *s* can be the four respective targets across four individuals. As long as the behaviors of participants who are not yet treated do not change from the baseline, the design can demonstrate that the treatment is effective.

Another variation of the multiple baseline design across subjects is to apply treatment sequentially to groups of participants. For example, three groups of children, all having language disorders, may be treated sequentially. The selected target behaviors are initially baserated in all participants in the three groups; then the treatment is applied to the participants in the first group. After repeating the baselines on the two remaining groups, the treatment is given to participants in the second group. After an additional baseline, the third group receives treatment in the final stage of the experiment. If participants in each group change only when treated, potential external variables are ruled out.

When groups of participants are used in the multiple baseline format, it is necessary to present evidence of change in individual participants as well. The philosophy of single-subject designs does not allow a mere reporting of statistical means based on group performances. For this reason, large groups are not practical in this format.

It is recommended that the participants selected for a multiple baseline across participants be similar to each other and that they be living in the same or similar environmental conditions. If one follows these recommendations, the design presents some of the same problems of a majority of group designs that require matching in the absence of randomization. Finding matched clients living in the same environment or similar environments can be difficult. Moreover, "environmental similarity" is not easy to determine. However, when the individuals can be described separately and the treatment effects are evaluated in relation to an individual participant only, the need for matching is not as strong as in a group design. The behavior that changes in an untreated participant affects the control of the design negatively, but such changes can be observed in homogeneous as well as heterogeneous participants. The assumption that such changes are more likely in heterogeneous participants is logically appealing, but its empirical status is not clear.

Demonstration of an experimental effect in individuals who are different from each other in terms of the clusters of problem behaviors (symptoms) or in terms of one or more of assigned variables (participant characteristics) can actually enhance the generality of experimental data. Therefore, unmatched participants can be used as long as the experimenter is aware of the potential risk involved. The risk of having a behavior change in a participant who is still in baseline must be weighed against the potential of producing data with enhanced generality. However, as noted earlier, the risk is logically justified, but it may be empirically weak enough to allow some creative risk-taking on the part of the experimenter.

Multiple Baseline Across Settings

When a given behavior of a single participant is measured in different settings and when the treatment is applied sequentially in those settings, the design is called multiple baseline across settings. In the most typical version of this design, the same behavior of the same participant exhibited under different settings provides the multiple baselines. The treatment is applied in one of the settings. When the target behavior shows the treatment effect in this setting, the baselines are reestablished in the untreated settings. The treatment is extended to the second setting, and so on until the behavior is independently established in all of the settings.

The design can be illustrated in the treatment of an articulation disorder. A child's misarticulation of a given phoneme may be measured in different settings such as the office of the clinician, the classroom, the school cafeteria, and the playground. The treatment contingency may be positive reinforcement of correct production of the phoneme in single words. After the initial baselines have been established in those settings, the treatment may be started in the clinician's office. When the treatment is successful in this setting, the behavior is baserated in the untreated settings. The treatment is then applied in the classroom setting with the cooperation of the teacher. Baselines are repeated in the cafeteria and the playground. In this manner, the clinician applies treatment sequentially in different settings, showing that in each setting, the correct production of the phoneme increases only when treated in that setting.

The correct production of the phoneme in one or some of the untreated settings creates design problems. Such a production may be due to generalization of the treatment effect or to some uncontrolled variables. Therefore, just as in the other versions of the multiple baseline design, independence of baselines is necessary for unambiguous interpretation of data. The design depends upon the discriminated responding in different settings. It assumes a lack of generalization of treatment effects across settings until treatment is applied in those settings. This assumption may or may not hold in given situations. In some cases, behaviors established in one setting can generalize to other settings although they may or may not be maintained over time. In other cases, the production of target behaviors may be restricted to the setting in which it is supported. Speech–language clinicians typically find that, at least in the initial stages, target behaviors are situation specific. The stuttering client who is fluent in the clinic may still be very dysfluent at home, in the office, or at the supermarket. In such cases, the design can demonstrate experimental control by showing that changes in the target behavior are associated with treatment in different settings.

The application of treatment in different settings can pose practical problems. Treatment may be inefficient or even impossible in some settings, such as the cafeteria or the playground in our example. The design is probably more efficiently used in certain institutions such as those for people with mental or neurological disabilities. In such institutions, different settings may all be under the control of the researcher to an extent necessary to carry out the experiment.

Typically, multiple baseline across settings involves single participants, but it can be used with a group of participants whose behavior is measured and treated in different settings. In this variation, it must be possible to apply the treatment contingency to the group as a whole. For example, a special educator may be able to apply a group token system for "quiet behavior" during the class, in the library, or in the cafeteria. When a group of participants is used, the clinician must still present data on individual participants to show that changes reported are not based on the group averages that mask individual differences. For this reason, a large group may be impractical from the standpoint of data analysis and presentation.

Problem of Repeated Baselines

As noted throughout our discussion, multiple baseline designs require repeated measures of target behaviors. This is a cumbersome aspect of the design. The last behavior, subject, or setting will have been measured repeatedly. The greater the number of series in a design, the more often the baselines need to be measured. Most behaviors studied within the designs are not reactive, but those that are can pose problems because of the repeated baseline measures. Obviously, reactive changes make it difficult to isolate the effects of treatment.

A partial solution offered to the problem of repeated measures is to treat more than one behavior in the multiple baseline across behaviors. For example, if six phonemes are targeted for treatment within a multiple baseline across behaviors, two phonemes may be simultaneously treated, resulting in only three sets of phonemes to be baserated instead of six individual phonemes. This limits the number of baseline measures. Similarly, in the multiple baseline across participants involving eight participants, baseline and treatment may be alternated with sets of two participants. In the multiple baseline involving multiple settings, treatment may be given in two settings while two sets of two settings each are kept in baseline.

Another solution offered to the problem of the repeated baseline measures is known as the multiple probe technique (Homer & Baer, 1978). This technique was originally described as a means of verifying the status of untreated target responses that are a part of a behavioral chain. Complex skills, such as the use of a hearing aid, for example, need to be taught in terms of specific target responses that are chained (Tucker & Berry, 1980). The child may be taught to remove the hearing aid from its box, place it behind the ear, turn the power on, adjust the volume, and so on. Each of these responses constitutes a chained element in the total behavior under training. In cases such as this, it is not necessary to spend much time measuring the subsequent behaviors of the chain when the responses that need to be mastered earlier have still not been learned by the client. For example, trying repeatedly to measure the response of adjusting the volume of the hearing aid when the client has not even learned how to put the aid on is a waste of time.

The probe technique, however, can be used in the treatment of independent behaviors as well. Instead of continually measuring behaviors yet to be trained, the behaviors may be probed periodically to see if they are stable. A probe is a quick test of a given response, usually used to assess generalization of treatment effects. A more detailed measure of a particular behavior just before treatment is considered the baseline. If there are additional behaviors in the baseline, they can be probed without detailed measurement. For example, in the treatment of four grammatical features, the clinician may establish baselines (more detailed measurement) on all of them. Each feature may be baserated in the context of 20 sentences, each presented on a modeled and evoked trial. The first feature is then trained. Then the second feature is baserated with the 20 sentences whereas the third and the fourth features are probed with only a few sentences. The second feature is then trained. The baseline is repeated on the third feature, but the fourth feature is only probed. Finally, the fourth feature is trained after a full baseline measure on it has been obtained. Especially in the treatment of language and articulation disorders, periodic probes are all that are needed to retain the control function of the design. Full baseline measures must be established initially on all behaviors and on every behavior just before it is treated.

Additional Control Within the Multiple Baseline Designs

As noted previously, the multiple baseline designs arrange a series of *AB* conditions. Control is demonstrated by either the untreated behaviors, the untreated participants, or the untreated settings. Each participant, however, experiences only two conditions: the baseline and the treatment. Therefore, multiple baseline designs are considered somewhat weaker than reversal or withdrawal designs.

A multiple baseline design can be combined with either reversal or withdrawal, however. When this is practical, the control aspect of the design is increased significantly. In the multiple baseline design across behaviors and subjects, treatment can be withdrawn for a brief period of time as soon as a particular treated behavior or participant shows a considerable change from the baseline. The treatment can then be reinstated. Reversal and reinstatement can be used in the same manner. In the multiple baseline across settings, treatment can be reversed or withdrawn in each of the treatment settings and then reinstated in each setting.

Although withdrawal (or reversal) and reinstatement can provide additional control to the multiple baseline designs, they also neutralize many of the advantages of these designs. The designs are thought to be more suitable for clinical purposes precisely because they do not require reversal or withdrawal to demonstrate experimental control. When a multiple baseline design includes four or more baselines (behaviors, subjects, or settings) and each baseline changes only when treatment is applied, the experimental control so exhibited can be considered reasonably satisfactory.

Changing Criterion Design

By now it must be clear to the clinician that a critical element of the experimental strategy is to demonstrate that the behavior varies in accordance with a specific experimental manipulation. A design that retains this feature but does not use the control features of the previously described designs is known as the changing criterion design (Hartman & Hall, 1976). In this design, the clinician tries to have a behavior repeatedly approximate a preset criterion. Whenever the clinician changes the criterion to which the behavior is held, the behavior changes and approximates that criterion. The previously discussed criterion-referenced change is the control mechanism in the changing criterion design.

The design has not been used in communicative disorders, and has had limited use in behavioral research. Still, the best example of the design comes from the original Hartman and Hall (1976) study on controlling smoking behavior with response cost based on the number of cigarettes smoked and a bonus awarded for reduced smoking. A baseline level of smoking was established over several days, and then the multiple treatment phases were initiated. In each phase of the treatment, a new criterion was imposed. A criterion allowed the client a certain number of cigarettes a day. In successive phases, the criterion was lowered so that the client was asked to smoke less and less. The study showed that every time a new (and lower) criterion was imposed, the client's rate of smoking approximated the criterion in force. The smoking behavior changed only at times when the criterion was changed. This fact helped rule out the influence of extraneous variables.

The changing criterion design is helpful when the behavior changes slowly and over a period of time. The design may be useful in the reduction of such behaviors as dysfluencies and errors of articulation, and of vocally abusive behaviors. In fact, the design can be used in any experiment in which a behavior or skill is either shaped up or shaped down. After the establishment of a baseline, the clinician requires a certain reduction in the frequency of undesirable behaviors over the next several days and uses appropriate reinforcement procedures to help the client move toward the new criterion. When the behavior approximates the criterion, a new criterion with a lower frequency of the undesirable behavior is established. Such progressive reduction in the behavior in accordance with changing criteria helps establish experimental control. Figure 9.8 shows hypothetical data from a changing criterion design in which the percentages of correct articulation are increased by escalating criteria. The data show how a behavior being shaped up comes under experimental control.

In the use of the changing criterion design, the clinician must make sure that the baseline phase is not too short when compared with any of the single treatment phase. Also, the clinician must implement multiple criterion changes to demonstrate the experimental control. If additional control procedures are considered necessary, the treatment can be totally withdrawn in one of the phases to show that the behavior returns to the original baseline. A more practical strategy is to return the client to an earlier criterion. In this case, the target behavior would reverse and approximate the earlier criterion. Following this, the new criterion may once again be imposed.

Periodic Treatments Designs

The periodic treatments design (Hayes, 1981) has not been used frequently, but it offers an interesting opportunity to assess treatment effects in such settings as private practice and in any settings where more stringent control procedures are not practical. The periodic treatments design is based on the logic that, in comparison with the times preceding treatment, a greater

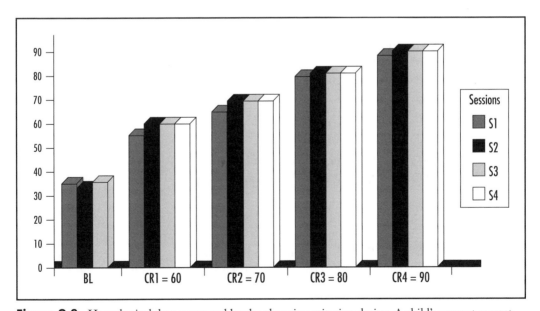

Figure 9.8. Hypothetical data generated by the changing criterion design. A child's percent correct response rate in articulation therapy is baserated (BL) and then subjected to four changing criteria (CR1 through CR4) across four sessions (S1–S4) for each criterion; the correct response rate increases to the set criteria.

change in behavior would be evident following treatment. If the treatment sessions are scheduled once a week or less often, it is possible that the treatment effects are most visible soon after therapy and may show a gradual decline until the next therapy session. Once again, following the therapy session, the treatment effects would be clearly evident.

During the session scheduled after a break in services, most clinicians probably notice some deterioration in their clients' target behaviors. Sometimes, differential changes of smaller magnitude may be noticed when the treatment sessions are scheduled twice weekly, say on a Monday–Wednesday schedule. During the very first portion of the Monday session, the behavior may be at a relatively lower frequency compared with the initial portion of the Wednesday session. However, the periodic treatments design requires that the target behaviors be measured more often than treatment is provided. That is, measures of the dependent variable must be obtained on a continuous basis.

Continuous measures can be obtained with the cooperation of parents or clients. When parents tape-record the speech of the child at home on a daily basis and submit the tapes for the clinician's evaluation, the measures are continuous. The clinician has data to track the differences in the dependent variable before and after therapy and anytime in between. It may become evident that soon after therapy, the target behaviors are produced at a high level at home and that they begin to decline with the passage of time until the next therapy session. Again, after the next therapy session, the frequency of target behaviors may increase noticeably. If such changes are replicated several times, the clinician has a basis on which to conclude that the treatment was probably responsible for the changes.

The control feature of the design is rather weak. Practicality also is a serious concern in using the periodic treatments design; continuous measurement of client behaviors during periods of no treatment can pose problems. Also, the design is perhaps more appropriately used in evaluating treatments whose effects are documented in designs with stronger control procedures.

EXPERIMENTAL DESIGNS FOR MULTIPLE-TREATMENT COMPARISON

A basic question about treatment procedures is whether they are effective when compared with no treatment. Within the single-subject strategy, the *ABA*, the *ABAB*, and the multiple baseline designs are useful in answering that basic question. However, these designs can evaluate only one treatment at a time. Chapter 8 shows that within the group design strategy, options are available to evaluate multiple treatments in a single study. Factorial designs are especially useful in this regard. Within the single-subject strategy, there are some designs that permit an experimental evaluation of multiple treatments.

Generally speaking, a study compares two treatments only when independent evaluations of them have produced some evidence that each is effective to a certain degree. When nothing is known about the effects of a given treatment, a logical start is to find out if it is effective at all. In this case, the design is more likely to be an *ABA*, *ABAB*, *BAB*, or multiple baseline. In the next stage of the experiment, the two treatments that have produced favorable effects in separate studies may be evaluated within a single study. I shall describe two methods of evaluating the effects of two or more treatments within the single-subject strategy.

ABACA/ACABA Design

A clinician may be interested in evaluating the effects of two treatments on a single behavior produced by one or several participants. For example, a clinician may be interested in evaluating the effects of two methods of teaching alaryngeal speech, articulation, or language responses. The two procedures, X_1 and X_2, may be applied to the same participant or participants interspersed by baselines *A*. The resulting design is known as the *ABACA/ACABA* design. The two portions of the design are needed to counterbalance the two treatment variables. Each portion of the design (*ABACA* or *ACABA*) is applied to one or more participants. For a given participant or set of participants, either the *ABACA* or the *ACABA* design applies. The first treatment, X_1, is represented by *B* in the design and the second treatment, X_2, is represented by *C*. The design is illustrated in Figure 9.9 with its two sequences of treatment presentations (Graphs 1 and 2).

The two sequences (*ABACA* and *ACABA*) counterbalance the order of presentation of the two treatments. If only one of the two sequences is used in a study, potential order effects cannot be ruled out. If the investigator were to use four clients in a study designed to evaluate the effects of two treatment procedures, the first two participants would undergo the first sequence, and the second two participants would undergo the second sequence. This way, each treatment precedes and follows the other treatment. It may be noted that the counterbalanced crossover group designs are similar to this single-subject design.

In this design, baselines separate the treatments. Therefore, the design can incorporate withdrawal or reversal. Either version of the design can demonstrate whether one or both the treatments are effective. Once it becomes clear that one or both of them are effective, the clinician can reinstate a treatment to achieve the clinical goals.

The results generated by the design can be suggestive of the relative effects of the two treatments but do not permit firm conclusions. In other words, whether one treatment is more effective than the other is a difficult question to handle within this design. Any suggestion regarding the relative effects of treatments from this design must be evaluated within other design formats. In the single-subjects strategy, the relative effects of two or more treatments

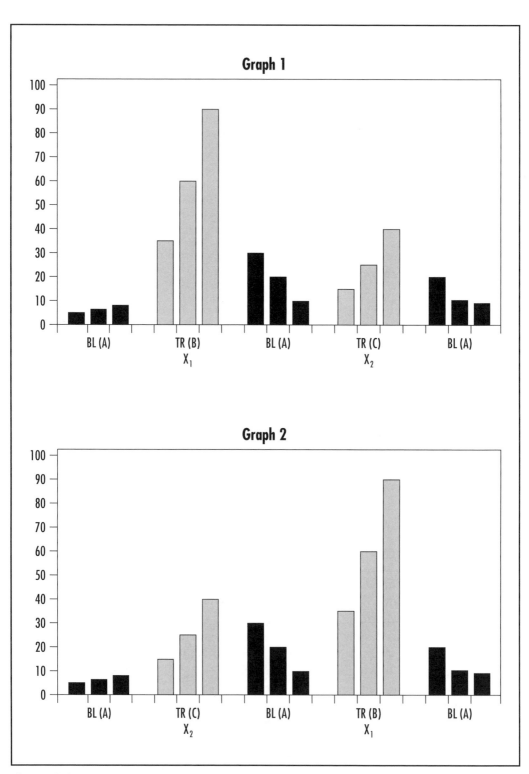

Figure 9.9. The *ABACA/ACABA* design. The first sequence (Graph 1) shows the administration of Treatment 1 (X_1) followed by Treatment 2 (X_2) with an interspersed baseline. The second sequence (Graph 2) is opposite to the first. In both cases, Treatment 1 had a larger effect than Treatment 2.

are compared only when they are administered in *adjacent* conditions. Interspersed baselines result in treatments that are separated in time, and data points that are separated in time are not considered reliable for analysis of the relative effects of two or more treatments (Barlow, Hayes, & Nelson, 1984). For this reason, the alternating treatments design, to be described shortly, is considered the most appropriate strategy to analyze the relative effects of two or more treatments.

A potential problem with the *ABACA/ACABA* design is that the first treatment may be so effective as not to leave any opportunity for the second treatment to show its effects. This is the ceiling effect described in Chapter 7. The clinician should know when this happens, however. When the wrong response rate is reduced dramatically to near-zero levels by the first treatment, the application of the second treatment may not serve any purpose. The design may also suffer from some carryover effects in spite of the interspersed baselines. In other words, some of the effects of the first treatment may be carried over to the second treatment. The second baseline may give some indication of a carryover, however.

Alternating Treatments Design

Once it has been determined that several treatment techniques are all effective with a given disorder, the clinician faces a different question. Can it be that one treatment technique is *more* effective than the other? The question, then, does not concern the absolute effects of a given treatment, but the relative effects of two or more treatments. Alternating treatments design offers a strategy to answer such questions.

The design can also help answer other questions of relativity. For example, is one therapist more effective than the other? In answering this question, a single treatment may be administered by two different therapists whose participation is alternated across sessions. Or two treatments may be administered by both the therapists alternately. Another question that can be answered by the alternating treatments design is whether the time of treatment can make a difference. The design can help answer this question by arranging treatments at different times of the day, while making sure that each treatment is administered in all of the selected time periods equally often.

The alternating treatments design has also been called *multiple schedule design, multi element baseline design, randomization design,* and *simultaneous treatments design* (Barlow & Hersen, 1984). Of these, simultaneous treatments design is clearly inappropriate because there is another design by the same name that does not involve alternation of treatment. The term *alternating treatments* (Barlow & Hayes, 1979) seems to describe the logic and the strategy of the design accurately. The basic arrangement of the design involving two treatments is illustrated in Figure 9.10.

The design is based on the logic that when two or more treatments are alternated rapidly in the treatment of the same participant, the relative effects

A. Alternating patterns for one set of participants (starting with Treatment 1)

Session	1	2	3	4	5	6	7	8
Treatment	X_1	X_2	X_2	X_1	X_2	X_1	X_1	X_2

B. Alternating patterns for another set of participants (starting with Treatment 2)

Session	1	2	3	4	5	6	7	8
Treatment	X_2	X_1	X_1	X_2	X_1	X_2	X_2	X_1

Figure 9.10. Counterbalanced arrangements (A and B) of experimental conditions of an alternating treatments design involving two treatments and two sets of participants.

of the treatments can be determined in a fairly short time. The treatments may be alternated in a single day with the number of daily treatment sessions corresponding to the number of the treatments being compared. However, as pointed out by Barlow et al. (1984), rapidity of alternations is determined by the nature of the clinical phenomenon under investigation. If daily measurement of the phenomenon is not appropriate and weekly measurement is most likely to reveal changes, weekly alternations may be acceptable.

In the treatment of stuttering, for example, a clinician may examine the relative effects of stuttering-contingent aversive noise and a verbal "no." Let us assume that both the procedures have been evaluated in separate studies showing that they are capable of reducing the frequency of stuttering to varying extents. The clinician can then evaluate the relative effects of the two procedures by applying both to the same client or clients. The two punishment procedures are alternated in the treatment sessions. In the analysis of the results, the rates of stuttering observed in the treatment sessions are separated according to the two procedures. The stuttering rate under the aversive noise sessions are compared with those under verbal stimulus.

Typical results of an alternating treatments design are represented in Figure 9.11, which shows that the first treatment, X_1, was more effective than the second treatment, X_2.

Order Effects and Counterbalancing

The reader may have noticed that in Figure 9.10 the treatments were not alternated systematically. If one treatment systematically follows another treatment, treatment effects may be confounded by the **order effect,** which is the influence of sequence with which multiple treatments are presented to

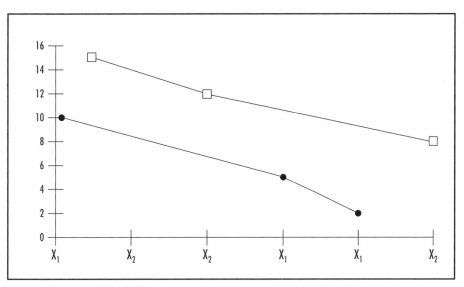

Figure 9.11. Typical graphic representation of the results of an alternating treatments design. The graph shows a larger effect for Treatment 1 than for Treatment 2.

the same individuals. Therefore, the order of treatment presentation is semirandomized.

The two treatments also should be counterbalanced across participants so that each treatment precedes and follows every other treatment applied in the design. To accomplish this, the design requires two sets of participants. One can use, for example, two sets of 3 participants, for a total of 6 participants. In the first session of the experiment, Treatment 1 will be offered to the participants in the first set and Treatment 2 will be offered to those in the second. In this arrangement, each treatment appears in the first and the second position. From then on, the order of treatment is semirandomized.

Each treatment can be made to precede and follow every other treatment equally often, although this is not always done, nor is it always necessary. As long as the treatments precede and follow more than once and the sequences are roughly comparable in number, the order effects can be minimized.

When two or more clinicians administer the same treatment, the order in which the two clinicians treat the client must be counterbalanced. When two clinicians administer two or more treatments, both the treatments and the clinicians must be counterbalanced. When two treatments are evaluated by the same clinician, it is possible that the sessions are held during a morning and an afternoon session; in this case, each treatment must be administered in roughly the same number of morning and afternoon sessions. Such counterbalancing avoids the potential for a given treatment to be more effective because it is administered by a particular clinician or at a certain time.

Counterbalancing requires multiple participants. For example, if the clinician counterbalances the time of treatment, he or she may apply the first treatment to the first participant in the morning session and the second treatment to the same participant in the afternoon session. From then on, the order of presentations is semirandomized and counterbalanced. In a second participant, the second treatment may be given in the first morning session and the first treatment in the first afternoon session. As in the first participant, the treatment presentations from then on are counterbalanced. In this case, the two treatments and time periods for presentation also are counterbalanced across the two participants.

Carryover and Contrast Effects

In addition to a potential order effect, the alternating treatments design can pose two other problems: carryover and contrast effects. Both these effects create problems for an unambiguous interpretation of data. In either case, the effects of a second treatment are partly determined by the effects of the first treatment.

As described in Chapter 7, the term **carryover effects** refers to generalization of the first treatment effect to the second treatment. In this case, the observed effects of the second treatment are larger than what might be expected if the second treatment were administered alone. In terms of our earlier example of the relative effects of aversive noise and verbal "no," a stutterer's fluency in the verbal punishment condition may be higher because of the carryover effects of the aversive noise condition.

Contrast is evident when the effect of a subsequent treatment is opposite to that found during the prior treatment. In other words, a behavior that decreases under the first treatment condition increases under the adjacent condition, and vice versa. Some punishment studies have shown the contrast effects in human participants (Newsom, Favell, & Rincover, 1983). For example, a mild punishment may be effective when administered alone. However, when it is alternated with a stronger punishment, the behavior may decrease under the stronger punishment procedure and increase under the milder procedure.

It is evident that contrast and carryover are opposite effects. In spite of this, some authors have described contrast as a variety of carryover effect (Ulman & Sulzer-Azaroff, 1975) and both often are subsumed under the term *multiple-treatment interference* (Barlow & Hersen, 1984). Carryover effect has also been described, quite appropriately, as *induction* or *generalization*.

In applied human research, it is thought that the carryover and contrast effects are not as great a problem as they might initially appear. Barlow and Hersen (1984) and Barlow et al. (1984) have suggested that multiple-treatment interference is not as serious a problem in applied research as in basic research. Nevertheless, the clinician wishing to use the alternating treatments design should take at least two steps to counteract its potential problems. First, the clinician should counterbalance the treatment conditions. This will help minimize both the order effects and the carryover effects. Second, the treatment sessions must be separated in time, and only one treatment must be administered in a given session. Originally, it was suggested that within a single session, two treatments may be alternated.

It is possible that even when there is a carryover effect from one treatment to the next, the relative effectiveness of the two treatments may still be the same as it would have been in the absence of carryover effects (Barlow & Hersen, 1984). In any case, should an investigator be concerned with the carryover effects in a particular study, he or she can proceed to analyze such effects by making them the object of further experimental inquiry. Procedures to analyze the carryover effects are described in Sidman (1960) and Barlow and Hersen (1984).

One issue raised in early discussion of the alternating treatments design was whether the clients should discriminate the two treatment procedures that are alternated in order for a differential effect to appear. It was originally suggested that some external stimulus must clearly signal the particular treatment in effect in any given session. The current thinking, however, is that the clients may be simply told what treatment is going to be applied in a given session. At the beginning of each treatment session, the clinician can tell the client, "In this session, we will be using the treatment procedure _____." No additional steps to ensure discrimination are considered necessary (Barlow & Hersen, 1984; Barlow et al., 1984). In laboratory research, when similar treatment variables (reinforcement schedules that are close to each other) are alternated rapidly (often by the minute), differential effects may not emerge because of a lack of discrimination. This has not been a major problem in applied research, in which clients are usually able to discriminate treatment procedures.

The alternating treatments design does not require a formal baseline before the treatment variables are introduced. For this reason, it is thought that the alternating treatments design is especially useful in case of behaviors that are inherently variable (Ulman & Sulzer-Azaroff, 1975). The alternating treatments design is considered to be relatively insensitive to background variability in behaviors. True differences between treatments can emerge against a background of variability.

Most investigators do establish baselines of target behaviors before introducing treatment. That is still a desirable, though not required, feature of an alternating treatments design. Such baselines give an opportunity to analyze the effects of different treatments in relation to baselines as well.

Simultaneous Treatment Design

A design available to evaluate the client preference for a treatment when multiple treatments are concurrently available is known as the simultaneous treatment design. Although the design was developed to study client preference for treatments, it can offer some initial data on the relative effects. Whereas the alternating treatments design helps evaluate the relative effects of multiple treatments to their fullest extent, the simultaneous treatment design may do it up to a point. Simultaneous treatment design is a strategy in which, after establishing the baselines, two or more treatments are simultaneously offered to clients in the beginning; subsequently, only the one the client prefers is offered. From the point at which the client preference emerges in a study, administration of multiple treatments is discontinued. Only the preferred (or more effective) treatment is offered.

Browning's study (1967) on decreasing the frequency of grandiose bragging in a 9-year-old boy is the first in which the simultaneous treatment design was used. Six therapists, forming three teams of two each, administered the three treatments in a counterbalanced order. They either offered positive reinforcement, verbal admonishment, or extinction (ignoring) for bragging. All therapists were simultaneously available to administer the treatments. Three weeks of simultaneous treatments showed that the boy preferred verbal admonishment and sought out those who administered it. Preference in this case meant that the boy's bragging increased when verbally admonished. His least preferred treatment was extinction (fewer bragging instances); he soon began to avoid the teams that administered it. Browning then applied extinction as the only treatment available and reduced the boy's bragging.

The design, though not used frequently, has excellent potential in communicative disorders. For instance, in the treatment of stuttering, syllable prolongation (stretching the syllable durations to reduce the rate of speech), time-out from speaking made contingent on stuttering, and response cost (reinforcing fluent speech with a token and withdrawing a token for stuttering) are known to be effective. An unanswered question, however, is whether clients would have a preference when they experience beneficial effects of all three procedures. One might design a study in which different therapists offer the three treatments in a counterbalanced manner to persons who stutter. All therapists would offer all three treatments, available for the clients to seek them out, but at any given day or week, the clients would know who offers what treatment. The clients would be free to choose the therapist who administers their preferred treatment on any given day. After experiencing similar reductions in stuttering under all three treatments, the clients might prefer one of the three treatments because of personal liking, minimum aversiveness, reduced task demand, and other such factors. The clients would reject therapists who offered unattractive treatments on scheduled days or weeks. The study would generate some limited data on relative effects and convincing data on preference. Hypothetical data from such a study are presented in Figure 9.12.

The simultaneous treatment design is not the method of choice to evaluate the relative effects of multiple treatments because the participants are not offered all treatments equally often. Once the preference or relative effectiveness emerges in the design, only one of the treatments will be continued. The effect is that the frequency of different treatment administration will have been unequal. It is for this reason that the design is not selected for

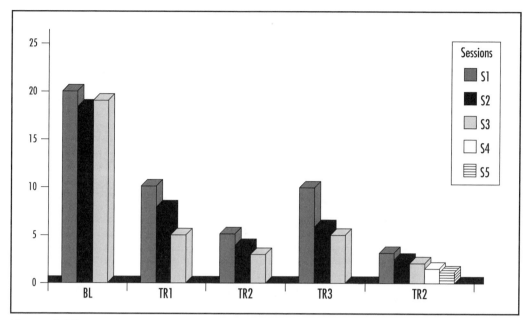

Figure 9.12. Hypothetical data generated by a simultaneous treatments design. Data show the percent stuttering rates under baseline, three stuttering treatments (TR1 through TR3) administered simultaneously for several days, and the final condition in which TR2, which was found to be the most effective (with the lowest frequency of stuttering) as well as the most preferred treatment, was offered. Note that data are shown for three sessions except for the last condition, which shows five sessions.

an evaluation of relative effects of treatments. Therefore, the alternating treatments design in which treatments are not simultaneously available, and all treatments are offered equally often remains the method of choice for this purpose. Similarly, because all treatments are offered equally often on a predetermined semirandomized sequence, the alternating treatments design does not help assess client preference.

It should be noted that client preference and effectiveness may be different matters, depending on the study. In the Browning study (1967), the preferred technique was the least effective in reducing the undesirable behavior; in fact, it increased that behavior. When young children are the participants in a simultaneous treatments design, the problem can be magnified. Most children, for example, love to go to speech clinics when it is fun-and-play, with no particular contingencies on any behaviors. More formal therapy procedures designed to produce systematic changes in children's behaviors may not necessarily be preferred. When the children are shifted from their preferred treatment to a more effective but less preferred one, their cooperation may be reduced. In such cases, additional incentives and reinforcers may be needed to make the shift smooth as well as effective.

On the other hand, in the hypothetical stuttering treatment study, preferred treatment might also be the most effective treatment. It is possible that certain individuals do not react that well to a certain technique, but still prefer it. Whether to offer a less effective technique than the client prefers or to convince the client to receive a more effective but less preferred technique is a clinical decision the investigator will have to make. On the other hand, as long as it is effective, a relatively less effective but preferred technique may be offered because of its potential extraclinical advantages. In the treatment of stuttering, for instance, a family member might find it easier to use the preferred but somewhat less effective time-out rather than the more effective syllable prolongation procedure at home. Or the time-out procedure may not produce unnatural sounding speech, which is a known negative side effect of syllable prolongation.

Ineffective Treatments in Multiple-Treatment Evaluations

Sometimes the clinician may find that one or more of the treatments in a multiple-treatment evaluation are ineffective. In an *ABACA/ACABA* design, for example, it may be found that Treatment *B* does not affect the behavior at all. In such cases, there is no point in returning the client to a period of baseline measurement. The *B* condition, for all practical purposes, is comparable to the baseline in that there were no changes in the response rate. The next treatment can then be introduced without the second, formal baseline. In such cases, the design is redesignated as an *A = BCA* design, which means that the first treatment was treated like a baseline because of lack of effect. If, in the second sequence, Treatment *C* is ineffective, Treatment *B* may be introduced without a preceding baseline, resulting in a *A = CBA* design.

Because ineffective treatments are functionally equivalent to baselines, single-subject strategies allow modifications in treatment procedures within a single study. Such modifications typically are not done within the group design strategy. Even when the experimenter realizes that the treatment is not producing changes in the behavior, the study is completed as planned. However, within the single-subject strategy, a clinician can introduce another treatment without baselines or make modifications in the original treatment. For example, if a 5-second time-out proves ineffective in reducing the frequency of stuttering, a 10-second time-out contingency may be applied. No baselines need to be interspersed between the treatment variations as long as the first treatment does not result in a changed baseline. If verbal praise does not act as a reinforcer for the correct production of target phonemes, a token system may be implemented. Of course, the treatment variable that produces changes in the baseline will have to be evaluated with such controls as untreated multiple baselines, withdrawal, or reversal.

EXPERIMENTAL DESIGN FOR INTERACTIONAL STUDIES

Clinicians know that, in most cases, what is considered a single treatment for a given disorder is actually a combination of several treatment components. For example, an articulation treatment program may consist of certain stimulus presentation, modeling, reinforcement for the correct production, and punishment for the incorrect production. In this case, the stimulus, modeling, reinforcement, and punishment constitute four components, each of which can be manipulated independently. Similar components are used in language treatment. In the treatment of stuttering, instructions, modeling, reduced rate, altered airflow, gentle phonatory onset, counseling, attitudinal changes, increased self-confidence, reinforcement of correct responses, and punishment of incorrect responses may all be treatment components. In fact, therapeutic packages that combine different components are quite popular in speech–language pathology.

In controlled studies, one can demonstrate the overall effectiveness of a treatment package. Such a demonstration, however, is no testimony to the effectiveness of the individual components included in the package. In our example of the stuttering treatment package, one or many of the components may contribute very little or nothing at all. There may be just one or two effective components, which then create the impression that all components are effective. When two or more treatment components within a package are effective to any degree at all, then the question of interaction, discussed in Chapter 8, emerges.

Interaction is not limited to components of a treatment package. Interaction between independent treatments that are not components of a package also is of interest. For instance, one might study potential interactions between two independent treatments for stuttering—psychological counseling and fluency shaping. In the rehabilitation of patients with traumatic brain injury, one might study the interaction between cognitive therapy and behavior therapy.

Single-subject interactional designs are strategies to study such interactional effects of two or more independent treatments or components of therapeutic packages. In addition, the design can help isolate treatment or treatment components that are effective to any extent from those that are not at all effective. The importance of such a design strategy in the task of developing a clinical science is obvious.

The single-subject interactional design has two variations. It is helpful to think of them as Type I and Type II interactional designs. In Type I interactional design, a single treatment (or component) is first applied and a second treatment (or component) is added and removed. In Type II interactional design, the combination of two treatments or the entire package is first applied and a treatment or a component is removed and added. Each type requires two experimental sequences, requiring two sets of participants. In any given study, only one of the two types need to be implemented.

The Type I interactional design, usually described as an *A-B-BC-B-BC* design in behavioral literature, is presented in Figure 9.13. However, because of the two sequences involved in it, it is more complete and less confusing to refer to it as *A-B-BC-B-BC/A-C-CB-C-CB* design. As can be seen in Figure 9.13, the first sequence of *A-B-BC-B-BC* is applied to one set of participants and the second sequence of *A-C-CB-C-CB* is applied to another set of

Sequence 1 (First set of participants)	A	B	BC	B	BC
	Baseline	X_1	$X_1 + X_2$	X_1	$X_1 + X_2$
Sequence 2 (Second set of participants)	A	C	CB	C	CB
	Baseline	X_2	$X_2 + X_1$	X_2	$X_2 + X_1$

Figure 9.13. Type I interactional design in which a single treatment (X_1 or X_2) is constant and another treatment is added and removed; in the first set of participants, Treatment 1 (*B*) is constant (*A-B-BC-B-BC*); and in the second set of participants, Treatment 2 (*C*) is constant (*A-C-CB-C-CB*).

participants. Each set may have three or more participants. These two sequences counterbalance the two single treatments and the two combinations; each single treatment appears in the first position once, followed by the combination. Furthermore, in the first sequence only Treatment 1 is tested in isolation and in the second sequence, Treatment 2 is tested in isolation. In each sequence, statements cannot be made about the independent effects of the treatment untested in isolation.

The Type II interactional design, usually described as an *A-BC-B-BC-B* design, is presented in Figure 9.14. This variation, too, is better represented as *A-BC-B-BC-B/A-BC-C-BC-C* because of the two necessary experimental sequences. It may be noted in Figure 9.14 that in the first sequence, the investigator offers the combined treatments to both the sets of participants in the initial condition of the experiment. Subsequently, the investigator removes the second treatment, adds it, and removes it again. Thus the first sequence has only Treatment 1 in isolation. If only this sequence is implemented, the study cannot answer the question of independent effects of Treatment 2. On the other hand, the participant in the second sequence experiences Treatment 2 as the isolated condition. If only this sequence is implemented, the study cannot evaluate the independent effects of Treatment 1. When both the sequences are implemented in the counterbalanced fashion, the independent and interactive (combined) effects of both the treatments can be evaluated.

Sequence 1 (First set of participants)	A	BC	B	BC	B
	Baseline	$X_1 + X_2$	X_1	$X_1 + X_2$	X_1
Sequence 2 (Second set of participants)	A	BC	C	BC	C
	Baseline	$X_1 + X_2$	X_2	$X_1 + X_2$	X_2

Figure 9.14. Type II interactional design in which a combination of two treatments (X_1 and X_2) is constant and one treatment is removed and added. In the first set of participants, Treatment 2 (*C*) is removed and added (*A-BC-B-BC-B*); in the second set of participants, Treatment 1 is removed and added (*A-BC-C-BC-C*).

An example will help clarify the actual implementation of this design. Suppose that a clinician wishes to study the independent and interactive effects of two treatment components in remediating stuttering: reduced speech rate X_1 and modified airflow X_2. Let us further suppose that the clinician wishes to use the Type I interactional design with its two sequences. The clinician selects 6 adults who stutter and creates two sets of 3 participants each. In the first experimental sequence, the clinician establishes the baselines of stuttering, A, and then applies the speech rate reduction strategy (X_1) in the initial treatment B condition to the first set of 3 participants. After several sessions of rate reduction, the clinician *adds* the modified airflow component (X_2) to the existing speech rate reduction component. This combined treatment condition (BC or $X_1 + X_2$) will be in effect for a certain number of sessions. In the next condition, the clinician withdraws the modified airflow procedure, leaving only the speech rate reduction as the treatment (the second B, or X_1, condition). Finally, the clinician adds the modified airflow a second time to the speech rate reduction component (the second BC or $X_1 + X_2$ condition). In this sequence, the independent effects of speech rate reduction, but not that of modified airflow, can be assessed along with the combined (interactional) effect.

In the second experimental sequence, the clinician applies the modified airflow to the second set of participants in the first treatment condition. The clinician then adds the speech rate reduction in the next condition and subtracts it in the following condition. In the final condition, the clinician once again adds the speech rate reduction to the modified airflow component. In this sequence, the clinician can evaluate the independent effects of modified airflow, but not that of speech rate reduction.

Assuming that the speech rate reduction results in some decrease in stuttering frequency, the addition of airflow may show a further decrease. When the airflow is subtracted, the stuttering frequency may increase; frequency may once again decrease when the airflow is added. Similarly, addition of speech rate reduction to the airflow may enhance the treatment effect on stuttering, and the magnitude of this effect may decline when the component is withdrawn. On the other hand, it may be evident that one of the components has a greater effect than the other. Adding one component may not make a big difference, whereas adding the other component may result in a more dramatic decrease in stuttering. In essence, the results may show that both the components are equally effective or equally ineffective, or that one is more effective than the other. The results may also show that each of the two components is weak by itself but that the two in combination can produce notable effects (interactional effect).

The same experiment may be conducted with Type II interactional design in which the application of both treatments is common to the first treatment condition in the two sequences. Subsequently, in the first sequence, Treatment 2 is removed, added, and removed again (*A-BC-B-BC-B*), thus testing the combination and Treatment 1 in isolation. In the second sequence, Treatment 1 is removed, added, and removed again (*A-BC-C-BC-C*), thus testing the combination and Treatment 2 in isolation.

The two types of interactional design differ in terms of whether in the initial stage of treatment the entire package or only one of the components is applied. If the entire package is applied, one of the components is first *subtracted* then added in subsequent conditions. If only one of the components is applied initially, another component is *added* and then subtracted in subsequent conditions. As noted before, any one type is satisfactory when both the experimental arrangements are used. However, both types, when applied with both the sequences, can strengthen the conclusions.

In using either of the sequences, it is important to remember that the same variable is added or subtracted. For example, if the clinician starts with the rate reduction as the first treatment condition, then the airflow is added and subtracted. One cannot add airflow in one condition and subtract rate reduction in the other. In other words, the first treatment component stays constant; the second component is added or subtracted. When the clinician starts with the airflow component, rate reduction is added and subtracted; airflow stays constant. When both the components are applied in the initial treatment condition, only one of them is subtracted and added in any one or a set of participants. The other component is subtracted and added only in another participant or set of participants.

Interactional designs have not been used frequently in communicative disorders. The design deserves greater application because many untested treatment packages exist in the treatment of articulation, speech, language, voice, and fluency disorders. Even when a total package is known to be effective, the independent and interactive effects of each of the components of the package need to be determined so that ineffective components can be discarded and more effective components can be combined.

DESIGNS TO ASSESS RESPONSE MAINTENANCE

An important clinical question concerns the durability of treated behaviors. Whether the target behaviors established in the clinical and educational settings are produced in other situations and over time is an important question, the answer to which determines the eventual success of treatment. Within the clinical tradition, the follow-up procedures are designed to assess the maintenance of treated behaviors over time. Follow-up, however, can only demonstrate whether the response is maintained. Variables that are responsible for either the loss of established behaviors or variables that are responsible for the maintenance cannot be determined in a follow-up assessment.

In clinical literature, the question of maintenance often is confused with that of generalization. Generalization is a temporary phenomenon of declining response rate when the independent variable is suspended (Hegde, 1998a). As a treatment consequence, generalization is measured in relation to situations, persons, and responses that are not a part of treatment in a given study (see Chapter 4). Generalization, however, is not the same as maintenance. A response that shows an initial generalization may not be maintained over time. For example, the client who is initially fluent in the home may not maintain that fluency 6 months after the treatment is terminated. Whether treatment effects are maintained over time in different settings, in interaction with different individuals, and in the kinds of responses that were not specifically trained by the clinician calls for a different approach.

An experimental analysis of response maintenance requires an identification of the independent variables that are responsible for such maintenance. Some clinicians seem to assume that the maintenance of target behaviors subsequent to the termination of treatment is still due to the treatment effects. However, there is no evidence to support this view. To assume that an absence of treatment variables is the required condition of response maintenance is to assume that effects are produced without causes. Perhaps there is an absence of the treatment variables manipulated by the investigator, but not necessarily an absence of any kind of independent variables because no dependent variable can exist without independent variables. Therefore, response maintenance is a question of transferred control. Initially, the response is controlled by the independent variables manipulated by the clinician, and this fact can be documented by any one of the several group or single-subject designs described so far in this book.

When the treatment is discontinued, the target responses must be maintained by independent variables that are operative in the client's everyday environment. Those variables may be similar to the ones manipulated by the clinician, or they may be of entirely different kinds. In any case, those variables are a part of the client's living environment, and they are knowingly or unknowingly administered by the people surrounding the client. An experimental analysis of maintenance should look at the independent variables that are operative in the client's natural environment and administered by persons that interact with him or her.

The technology of response maintenance is at its earliest stage. Rusch and Kazdin (1981) have proposed three design strategies that they believe will help assess response maintenance. First, when a treatment procedure consists of multiple components, such as modeling, reinforcement, informative feedback, and tokens, the clinician can withdraw each of the components, one at a time and in sequence. Any time a given component is withdrawn, whether the response is maintained is carefully assessed. If it is, the next component is withdrawn. In this manner, all the components are withdrawn while care is taken to ensure that the target behavior is not lost. This design is known as the **sequential-withdrawal design.**

Second, when a clinician is using a multiple baseline design to evaluate the effects of a treatment package, either the entire package or one of the components can be withdrawn from one of the participants, behaviors, or settings used in the design. This is known as the **partial-withdrawal design.** Of course, the treatment is withdrawn only after the behaviors show change under treatment. In the multiple baseline across participants, if the participant for whom the treatment is withdrawn continues to respond appropriately, the treatment is withdrawn from other participants as well. In the multiple baseline across behaviors, if a particular response in the same participant continues at a high rate in spite of treatment withdrawal, then the treatment can be withdrawn from other behaviors of the same client. Similarly, if the withdrawal of treatment in one setting proves to have no negative effects, then it can be withdrawn in other settings when the design is the multiple baseline across settings.

Third, a treatment component or a package can be first removed from one behavior, participant, or setting and then if the data warrant, removed from all of the behaviors, participants, or settings. Once again, the basic design used to demonstrate the treatment effects will be the multiple baseline design. This strategy is a combination of the first two strategies, and therefore it is known as the **partial-sequential withdrawal.**

The strategies suggested by Rusch and Kazdin (1981) do not necessarily address the issue of response maintenance as described here. Obviously, when a treatment is withdrawn, the response rate may or may not be sustained. If it is not sustained, the treatment is clearly still needed for the response to be made, and no other variable has come to control it. If the response rate is sustained when the treatment variable is withdrawn, then either the response is under the discriminative stimulus control, which may fade in time, or independent variables other than the one manipulated by the clinician are controlling the response. The withdrawal strategies described by Rusch and Kazdin (1981) are not able to make a discriminative experimental analysis of these possibilities.

Further developments in the technology of response maintenance may be possible when research attention is focused on the mechanisms by which the response controls initially exerted by the clinician are transferred to other individuals and other settings. It may be a mistake to assume that the end of a clinician's treatment is the end of response control. This assumption implies that once created, an effect does not need a cause to sustain itself.

It would appear that no new technology is needed to begin an experimental analysis of response maintenance in nonclinical settings. What is needed is a study of contingencies managed by other individuals in natural settings and over time. Existing experimental methodologies are capable of handling these concerns.

SINGLE-SUBJECT DESIGNS IN CLINICAL RESEARCH

In many clinical disciplines, including communicative disorders and special education, the application of single-subject designs has increased in the past few years. Many clinicians and special educators have found that the method is more applicable than group designs in evaluating treatment effects.

Although single-subject experimental designs were fully developed in the context of behavioral research, the approach has medical and clinical roots, as I noted in the first part of this chapter. In recent years, single-subject studies and overview of designs have begun to appear in medical journals as well. Generally speaking, the single-subject strategy is more relevant to clinical research because it frees the clinician from seeking the unattainable random samples of clients and from the pursuit of the unrealistic goal of inferential generality through a single large-sample study.

Single-Subject Designs in Behavioral and Educational Research

Single-subject designs have been extensively used in evaluating behavioral treatment methods. Most of the basic procedures of behavioral treatment, including positive reinforcement, negative reinforcement, extinction, discrimination training, response reduction through corrective feedback (punishment), and others have been evaluated in single-subject designs. Because of their emphasis on controlled experimental data, behavioral scientists have produced a wealth of data on the efficacy of behavioral treatment methods in teaching appropriate behaviors and skills and in reducing inappropriate behaviors in a variety of clinical populations, including those with communicative disorders (Hegde, 1998a).

Single-subject designs also have played an important role in documenting the effectiveness of various teaching methods used in regular and special education. Single-subject designs, such as multiple baselines, have been developed largely in the context of evaluating behavioral instructional methods used in special education. Methods of teaching skills to children with autism, developmental disabilities, and various behavior disorders have largely been evaluated with single-subject designs (Hegde, 1998a).

An advantage of single-subject designs is that the clinicians and educators can integrate their service delivery with experimental evaluation of their techniques. While providing services, clinicians and educators can answer questions of practical significance. Because the single-subject method does not require random sampling of participants and accepts small numbers of available participants, clinicians and educators can collect data as they work with their clients and students. Because the designs avoid control groups, treatment or teaching need not be denied to anyone who needs it. Therefore, single-subject designs help bridge the gap between research and clinical or educational services.

If practicing clinicians were to use the single-subject designs on a large scale, the amount of in-house knowledge regarding the effectiveness of treatment procedures would be greatly increased. There is an urgent need to use the experimental methods of science and an equally urgent need to establish the treatment effects under controlled conditions. Although theoretically the group designs can offer the same opportunities for experimental–clinical research, it is the single-subject strategy than can actually make it happen.

Single-subject designs help generalize from research studies to individual clients. Thus, they provide for the much-needed logical generality. Detailed descriptions of individual client characteristics and treatment effects can help establish the generality of treatments across a wide variety of clients.

Behavioral and educational methods that have been evaluated by single-subject designs have often been replicated. This is because clinicians and educators find it easier to replicate single-subject design studies than group design studies. This ease of replication has contributed to a faster accumulation of experimental data on many behavioral treatment and instructional methods.

Single-Subject Designs in Medical Research

Single-subject designs have great potential in evaluating the effects of medical and medically related procedures. Pharmaceutical effects of drugs, although traditionally evaluated through randomized clinical trials in medicine, may be evaluated with single-subject designs with some distinct advantages (Barlow & Hersen, 1984). Various surgical procedures, too, may be evaluated with single-subject designs. The usefulness of the single-subject designs approach in evaluating the effects of drugs on psychiatric behaviors as well as in studying interaction between drugs and environmental contingencies is well established (Branch, 1991; Higgins & Hughes, 1998; McKim, 1986). Effects of physical rehabilitation procedures, including most procedures used in physical therapy, are amenable to single-subject design evaluation. Similarly, procedures designed to promote health, fitness, and well-being may be evaluated with single-subject designs. Research on treatment of neurological and neuropsychological problems also can effectively use single-subject designs (B. Wilson, 1987). Furthermore, assessment and treatment research on psychophysiological variables including heart rate modification, stress management, and blood pressure reduction have used the single-subject strategy (Kazdin, 1982; Tomarken, 1999).

The basic *ABA* design format may be modified to suit studies that evaluate various medical and medical rehabilitation procedures. Barlow and Hersen (1984) described 15 extensions of the *ABA* structure that may be used as preexperimental and experimental designs in medical research. The designs allow baselines (no intervention or placebo), placebo controls, single or double blind conditions, and withdrawal and reinstatement of the medical procedure. Table 9.1 presents selected single-subject designs that may be used in evaluating drug effects.

The designs Barlow and Hersen (1984) suggest are all applicable to medial (not surgical) treatment evaluation. Although the authors discuss designs for behavioral pharmacology in which the drugs are evaluated for their behavioral effects, the same designs can help evaluate chemical and physiological effects as well. In several (but not all) single-subject designs, placebo

TABLE 9.1

Selected *ABA* Design Variations for Drug Evaluations

Design	Description	Comment
A-A_1-A	Baserate–Placebo–Baserate	A placebo condition compared with two baserate conditions
A_1-A-A_1	Placebo–Baserate–Placebo	Two placebo conditions compared with a baserate condition
A-B-A	Baserate–Treatment–Withdrawal	Treatment compared with baserate and withdrawal conditions
A_1-B-A_1	Placebo–Treatment–Placebo	Two placebo conditions compared with a treatment condition
B-A-B	Treatment–Withdrawal–Treatment	Two treatment conditions compared with a withdrawal condition
B-A_1-B	Treatment–Placebo–Treatment	Two treatment conditions compared with a placebo condition
A-B-A-B	Baserate–Treatment–Withdrawal–Treatment	Two treatment conditions compared with a baserate condition and a withdrawal condition
A_1-B-A_1-B	Placebo–Treatment–Placebo–Treatment	Two treatment conditions compared with two placebo conditions
A_1-B-A_1-C-A_1-C	Placebo–Treatment 1–Placebo–Treatment 2–Placebo–Treatment 2	Two drugs compared with three placebo conditions

Note. The designs are based on Barlow and Hersen (1984).

condition may be compared with a no-treatment condition. For instance, in the preexperimental A-A_1 design, the initial baseline condition (A) is compared with a placebo condition (A_1). In the preexperimental A-B design, a baserate condition is compared with a treatment (B). In another variation, a placebo may be compared with treatment (A_1-B).

Controlled single-subject experimental designs that help evaluate drug effects include variations of the *ABA* and *ABAB* designs. The control condition may be either a placebo (A_1), traditional baserate (A), or both. Treatment may be single (B) or multiple (B, C, and so forth). All combinations of control and experimental conditions are possible. For instance, placebo may be compared with baserates, and treatment may be compared with either placebo, baserates, or withdrawal conditions, or with all of these control conditions. However, single or double blinding (see Chapter 4 for details) is possible only when a placebo and treatment are both involved. Blinding is not possible when baserate conditions are compared with treatment and withdrawal conditions.

The basic strategy of baserating, treatment application, withdrawal, and reapplication is applicable to most pharmaceutical treatment research. The strategy does not work with surgical procedures because once performed, surgical treatment cannot be withdrawn. The *AB* strategy (baserate-surgical treatment) will work fine, but that would be preexperimental. To evaluate surgical procedures experimentally, multiple baseline across participants design will probably work well. When multiple baselines include sets of participants, the effects of surgical procedures may be evaluated in a fairly large number of participants. Even within the group design strategy, the number of participants involved in surgical treatment studies is much smaller than those in pharmaceutical treatment studies.

Although randomized group clinical trials are the established method of evaluating medical and surgical procedures, many medical researchers as well as practitioners have expressed dissatisfaction with the group approach (see Chapter 4). There has been a search for alternative, better ethically justified methods for evaluating medical treatment procedures. There are suggestions to physicians to consider single-subject designs in evaluating their practice in a practical and efficient manner (Marvel & Amodei, 1992). The importance of using single-subject designs in evaluating medical educational techniques also has been pointed out (Bryson-Brockmann & Roll, 1996).

SUMMARY

Single-subject designs are experimental designs that help establish cause–effect relations based on individual performances under different conditions of an experiment. They permit extended and intensive study of individual participants and do not involve comparisons based on group performances. Instead of the pretests and posttests of the group designs, single-subject designs measure the dependent variables continuously. The participants are not necessarily selected with the random procedure, and the results are not always analyzed statistically. Typically, the magnitude of effects produced within single-subject designs are large enough to be appreciated via visual inspection.

Single-subject designs use a variety of control mechanisms to rule out the influence of extraneous variables, including replication, withdrawal of treatment, reversal of treatment, reinstatement, criterion-referenced change, rapid alternations, baselines, and simultaneous multibaselines. Table 9.2 summarizes information on the major single-subject designs along with the kinds of questions they can answer and their strengths and limitations.

The *AB* design is a preexperimental single-subject design that lacks internal validity. It is similar to the traditional case studies. The prototype of the experimental single-subject design is the *ABA* design, which involves a baseline, treatment, and either withdrawal or reversal of treatment. It can demonstrate the effects of a treatment variable clearly, but it is not a clinical design because it does not end with treatment. A variation of this design is the *BAB* design, which does end with treatment.

The *ABAB* design is an extension of the *ABA* design and is useful in clinical research. The conditions of this design are the baseline, treatment,

TABLE 9.2
Summary of Major Single-Subject Designs and Their Applications

Design	Research Questions	Strengths and Limitations
AB design (case studies)	Is there an apparent change due to treatment?	Clinically useful; results only suggestive; lacks internal validity
ABA design	Is a treatment effective? Is there a cause–effect relation?	Controlled experimental design; can assess treatment effects and isolate cause–effect relations; not for producing lasting treatment effects
BAB design	Is a treatment effective? Is there a cause–effect relation?	Controlled experimental design; can asses treatment effects and isolate cause–effect relations; may produce lasting treatment effects
ABAB design	Is a treatment effective? Is there a cause–effect relation?	Controlled experimental design; can assess treatment effects and isolate cause–effect relations; may produce lasting treatment effects
Multiple baseline across behaviors	Is a treatment effective? Do only treated behaviors change? Do untreated behaviors remain at baseline?	Fairly well controlled; clinically useful; may produce lasting treatment effects; problems of repeated measurement
Multiple baseline across participants	Is a treatment effective? Do only treated participants change? Do untreated participants remain at baseline?	Fairly well controlled; clinically useful; may produce lasting treatment effects; problems of repeated measurement
Multiple baseline across settings	Is a treatment effective? Does the behavior change only in the treatment setting? Does the behavior remain at baseline in untreated settings?	Fairly well controlled; clinically useful; may produce lasting treatment effects; problems of repeated measurement
ABACA/ACABA design	Are two or more treatments effective? Is one treatment more effective than the other?	Well-controlled design; can assess the independent and relative effects of two treatments; need to use counterbalancing
Alternating treatments designs	What are the relative effects of two or more treatments?	Somewhat weak control; can identify effective and ineffective treatments; may produce lasting treatment effects
Interactional design	Is there an interaction between two or more treatments? What are the relative effects of different treatment variables?	Fairly well-controlled design; clinically useful; can show interactive effects; can separate ineffective treatment components from effective ones
Changing criterion design	Is a treatment effective? Do behaviors approximate changing treatment criteria?	Somewhat weak control; useful only for certain kinds of behaviors

either withdrawal or reversal, and reinstatement of treatment. An effective treatment can be continued until certain clinical objectives are met.

A set of clinically appropriate designs that do not involve either the withdrawal or reversal of treatment is known as multiple baseline designs. These designs are based on the logic that multiple dependent variables change only when each of them is brought under the control of an independent variable, then the extraneous variables are ruled out. The multiple baselines may be either behaviors, individuals, or physical settings.

Single-subject designs that permit evaluations of multiple treatments include the *ABACA/ACABA* design and the alternating treatments design. In both the designs, treatment conditions are counterbalanced. In the *ABACA/ACABA* design, the effects of two treatments (*B* and *C*) are compared. The treatment sequence is counterbalanced so that each treatment is preceded as well as followed by the other treatment. The treatments are separated by baselines. In the alternating treatments design, two (or more) treatments are rapidly alternated with the same participants to evaluate the relative effects of those treatments. Most single-subject designs that expose the same participants to multiple treatments have the potential problems of order effects and carryover effects.

The interactional design permits the assessment of interaction between two or more treatment components included in a treatment package. The design can also help isolate effective components from ineffective or less effective components.

In the changing criterion design, behaviors are forced to approximate changing criteria of performance. The design seeks to demonstrate that whenever the performance criteria change, the behavior also changes to fulfill the criteria in force. Such systematic criterion-referenced changes help establish control within the design.

Designs that help assess response maintenance after successful treatment include the sequential-withdrawal design, the partial-withdrawal design, and the partial-sequential withdrawal. However, these designs do not necessarily shed light on the mechanisms of response maintenance in natural environments.

Single-subject designs are eminently practical in clinical settings. Their philosophical bases are compatible with clinical philosophies. They permit the assessment of treatment effects with individual clients who seek clinical services. The designs help blend the needs of science with needs for clinical services.

STUDY GUIDE _____

1. Distinguish between case studies and single-subject design studies.

2. In the single-subject strategy, what kinds of measures are substituted for the pretests and posttests of the group design strategy?

3. What are the six control mechanisms used within the single-subject strategy?

4. Illustrate how in a given study, more than one control mechanism may be used to demonstrate the experimental effects.

5. Distinguish intrasubject replication from intersubject replication.

6. Distinguish between reversal and withdrawal of treatment.

7. What are the limitations of withdrawal and reversal when used in clinical treatment research?

8. Design a study in which you would use the reversal procedure to demonstrate the effects of an articulation treatment program.

9. What is a conservative use of the reversal strategy?

10. Why is reinstatement a contingent control condition?

11. How many times is a treatment effect demonstrated when that treatment is reversed and reinstated once?

12. Why is criterion-referenced change the weaker of the control strategies?

13. Describe how rapid alternations can demonstrate the controlling effects of an independent variable.

14. Define baselines. What are the baseline criteria?

15. Describe how a good potential for contrast can make it possible to use a variable baseline in evaluating treatment effects.

16. In an *ABA* design, what conditions are not supposed to show contrast?

17. How do simultaneous multibaselines help rule out the influence of extraneous variables?

18. What are the limitations of an *AB* design?

19. Suppose you wish to evaluate the effects of delayed auditory feedback on stuttering. Describe a study with the *ABA* design. Specify the design aspects of the study.

20. In evaluating the effects of a treatment procedure, what design will permit you to start with the treatment condition?

21. Describe the *ABAB* design and point out its advantages and disadvantages from the clinical research standpoint.

22. What kinds of research questions require the use of the *ABAB* design?

23. Describe the three variations of the multiple baseline design.

24. What problems do you face when the multiple behaviors used in a multiple baseline design are not independent of each other?

25. What additional controls can you introduce to a multiple baseline design? What problems do these additional controls create?

26. Suppose you wish to evaluate two methods of teaching basic vocabulary to clients with mental retardation. What design would you use? Justify your answer.

27. Compare and contrast the *ABACA/ACABA* design with the alternating treatments design.

28. Why do you need both the *ABACA* and *ACABA* sequences?

29. What kinds of questions are answered by the alternating treatments design?

30. Describe the carryover and contrast effects.

31. What is an *A = BCA* design? When do you use it?

32. What is an interaction? How do you study it within the single-subject strategy?

33. Find two methods of teaching correct articulation in young children. Then design a study to evaluate the independent and interactive effects of the two methods with a single-subject interactional design. Use both the sequences described in the text.

34. Describe the difference between the *A-B-BC-B-BC* design and the *A-BC-B-BC-B* design.

35. In an interactional design, should you change more than one variable at a time while moving from one experimental condition to the other? Why or why not?

36. Describe the changing criterion design. Illustrate the design with a hypothetical study.

37. What kinds of behaviors are especially suited for the changing criterion design?

38. Distinguish between generalization and maintenance.

39. When can you say that you have made an experimental analysis of response maintenance?

40. What is the sequential-withdrawal design? What is its purported use?

41. What is a partial-withdrawal design? How would you use it in clinical research?

42. Do the strategies suggested by Rusch and Kazdin (1981) necessarily address the issue of response maintenance? Justify your answer.

43. Suppose you wish to study whether clients prefer one treatment over the other, assuming that both are equally effective. What design would you use?

44. What is a periodic treatments design? What are its limitations?

45. Summarize the advantages of single-subject designs in clinical research.

Chapter 10

◆◆◆◆◆◆◆◆◆◆◆◆◆◆◆◆◆◆◆◆◆◆◆◆◆◆◆◆◆◆◆◆◆◆

Generality Through Replications

The various group and single-subject designs described in the previous chapters help establish cause–effect relations between independent and dependent variables. Necessarily, any experimental study is done in a given setting, by a single or a few investigators, and with selected participants. A laboratory study may isolate a cause–effect relation between two variables. A clinical study may show that a treatment technique was effective in a few clients, as in single-subject design studies, or a larger number of clients, as in randomized clinical trials. Such experimental treatment studies also demonstrate a cause–effect relation. When cause–effect relations are demonstrated under well-controlled conditions, internal validity (described in Chapter 7) is assured. Once a cause–effect relation emerges within a single study, the next question to be asked is whether the same relation holds good when other investigators in other settings and with other participants or clients investigate the same variables. As noted in Chapter 7, this is the question of generality of research findings.

In Chapter 7, various types of generality were described. In this chapter, the procedures used to establish generality of research data will be discussed. The emphasis will be on the generality of data relative to clinical treatment research. **Generality** is the extent to which conclusions of a research study can be extended to persons who have not been included in the study; like reliability, generality is quantitative. There is more or less generality for otherwise valid and reliable data.

The clinical importance of the question of generality is obvious. Clinicians wish to know whether a given procedure, demonstrated to be effective in a particular study, will be equally effective when other clinicians in other settings use it to treat their clients. The question of generality is related both to reliability and to the range of conditions under which a demonstrated cause–effect relation holds good.

Replication, which is the repetition of a study with or without variations, is the method of establishing generality of research findings. A single study, no matter how well done, cannot establish generality. This is true even of group designs that draw random samples from the population, because sampling equivalence should not be equated with generality. A study must be repeated to find out if the evidence holds under different circumstances. A study can be replicated in different ways, and different replication strategies are used in different stages of research. The questions and strategies of replication have received much attention from behavioral scientists, who have described two major kinds of replications: direct and systematic (Barlow & Hersen, 1984; Sidman, 1960).

In Chapter 9, it was pointed out that single-subject designs replicate the treatment effects within the same study; this is known as **intrasubject replication,** which is typically done with similar participants. Such replications help increase the confidence one can place in the experimental findings, but they may not suggest generality. Both direct and systematic replications are necessary to establish generality.

DIRECT REPLICATION

In **direct replication,** the same researcher repeats the same experiment in the same physical setting. Only the participants are new, though they are similar to those in the original study. Because different but similar participants are used, direct replication is **homogeneous intersubject replication** by the same investigator in the same setting.

When a treatment is found to be effective with a set of clients with a particular disorder, direct replication should be initiated. It does not matter whether the single-subject or group design strategy was used in the original study because generality is not a matter of design; it is a matter of repeating the experiment with some variation, minimally with new participants. Therefore, the investigator finds new participants who are similar to the original participants and repeats the experiment. If the treatment shows similar effects with new participants, generality of findings begins to emerge.

In clinical research, there is no 100% replication of an experiment. Even if the same original participants are used in the first replication, the experiment is not a 100% replication because of the prior exposure to the treatment variable. Therefore, direct replication of treatment effects requires that the treatment procedure be the same as in the original experiment. The treatment, the client disorder or behaviors, the physical setting, and the clinician–experimenter all stay constant through the direct replication series. Generally, the experimental design is also the same although variations in design are possible.

The new participants used in a direct replication must be similar to those in the original study. The clients selected for replication of a treatment method should have the same disorder and be similar on relevant assigned variables. For example, when a language treatment procedure is found to be effective with four to six patients with aphasia, the research clinician may find other patients who are similar to the original ones and repeat the experimental treatment program.

Homogeneous intersubject replication is a safer initial strategy than the **heterogeneous intersubject replication** in which different kinds of participants are used in replication. If the method does not work with a heterogeneous set of participants, it is difficult to determine the source of the problem. Continuing our example of treatment evaluation involving patients with aphasia, it is possible that compared with those in the original study, a replication study may have patients who have a different kind of aphasia, different preonset educational and intellectual levels, different postonset duration before therapy is introduced, different ages, and such other variables. In this case, if the investigator fails to replicate the original effects of the treatment procedure, it is difficult to know whether the failure was due to differences in one, some, or all of the variables that were different in the second set of participants. Thus, the initial replication of a study should use participants who are similar to those in the original study.

Problem of Finding Homogeneous Participants

Homogeneous participants are similar on measured variables; **heterogeneous participants** are different. The requirement that direct replication involve participants who are similar to those used in the original investigation can pose a difficult problem for the clinical researcher. In some respects, this requirement is based on an ideal and theoretical progression of research through various stages of original and replicated series of investigations.

Ideally, the investigator has either strictly homogeneous or strictly heterogeneous participants in the original investigation. In practice, participants in most experiments are more or less homogeneous. In the single-subject strategy, the participants are expected to be homogeneous; in the group strategy, they are expected to be heterogeneous. When the participants in the original study were homogeneous, the participants in direct replication are expected to be similar to those in the original study and homogeneous among themselves. When the participants in the original study were heterogeneous, the participants in the direct replication are expected to be similarly heterogeneous.

It is somewhat easy to find the particular kinds of animal subjects—homogeneous or heterogeneous. The investigator can control the animal subjects' genetic and environmental history to produce similar or different animal subjects that can then be used in the original, direct, and systematic series of experiments. In human research, especially in human clinical research, this ideal sequence of original, direct, and systematic research is difficult to achieve. Therefore, those sequences are not as well distinguished in human clinical research as they are in animal research. Practical exigencies of direct and systematic human clinical research replications create an interwoven sequence.

In practice, neither a single-subject design study nor a group design study is likely to have the kinds of participants they are supposed to have. The participants in a single-subject design study, though few, may be more heterogeneous than expected. The participants in a group clinical study, though many and randomly selected, may be less heterogeneous than expected. In essence, clients in clinical research are neither ideally homogeneous nor ideally heterogeneous. If the target is a heterogeneous sample, the clinician does his or her best to increase the diversity of participants. If the target is a homogeneous sample, the investigator tries to minimize differences in participant characteristics. In either case, the eventual participant sample is not likely to be ideally homogeneous or heterogeneous.

Another difficulty with participant selection for either an original or a replicative study is that the researcher who can strive for an ideal sample may not know what makes an ideal sample. Homogeneity or heterogeneity of participants is a matter of judgment based on past research and clinical experience. Investigators judge the similarities and differences between individuals on known variables, but unknown variables may make participants either similar to, or different from, each other. Assume, for example, that the age at which schooling is started affects the outcome of aphasia treatment but no researcher is aware of this. Therefore, researchers will not consider that variable in judging homogeneity and heterogeneity of participants for a study on aphasia treatment. Consequently, participants who are similar on this variable may be considered different, and vice versa.

Practical difficulties in obtaining participants for a study often lead to compromises in the application of adopted participant selection criteria. Age ranges may be extended or restricted to accommodate available participants. Differences in health history may be ignored. Although the initial plan may be to have participants of only one gender, the eventual sample may contain females and males. Most investigators make these and other compromises sooner or later. Though justified on practical grounds, such compromises may create difficulties for interpreting data and for planning replications.

When the participants in the original study were about as homogeneous as expected, and all of them reacted the same to the treatment variable, the investigator may search for similar participants for a direct replication. There is no guarantee, however, that the participants selected for the direct replication will be similar to those in the original study. They are likely to be more or less homogeneous among themselves and more or less similar to the participants in the original study. If the participants selected for direct replication are about as similar to those in the original study as can be expected, another replication may be attempted. In some cases, the investigator may decide that it is time to initiate systematic replications, which involve participants who differ from those in the original, as well as direct replication studies.

To a certain extent, an original study that contains heterogeneous clients and produces consistent data is already a systematic replication. In other words, an initial study may have produced data showing effectiveness for a procedure in spite of failed attempts to obtain homogeneous participants. For example, the investigator wishing to evaluate the effects of a new treatment for patients with aphasia may not have been able to select patients of the same age, health history, and severity of aphasia. Instead of not doing a study because it may be imperfect, the investigator, trying his or her best to minimize the differences between participants, may go ahead with the study. If the results are consistent across those somewhat different participants, the original study itself can be considered a systematic replication. Such a study will have demonstrated that different participants react the same to the same treatment variable. In effect, a risky original treatment evaluation involving heterogeneous participants may produce the same results as a subsequent systematic replication.

Research philosophies generally discourage such studies in the initial step because when the results are not uniformly good or bad, an unambiguous interpretation of results is not possible, although those who use the group design approach are generally not as concerned about individual variability in response to treatment as are single-subject design users. However, when practical considerations force the selection of available clients for an initial study, the next attempt often depends on the judgment of the investigator. If the sample is thought to be relatively heterogeneous and the results are consistent, replications may be either direct or systematic. However, when the results are inconsistent across clients while there is reason to believe that the sample was heterogeneous in some respects, then the investigator will have learned a lesson. He or she will not try too hard to interpret the data in any global manner and instead will look at individual differences that might have accounted for divergent data. In further studies, a more serious attempt may be made to obtain homogeneous sets of participants. In essence, there are very few rigid rules that an investigator can follow in determining the exact nature and sequence of replication.

Direct replication need not be an endless series of studies. When the effect of an independent variable is replicated across a few participants, systematic replication may be initiated. Within the philosophy of single-subject designs, Barlow and Hersen (1984) recommend that when a procedure has been directly replicated in four participants or clients, systematic replication should be started. Continued direct replication may not be productive beyond that point. This recommendation is especially acceptable when the demonstrated treatment effects are strong and individual variability has been minimal.

SYSTEMATIC REPLICATION

Direct replication can demonstrate only that the causal relation found in the original study may have some homogeneous participant generality. That is, a treatment is effective in similar participants when the same investigator used the same treatment in the same setting with different but similar clients. However, direct replication does not tell whether the treatment will be equally effective when different investigators use the same treatment with different clients, in different settings, and perhaps with different response classes. In essence, to establish all the different kinds of clinical generality described in Chapter 7, one needs systematic replication.

In systematic replication, one or more variables or aspects of procedures are varied at a time to see if the results of the direct replication series can still be duplicated. For the sake of clear interpretations, it is necessary to vary only one or two variables at a time. If too many factors are varied simultaneously, a failure to replicate the findings of the direct replication series is difficult to understand, although success in such cases results in significant economy of effort.

It is possible that the same investigator makes the initial systematic replication. Once it has been determined that a given functional relation is reliable and that it has some degree of participant generality, the investigator may wish to find out if the same relation can be found in a different setting or with participants who are in some specific ways different from those in the earlier studies. A clinician who has found that a given treatment procedure is effective with several clients showing a particular disorder may ask the following kinds of questions:

1. Is the treatment effective in a different setting, involving similar clients?

2. Is the treatment effective in the same setting, but with clients who show a variation of the same disorder?

3. Is the treatment effective in the same setting with clients who have the same disorder but are different in other respects?

4. Is the treatment effective in a different setting, also involving clients who show a variation of the same disorder?

5. Is the treatment effective in the same setting, with clients who have an altogether different disorder?

6. Is the treatment effective in a different setting, also with clients who show a different disorder?

Those are not the only questions the clinician could ask. However, they illustrate the basic nature of systematic replication, which investigates the effects of one variable (treatment) when other variables come to play.

Systematic replication of clinical treatment effects is a time-consuming process because the diagnostic categories are not strictly homogeneous. There usually is notable intersubject variability among such clinical groups as persons who stutter, children who have hearing or language impairment, and patients with aphasia or dysarthria. The variability regarding such background variables as age, gender, education, premorbid health status, and socioeconomic status of clients within diagnostic categories is well known. Besides, clients within and across diagnostic categories vary in the severity of the disorder, subtypes within the disorder, the degree and types of prior treatment experiences, and so forth. A treatment procedure that works well with young individuals with language problems may or may not work with older persons having the same disorder. Clients with multiple misarticulations may not react as favorably to a treatment procedure as those with single-phoneme misarticulations. A procedure that is effective with persons who have mild stuttering may not be equally effective with those who have severe stuttering. A technique that is effective with people who stutter who have marked respiratory abnormalities may be useless with those who do not show such abnormalities.

On the other hand, certain treatment techniques may be effective within and across diagnostic categories. Obvious differences between clients in age, gender, and diagnostic categories and subcategories do not necessarily mean that they will react differently to the same treatment procedure.

Many behavioral treatment procedures including modeling, differential reinforcement, and response reduction work well across people with varied types of disorders, including communicative disorders (Hegde, 1998a).

Systematic replications help establish that a given treatment procedure works when other clinicians implement it. When other clinicians are equally capable of administering the treatment procedure, the results must be comparable to those of the original investigator. If other clinicians cannot replicate some dramatic results of a study, then those results must be attributed to some extraneous factors. Those extraneous factors may include such variables as the personality or the special interpersonal skills of the original clinician. What is more important is the possibility that the original investigator may not have described all aspects of the treatment procedure. Certain critical elements of the procedure may not have been included in the description, and hence those who try to replicate the study may not do precisely what the original clinician did.

It is likely that other clinicians will replicate a treatment procedure in a setting different from that of the original setting. In this case, successful replicative attempts demonstrate generality not only across participants and clinicians, but also across settings.

Successful replication across clients, clinicians, and settings is essential to a widespread practice of therapeutic techniques, although this has rarely been a condition speech–language pathologists require. A treatment procedure can be recommended for general application only when it is shown that a variety of clients can benefit from it. In speech–language pathology, many therapeutic practices are neither experimentally evaluated nor replicated.

When the treatment of a given disorder is effective and replicated, the question that arises is whether the technique can be equally effective with different disorders. A successful language treatment technique or components of the technique may be useful in treating articulation or voice disorders. For example, components such as modeling, shaping, and differential reinforcement are useful components of therapy for many different kinds of verbal and nonverbal behavior disorders.

Unfortunately, the fixed notions of nosology—the science of classifying disorders—discourage replication of a technique across disorders. There is an implicit assumption that different diagnostic categories necessarily require treatment techniques that are independent of each other. This assumption may not be valid in speech–language pathology, in which diagnostic categories are not strictly etiologic but often are descriptive. As a result, topographically different behaviors such as high vocal pitch or dysfluency may be susceptible to the same treatment variables. Furthermore, there is no compelling reason to believe that different instigating causes of communicative disorders necessarily dictate totally different treatment variables. For example, whether a language disorder is thought to be due to genetically determined mental retardation or some unexplained environmental events may not be critical in shaping specific verbal responses in a group of clients.

It is clear that systematic replication across clients and disorders will help reduce unnecessary diversity in treatment techniques. If there are a few core techniques whose limited variations can help treat a variety of communicative disorders, so much the better. Economy in treatment procedures that does not do any injustice to individual differences may be a desirable outcome of systematic replication.

Conditions Necessary for Systematic Replications

Systematic replications of research data are possible within a discipline only when that discipline meets certain criteria. The treatment techniques should be specific and well researched through experimental methods and direct replications. Procedures for measuring dependent as well as independent variables should be objective and standard. The dependent variables should be conceptualized on empirical (not just logical or theoretical) grounds and should be defined in such a way that reliable observations can be made. In addition, the treatment outcome criteria must be measurement-oriented. To realize these conditions, the discipline should have a long and strong experimental history.

Unfortunately, carefully planned and extensively conducted systematic replications are rare in speech–language pathology, which does not meet many of those criteria. As noted before, direct replication follows experimental analysis of treatment procedures, which in turn leads to systematic replication. Unfortunately, treatment techniques in speech–language pathology are generally not subjected to experimental analysis. They often are vague and riddled with controversies. For the most part, treatment techniques are justified on the basis of clinical judgment; speculative theories and presumptions; liberal recommendations coming from nonclinical disciplines, well-recognized authorities, and subjective preferences; tradition; dated training; and personal experience not supported by objective evaluations.

There is little agreement on the dependent variables and their measurement procedures. As will be discussed in Chapter 12, most of the dependent variables are conceptualized on logical, topographical, and speculative grounds. For example, what are the dependent variables in the case of language behaviors? Transformational grammar? Innate grammatical competence? Knowledge of language structures? Semantic notions? Pragmatic rules? Response classes? What are the dependent variables in stuttering treatment? Stuttering events? Dysfluency rates? Molar moments? Negative attitudes? And how can any one of these be measured? When there is much controversy about the dependent variables (compounded by disagreement on treatment—independent variables) and the controversies are debated by speculative opinions, experimental analysis becomes very difficult.

In the experimental evaluation of treatment, outcome must be specified in terms that different investigators can use. If the few treatment evaluation studies that are done do not report their treatment evaluation procedures in objective terms, other investigators cannot replicate those studies. The questions are these: How did the clinician determine the effectiveness of a treatment procedure? What magnitude of change in the clients' problem behaviors did the clinician require before concluding that the treatment was effective? Was it a statistical or clinical criterion? Did the investigator adopt generalization or maintenance of the target behaviors as the criterion, or both? Answers to questions such as these are important in treatment evaluations and their replications.

One may think that different clinicians should agree upon the evaluative criteria so that investigators can use the same criteria. However, agreement among investigators is not the issue. Whether some specified criterion is described in operational terms at all is the issue. Such a criterion can be used in evaluating treatment effectiveness regardless of agreement among investigators.

A discipline that does not have a strong tradition of experimental evaluation of its practices cannot even begin direct or systematic replications. Systematic replications are a sure sign of the advanced scientific status of a clinical profession. However, to achieve such a status, the members of a profession need to place a heavy emphasis on experimental evaluation of treatment procedures. Although a general agreement upon the dependent and independent variables and their measurement procedures is likely to cause more rapid progress, diversity of approaches, by itself, is not a hindrance to scientific progress. The hindrance is a lack of appreciation of the philosophy and methodology of science. What is crucially needed to achieve scientific progress is a commitment on the part of investigators to the experimental methodology of natural sciences. When such a commitment is made, the progress may still be slow, but it is inevitable. In the long run, it does not matter what theoretical orientation one takes. Some orientations may prove to be valid and others not so valid—many in between. Because science is a self-corrective method, things will be sorted out in the process of experimental research. However, what matters is whether one finds a way to experimental verifications and direct and systematic replications or whether one is satisfied with self-generated or other-generated theoretical pronouncements.

SAMPLE SIZE AND GENERALITY

The size of a sample used in a study is a significant issue in generality. There are two views on the relation between sample size and generality. The first view is that only large sample studies can hope to claim generality. Historically, group design advocates have argued that generality is possible only when the sample is large enough to represent the population. To represent a population, the sample must not only be large, but it also should be drawn randomly from that population. This argument is presented especially in the context of statistical (inferential) generality. Randomized clinical trials, described in Chapter 4, are based on this argument. Those who advocate the use of randomized clinical trials in medicine insist that there is no generality without large numbers of participants, in most cases, several thousand persons.

The second view is that large samples are unnecessary to claim generality and that a single study, no matter how large its sample, cannot demonstrate generality. Advocates of single-subject designs have argued that generality is achieved only by replication. They further argue that strong experimental effects produced in a few individuals under well-controlled conditions are more likely to be replicated than are weak effects demonstrated in large groups summed across individuals. Indeed, these two differing views on generality are at the heart of the skepticism typically expressed by group design advocates about the usefulness of single-subject designs. Skepticism turns into outright rejection when some group design advocates confuse single-subject experimental designs with uncontrolled case studies.

There is a long history of scholarly debate on the importance of the individual and the group in philosophy and, subsequently, in such sciences as biology, psychology, sociology, and medicine (Allport, 1962; Barlow & Hersen, 1984; Dukes, 1965; Valsiner, 1986a, 1986b). The perspectives in psychology and historical developments in the design of experiments in agriculture have greatly influenced this debate. In psychology, studying groups of individuals was seen as a method of understanding the individual as well. The counter argument has been that group averages do not teach us anything significant about the individual.

Rational arguments aside, behavioral scientists have provided plenty of experimental evidence that strong effects produced under tightly controlled conditions in just a handful of participants may be replicable. As pointed out elsewhere in the book, Skinner's (1953) principles of operant behavior and Pavlov's principles of classical conditioning have been initially formulated with a few animal subjects but later replicated in many human experiments. Behavioral treatment studies also have demonstrated that most treatment effects demonstrated in single-subject studies have been replicated (Barlow & Hersen, 1984; Kazdin, 1982). One of the early advocates of single-subject designs in clinical psychology, Shapiro (1961) demonstrated through his experiments that data supporting a scientific law discovered in the context of one or two participants are replicable across many participants. Other historically significant advocates of research with small number of participants have documented much systematic and replicated knowledge stemming initially from one or few participants (Bolgar, 1965; Dukes, 1965). Dukes has pointed out that if the objective is to study an individual's uniqueness, a single participant exhausts the population. He has further pointed out that when data generated from a single-subject study contradict previously established data with large numbers of participants, the negative evidence is extremely useful because it shows the limits of generality. In treatment research, it is important to understand individual response to treatment so that practitioners can make meaningful judgments about treatment application to their individual clients.

Large samples, while not so critical for establishing generality of treatment effects, may be necessary to predict group actions or opinions. Statistical generality is useful in such studies as sample surveys whose goal is to predict what a majority of people will do or say. Being nonexperimental, sample surveys do not try to change something, as experiments seek to do. Therefore, in sample surveys, the action of an individual does not matter. What matters is the action of a defined population. Therefore, a large number of heterogeneous participants who represent that population must be studied to achieve generality. Large numbers of participants also may be needed in clinical sciences when the goal is to predict the average number of people who will benefit from a treatment or clinical program. Finally, large numbers of participants may be needed in several other kinds of nonexperimental research (e.g., epidemiological studies).

Concentrating on generality of treatment effects, it is clear that the traditional argument for large samples is highly questionable. Beside the criticism that they may be unnecessary, large samples have other limitations that render them especially troublesome to clinicians who wish to generalize the data to particular patients or clients they serve. Both the treatment researcher and the practicing clinician wish to apply the results of a treatment study to individual clients. But this is exactly where the randomized large sample clinical trials fail. Not only single-subject design experts (Barlow & Hersen, 1984; Johnston & Pennypacker, 1993; Kazdin, 1982), but also psychologists (Valsiner, 1986b), and several medical statisticians and treatment research experts (Dekkers & Boer, 2001; Feinstein, 1970, 1995; Kaptchuk, 2001; Pringle & Churchill, 1995, among others) have pointed out serious limitations of randomized large-group medical treatment research. The group averages reported in randomized control trials may predict the parameter (average value) of the population, but they do not predict an individual's reaction or performance under the same treatment. Valsiner (1986b, p. 394) has stated that "Group data, statistically aggregated, may allow us to make generalizations about populations. . . . However, inference from the population system to its parts (individuals persons in the sample) is epistemologically questionable." Feinstein (1970), a medical expert in statistics and treatment research, has stated that a problem with randomized clinical trials in medicine "is the frequent claim that a large heterogeneous population gives the results 'wider applicability.' . . . The scientific effect of a diverse poorly identified mixture is to produce imprecision, confusion, and perhaps delusion, not generalizability" (p. 76). He further pointed out that the results of randomized clinical trials "will be meaningless because a clinician will not know how to apply them in the future; he cannot determine whether 'good risk' and 'poor risk' patients responded the same way to each therapeutic agent" (p. 289). Consequently, Feinstein has suggested that small-group treatment research will produce more meaningful data than large randomized clinical trials. Feinstein's argument is consistent with that of single-subject researchers who seek to produce logical generality on the basis of which clinicians can select researched treatment procedures for their individual clients.

FAILED REPLICATIONS: SOURCES OF TREATMENT MODIFICATIONS

A functional relation found in experimental research—whether in basic research or treatment research—may or may not be replicated. Several reasons may account for failed replications. When an investigator fails to replicate his or her own previous findings, the first consideration is the reliability of the original findings. It is possible that the functional relation found in the original study was mistaken in that extraneous variables, not the manipulated independent variables, were responsible for changes in the dependent variables. This is the question of internal validity. Findings of questionable internal validity are not replicable, but typically one does not know this until an effort to replicate has failed.

On the other hand, a study may have had good internal validity in that the external variables were ruled out and the results obtained were valid in the case of the original participants or clients. Direct replication of such a study across participants might still fail. Such a failure suggests a more complex situation than failures involving questionable internal validity. Failed direct replications are both challenging and interesting. In clinical treatment research, those failures can be a valuable source of treatment modifications that suit individual clients.

When a well-researched treatment procedure cannot be replicated across clients, several possibilities must be considered. Perhaps the participants used in the original and replicated experiments differed and this made a difference in treatment effects. The clients in the replication series may be thought of as belonging to the same diagnostic category as those in the original study, but in reality they may form a subcategory. For example, *children with language disabilities* may not be a homogeneous group in spite of commonly observed language problems. Past learning experiences, intelligence, or other important variables that differ across children who show the same type of language disorder may produce divergent data. The importance of some of these variables may not have been apparent to the investigator. In essence, all clients with language disorders may not benefit from the same treatment procedure. Similarly, all persons with stuttering or aphasia may not react the same way to a treatment procedure known to be effective with some of them.

In systematic replication, the investigator takes careful note of client differences, because establishing generality across different kinds of clients is the goal in this type of replication. In direct replication, on the other hand, the investigator tries to have clients who are similar to those in the original study, but this objective may not have been realized in a particular replication. When the replication fails, one must look for possible differences in clients' background variables or the special characteristics of the disorder some of them exhibited. In such cases, a modification in the technique or a totally different technique may be necessary. Patients with aphasia in a replication study may have additional health problems that were not present in the patients of the original study. Persons with stuttering in the replication series may have had marked breathing abnormalities associated with their stutterings, and this may render a pure syllable prolongation approach less useful compared with its use for those without such abnormalities. A modified breathing component may prove effective either alone or in combination with syllable prolongation. The researcher may then pursue this question and eventually offer suggestions on differentially treating persons with unique characteristics.

The source or sources of failure to replicate results in a systematic replication series can be more obvious than such failure in a direct replication series. The investigator knows the differences between the participants in the original study and those in the replication because such differences are built into a replicative study. A treatment procedure known to be effective with children exhibiting an articulation disorder may be evaluated with adult clients. Or a technique known to be effective with children who have language disorders may be tried with those who have an articulation disorder. There is no guarantee, however, that the known difference is the source of failure when it occurs; for example, failure with adults treated with a procedure known to be effective with children does not necessarily mean that age is the critical variable. Some unknown variable or variables may be responsible for the failure.

The influence of unknown variables can be suspected when replicative efforts are continued in spite of an initial failure and suddenly a success emerges even though the participants showed the same difference as in the earlier series. For instance, following a failure to replicate a study with clients older than those in the original study, an investigator may replicate the results in a subsequent effort, also involving older participants. This would then suggest that age may not have been the reason for the initial failure and that there are other, unsuspected variables that must be studied. An unsuspected difference in the family background of participants or hereditary differences may account for the initial failure.

Generally speaking, it is the success that must be replicated, but a single failure may also be replicated when there is reason to believe that the original findings were strong and reliable and that the initial replication may have failed because of some flaw in the study. A second failure, however, may convince the investigator that additional efforts are not worthwhile. In fact, in clinical treatment evaluations, repeated attempts to replicate failed treatments may be unethical.

What is done when a failure is considered genuine may depend on the investigator's dispositions. Personal views seem to have a strong influence on the course of action taken in such situations. The investigator who still believes that the overall approach evaluated in the original study is valid may proceed to modify the procedure. This modified technique then goes through the initial experimental evaluations, followed by its own direct and systematic replications. However, the investigator who has second thoughts about the effectiveness of the technique is unlikely to replicate it with or without modifications. Replications are done to support as well as refute certain existing practices. When replications done to refute a given approach succeed in the refutation, the investigator is likely to stop, although those who believe in its success may redouble their efforts.

In essence, failed replications are full of good lessons. They point out possible exceptions to a general rule. Clinically, failed replications suggest limitations of generally effective treatment procedures. Such exceptions are important in science because the scientist is interested in identifying the limits of known functional relations. Exceptions are equally important for clinicians because their philosophy and methodology are based upon individual uniqueness as well as human generalities. The instant a generally effective treatment procedure fails with a given client, the clinician has made an empirical contact with individual uniqueness. A responsible clinician may then think that the best course of action is to modify the procedure to suit the individual or to evaluate a totally new approach that may prove more successful. In this way, when the message of failed replications is heeded, a clinical science moves ahead.

TREATMENT VARIABLES AND TREATMENT PACKAGES

As noted in the discussion of the interactional design strategy, most treatment procedures are, technically, packages of different treatment components. It is not uncommon to teach multiple target behaviors with multiple treatment components. A treatment package may be more successful in treating such complex disorders as stuttering or dysarthria. In the treatment of stuttering, for example, such components as modified airflow, gentle phonatory onset, rate reduction through stretched syllables, and relaxed movements of the articulators are all a part of several treatment packages. When a disorder includes different classes of problem behaviors, different treatment components may be necessary to handle them. There is one method for developing treatment packages and another method for verifying existing packages. Both have implications for replications.

In the strategy of **developing a treatment package,** the clinician first individually tests each of the components to be included in a package and then replicates them separately in direct as well as systematic series. For example, if modified airflow, rate reduction, and gentle phonatory onset are to be included in a stuttering treatment package, then the independent effects of each of these components must be evaluated experimentally and replicated appropriately. When it is known that the three components are effective by themselves, they may be combined into a package and the total package can then be applied to clients. The process of combining treatment packages also may involve an analysis of the interactional effects of two or more components. With interactional analysis, only those components that yield the best possible results in combination may be included in the package. The total package itself then goes through direct and systematic replications.

In practice, however, the ideal of independent evaluation of components that are then combined into treatment packages is rarely achieved. For instance, neither the specific components nor the total packages of most stuttering treatment programs are experimentally evaluated. Some may have been evaluated in an uncontrolled series with the one group pretest–posttest design or case studies. Often, clinicians start with a treatment package—the components of which are selected on theoretical grounds or clinical traditions. The philosophy of eclecticism, which has been so popular in speech–language pathology, has also encouraged the use of untested components in treatment packages. Typically, though, the philosophy of eclecticism has been justified on the basis of the common sense idea that one selects what is good from every viewpoint. Unfortunately, the justification requires more than common sense, which is to say that experimental evidence is needed. Such evidence has been woefully lacking. As a result, the treatment packages may contain components whose effects are unknown, minimal, nonexistent, or even detrimental.

The method of **verifying an already existing treatment package** is to break it down into its components and experimentally evaluate each of the components for its independent effect. The components are then subjected to direct and systematic replications, and the components that prove effective are combined into a treatment package. In this process, the interactive effects of two or more components can also be determined. The final package that emerges through this kind of research may be different from the one that the clinicians used because some of the components that proved useless will not have been included in the package.

The proliferation of untested treatment packages creates a dilemma for the practicing clinician who cannot evaluate the effectiveness of those that need to be used. It behooves those who advocate the use of treatment packages to verify the effectiveness of independent components in isolation and in combination. The total package is then applied to a group of well-defined clients with multiple problems. Additional direct and systematic replications, when successful, enhance the generality of the treatment packages.

Economy of clinical practice is enhanced when a clinician does not use all components of a widely recognized but experimentally untested treatment package. The "do everything possible" strategy is considered the best because if some components fail, others may ensure success. But this strategy also encourages superstitious therapeutic practices. Therefore, an alternative practice is purposefully to eliminate some of the components and see what happens. If the clients improve, there will be no assurance that the treatment components used were indeed responsible for the improvement. Nevertheless, that the omitted components were indeed unnecessary will be loud and clear. In such informal evaluations, the clinician must make sure that the dependent variables are carefully monitored in every treatment session. Systematic measurement of the target behaviors will help clinicians make decisions to drop the components when they prove ineffective, or to add other components when the data warrant. Constant monitoring of the target behaviors will help clinicians make those decisions at the earliest possible time so that clients do not continue to receive ineffective treatment.

HOMOGENEITY AND HETEROGENEITY OF PARTICIPANTS

That people are similar and yet unique is a fundamental principle that, while advancing science, creates problems as well. This is the issue of homogeneity and heterogeneity of participants. The issue is relevant to animal as well as human research and to basic as well as clinical research. Within a single study, whether participants were homogeneous or heterogeneous can make a difference in internal validity and generality. Typically, investigators strive to have either homogeneous or heterogeneous participants, depending on the research design philosophies and the purposes of the experiment.

Within the philosophy of group designs, heterogeneous samples are considered ideal because such samples are expected to represent the necessarily heterogeneous population. Only when this is not practical would an investigator think of using homogeneous participants, hoping to show that a given variable has an effect in the case of individuals with known (and homogeneous) characteristics. Within the single-subject strategy, investigators usually try to select homogeneous participants. However, the single-subject methodology does not pose serious problems when heterogeneous participants are used because the data analysis is subject specific. Even so, heterogeneous participants may not be preferable, because if the results are different across participants, the investigator does not know why.

When the purpose of an experiment is systematic replication across participants, one would, of course, select participants who are in some specified way different from those in the original study. The tactic is to select homogeneous participants who are heterogeneous relative to those in the original study.

As noted earlier, homogeneity is more easily achieved in laboratory experiments involving animal subjects. And in human research, especially in clinical research, homogeneity of participants is a strongly wished-for but rarely achieved goal. This section takes a critical look at this concept because so many clinical researchers agonize over it.

There is no doubt that homogeneity of participants would make the life of the clinical researcher much easier. If all children with language disorders were the same, the problem of replication would be a minor one. If all persons who stuttered were the same, a single effective treatment would be sufficient and the burden of replication would be pleasantly light. However, people are just not as homogeneous as the methodology of research requires them to be. People are different, and they do not seem to care about the clinical researchers' pressing problem! Therefore, instead of searching for homogeneous participants that may not exist, it may be prudent to consider heterogeneity as a fact of life and design studies accordingly. In essence, people cannot be changed, but research tactics can be.

The basic problem is that the concept of homogeneity is difficult to define. When are clients homogeneous? Is it when they are of the same age? (Do all children of the same age behave the same?) When they are of the same social status? (Do people within the same social status necessarily behave the same?) When they come from similar family background? (Do the members of a family always behave the same?) When they have similar intelligence? (Do people with similar IQs behave the same?) When they have the same educational background? (Does a 4-year college education create similar individuals?) When they all have suffered the disorder for the same duration? (Does 2 years of stuttering make some individuals the same compared with those who have stuttered for 4 years?)

A set of converse questions can also be asked: Are there no behavioral patterns that are similar across age groups? Do people with different social strata ever share common behavioral patterns? Do the members of the same family—let alone those with similar family backgrounds—behave differently? Do people with different levels of intelligence ever behave similarly? Do people with the same level of education behave differently? Do clients with the same disorder, the same level of severity, and the same duration of history ever behave differently?

The questions raised here are not just rhetorical. The point is that there are no fixed answers to those questions. A bias one way or the other is not implied. In case of given individuals, the answer to any one question may be positive or negative. What is suggested here is that the goal of homogeneity, either in an original series of experimental evaluation or in direct and systematic replications, should not stultify research. If the available clients are somewhat different, then the investigator should carefully describe the differences among them and offer results separately for the individuals. As long as the investigator does not offer group means that mask individual differences, there is no major problem with individual differences in reactivity to treatment variables. An ensuing analysis of reasons for variability may be required, but the data generated by the study will be valuable. It is better to do research with differing clients than to wait for homogeneous clients that may never be found.

The foregoing discussion suggests that there are significant participant selection problems in conducting direct and systematic replications. Besides, research strategies themselves make replications more or less difficult. Generally speaking, the group design strategy, which is difficult to employ in many kinds of clinical treatment research, also is difficult to use in replication studies. The required number of participants may not be available for a series of direct and systematic replications. The single-subject strategy, on the other hand, encourages replications of treatment techniques in a variety of behavior disorders. In the treatment of language, articulation, and fluency disorders, the single-subject studies of behavioral treatment techniques have provided impressive replicative evidence. Comparable evidence has not emerged from the group design strategy. Every time a clinician uses a treatment procedure under controlled conditions with one or few clients, the cause of replication is advanced. This is made possible by the clinically practical single-subject strategy.

SUMMARY

- Generality is a quantitative concept that refers to the extent to which the conclusions of a research study may be extended beyond the limits of that original study. Generality is not a matter of research design or research strategy. It is a matter of replication. No matter what research strategy is used, a study must be replicated to establish its generality.

- Replication is the method of establishing or testing the limits of generality. Replication may be direct or systematic.

  — In direct replication, the same investigator duplicates the same procedure with different participants. For direct replications, investigators typically try to obtain participants who are similar to those in the original study. This is homogeneous intersubject replication.

  — Systematic replication is the method of establishing generality of findings beyond the original limits of the study. One or a few variables are systematically varied to see if the original findings may still be obtained. Systematic replication will test setting, researcher, and participant generality. Systematic replications typically involve heterogeneous participants, resulting in heterogeneous intersubject replication.

  — It often is difficult to find homogeneous participants for clinical treatment research evaluations. Both the single-subject and group design strategies may use participants that are less homogeneous or heterogeneous than desired. However, when heterogeneous participants show similar results, treatment generality is enhanced.

- There are two views on sample size and its relation to generality. Some claim that only large samples can demonstrate generality, and others claim that single-subject data are replicable, and hence can establish generality.

- Failed replications suggest that the original data may have been unreliable or that the replication was not methodologically sound.

- Effective treatment packages may be developed by either testing treatment components individually and then combining only those that are effective or by breaking down an existing package to test its components. Ineffective components of an existing package may then be discarded.

- The concepts of homogeneity and heterogeneity are so relative that they need to be examined critically. The similarities and differences between and among participants and the reasons for those similarities and differences are difficult to determine. Only relative answers that apply to individual studies may be given.

STUDY GUIDE

1. Why should a clinician be concerned with the generality of clinical and experimental data?

2. What kinds of generality are not established by a group design study even when the investigator has drawn and assigned participants randomly?

3. What is the method of establishing generality of research findings?

4. What is direct replication?

5. Suppose that you have just completed a study in which you evaluated a particular method of teaching correct production of speech sounds to 5-year-old children who exhibit disorders of articulation in the absence of any other communicative disorders. Now you wish to do a direct replication study. How would you do it? (You may make up whatever information you need to answer this question.)

6. What is considered to be the safest initial direct replication strategy? Why?

7. Define systematic replication.

8. Suppose you have completed a study in which you experimentally evaluated the effects of a treatment program designed to teach

morphological features to 5-year-old children with mental retardation. Now you plan to do a systematic replication study. How would you do it? Specify the variables that will be the same as in the original study as well as those that will be different. Use hypothetical information.

9. What are the different parameters of systematic replication in clinical research?

10. What conditions are necessary for conducting systematic replication?

11. Summarize the two arguments on the relation between sample size and generality of research findings.

12. What is the value of failed replications? Give a hypothetical example from clinical research.

13. Distinguish the strategy used in developing a treatment package from that used in verifying an existing package.

14. Assuming it is practical, what is gained by having homogeneous participants in clinical research?

15. Critically evaluate the concepts of homogeneity and heterogeneity of human participants.

16. In what kind of replication are participants selected who are heterogeneous relative to those in the original study?

Chapter 11

◆◆◆◆◆◆◆◆◆◆◆◆◆◆◆◆◆◆◆◆◆◆◆◆◆◆◆◆◆◆◆◆◆◆◆

Comparative Evaluation of Design Strategies

In Chapters 8 and 9, I described two major approaches to designing experimental research: the group strategy and the single-subject strategy. In this chapter, I shall discuss the strengths and weaknesses of the two approaches. The purpose of this chapter is to help researchers select appropriate methodological strategies for investigating a variety of research questions.

A research strategy is appropriate or inappropriate only for a particular investigation. Every design with a sound structure has its place in scientific research. However, a design that is perfectly suited to one kind of investigation may be somewhat inappropriate to another kind; it may be totally wrong for yet another kind. Therefore, the appropriateness of a design is judged in relation to the research question or questions the investigator seeks to answer.

Many research questions can be answered by two or more methods. In such cases, selection depends mostly on the training, experience, and philosophy of the investigator. Most investigators tend to use either the group or the single-subject strategy. When an investigator is inclined to use either of those strategies, the selection may depend upon practical considerations. For example, the number of participants available for a study may determine whether one selects a single-subject interactional design or a factorial group design. If many participants are available, the factorial design may be used. If only a few individuals are willing to participate, the single-subject interactional design may be selected.

RESEARCH QUESTIONS AND INVESTIGATIVE STRATEGIES

Though much attention is paid to them, research methods are subservient to research questions. An investigator may find a method fascinating and try to find a problem that can be investigated with it. Such a search for a problem can be intolerably long. More typically, scientists first have research questions and then look for methods to answer them.

Problems or research questions fall into different types of investigations, which were considered in Chapter 4. Taken together, the kind of question and the type of research determine the strategy selected for the study. I shall describe several kinds of research questions and suggest more or less appropriate strategies or designs to answer them. Of necessity, the questions described will be generic, not specific. It is not possible to describe all kinds of research questions one can investigate. Therefore, this discussion will be illustrative only; I shall not try to list every correct design one could use in answering particular types of questions. As you read these pages, you may wish to think of other types of research questions and appropriate strategies to answer them.

What Are the Dependent Variables?

This question is about the existence or description of variables. The investigator may ask, "Does it exist? If so, what are its characteristics?" The investigator may suspect a new disorder, a new disease, or a new effect, and proceed to find out if it exists.

The dependent variable suspected to exist is investigated mostly through descriptive research or case study methods. Once it is found out that a hitherto unknown dependent variable (effect) exists, causal variables may be investigated. Most pilot studies and descriptive studies of new phenomena fall into this category. For example, an investigator may research the communicative effects of a new genetic syndrome or a new disease that affects children's development.

How Are the Dependent Variables Distributed in the Population?

This type of question is a part of normative research. The investigator is interested in finding out the distribution of certain dependent variables in selected populations, such as children or adults. Studies designed to answer this kind of question are descriptive. They do not manipulate independent variables; instead, they describe either the characteristics of their participants or selected dependent variables. See the section covering normative research in Chapter 5 for details.

The distribution of dependent variables is the main concern in many kinds of research questions. For example, what are the language characteristics of 3- and 4-year-old children? How many phonemes can children at different age levels produce correctly? Do 5-year-old children produce more dysfluencies than 3-year-old children? Any kind of research that attempts to establish norms would ask questions of this kind.

Questions of the distribution of dependent variables are investigated without experimental designs. Generally speaking, the methods come from the group design strategy because a large number of participants, selected randomly, is needed to answer such questions. Typically, a large group divided into age levels is observed for somewhat brief periods with limited response sampling. The observed characteristics of participants of different ages are described. However, such descriptions rarely pertain to individual participants. The performance of individual participants in groups or subgroups of participants is averaged to obtain single scores that distinguish one group from the other. These studies seek inferential generality; therefore, the method includes statistical analyses of data.

How Are the Variables *Differentially* Distributed in a Population?

Questions concerning the *differential* distribution of a variable are researched in clinical sciences. The research involved is a combination of three types: ex post facto, normative, and standard-group comparison. Investigators typically ask such questions as whether people who stutter and people who do not stutter differ in their personality, or whether persons with and without laryngectomy differ in their smoking histories. Investigations into such questions seek to determine the differential distribution of certain variables in contrasting populations. Whenever clinical and nonclinical groups are compared on some variable that is not manipulated, the question is one of differential distribution of variables.

Questions of differential distribution of variables use the group methodology. No experimental designs are required to answer these questions; however, the methods are descriptive. The selected dependent variable is measured in groups that are different on some criterion, which is often a clinical diagnosis. The different values of the dependent variables in the two groups are statistically evaluated and reported. For example, it may be found that the scores on a test of intelligence are differentially distributed in misarticulating and normally speaking children. Children with and without language disorders may score differently on a test of pragmatic use of language.

What Factors May Have Contributed to this Effect?

This type of question is asked when the event under investigation has a history and the causes of the event have occurred in the past. The ex post facto method of research is used to answer this kind of question. Most case studies are of this type. The effect is directly observable, but the causes are not. The experimenter cannot manipulate the causes. The investigator makes a search of the factors that may have contributed to the effect under study. See ex post facto research in Chapter 5 for details.

Factors that may have contributed to an effect are widely investigated in clinical sciences. Questions about the causes of most disorders often fall into this category. Questions about what contributed to the onset of stuttering, language disorders, articulation problems, or voice difficulties in given clients are of serious clinical concern. These questions can be researched with either the group strategy or the single-subject strategy. Often, the history of a small number of clients or of single clients is investigated to determine if factors known in some cases to cause the observed effect were present. Whether it is a group or a single-subject study, this type of research is best described as a case study and does not have an experimental design in the technical sense of that term.

What Are the Effects of an Independent Variable?

An investigator may simply ask, what happens when I manipulate this variable? What effects follow when a factor is introduced, removed, or reinstated? Questions of this kind attempt to find out the unknown, or not well-understood, effects of independent variables. For example, one may ask several questions: What happens when the auditory feedback for speech is presented to the speaker with a delay? What happens to the electroencephalographic patterns when meaningful linguistic stimuli are introduced? What are the effects on children's language of training mothers to read stories aloud? What are the effects of reducing the rate of speech in people who stutter? Questions such as these concern the effects of selected independent variables. Evaluation of clinical treatment procedures involves these kinds of questions.

The evaluation of the effects of independent variables requires the experimental method. Questions about the effects of independent variables can be investigated through either group designs or single-subject designs. To control for potential extraneous variables, the investigator must select one of the true experimental designs. Within the group strategy, the pretest–posttest control group design or the posttest-only control group design may be selected to investigate the effects of independent variables. Among the within-subjects designs, the two-group single-treatment counterbalanced design is appropriate. Among the time-series designs, a nonequivalent two-group design may be used with the understanding that there is no sampling equivalence of the groups. Within the single-subject strategy, an *ABA* reversal or withdrawal design would be appropriate. The *BAB* single-subject design may also be used along with *ABAB* reversal or withdrawal designs. Although they are used more frequently in answering clinically oriented questions, the *ABAB* and multiple baseline designs also can be used.

Is a Treatment Associated with Improvement?

In clinical sciences, treatment procedures may be initially evaluated informally. A clinician may try a new procedure by carefully measuring the behaviors before and after treatment. If systematic changes are seen after treatment, it is considered possible that the treatment worked.

Obviously, evaluations of this kind lack appropriate controls. Conclusions are tentative and based on the mere association between treatment and improvement because the extraneous variables are not ruled out. Therefore, the studies lack internal validity, and the clinician cannot assert that the treatment was indeed effective. Nevertheless, research of this type may be useful because many clinicians may be willing to try new ideas informally. Improvement in client behaviors, when documented systematically, may suggest that it is worthwhile to design a more controlled study to evaluate the treatment procedure.

Uncontrolled treatment studies can be more or less useful depending upon the thoroughness of measurement. Repeated and reliable pretreatment measures, measurement during treatment sessions, and posttreatment measures that show a convincing change in client behaviors help establish the value of case studies. Missing pretreatment measures, lack of measures during treatment, and small changes after treatment invalidate most studies of this kind.

Uncontrolled treatment studies can use either a single-subject or a group design. The one-group pretest–posttest design of the group strategy or the *AB* design of the single-subject strategy would be appropriate for this kind of research.

Is a Treatment Effective?

Questions about the effectiveness of clinical treatment procedures are similar to those concerning the effects of independent variables because both are experimental. However, questions about treatment effects are a part of clinical research. Therefore, in answering such questions, some investigators avoid certain designs that are appropriate to investigate the effects of independent variables within basic research.

Effects of treatment procedures can be assessed with either the group strategy or the single-subject strategy. To go beyond a seeming association between treatment and improvement, the investigator must use an experimental design. The pretest–posttest control group design or the posttest-only control group design can help evaluate the effects of single treatment variables. Among the within-subjects designs, the two-group single-treatment counterbalanced design can be used. One of the quasi-experimental designs, such as the nonequivalent two-group time-series design, also can be used, but with some loss of rigor because of the lack of randomization.

Among the single-subject designs, the *ABAB* reversal or withdrawal design; the multiple baseline design across subjects, settings, or behaviors design; and the changing criterion design are all available for selection. If the investigator does not wish to neutralize the treatment effects, the multiple baseline and changing criterion designs are preferable. Of the two, the multiple baseline design is probably more powerful and versatile. If there is no clinical concern about using reversal or withdrawal as a part of treatment evaluation, the *ABAB* design with either reversal or withdrawal can produce the most convincing evidence.

Is One Treatment More Effective than the Other?

The relative effects of two (or more) treatments become an issue when it is known that, compared with no treatment, all of them are effective to some degree. Is reinforcing fluency more or less effective than counseling people who stutter for their emotional problems? In teaching language response classes, is modeling without client imitation more or less effective than modeling that requires client imitation? Is informative feedback on performance accuracy in articulation therapy more or less effective than reinforcement in the absence of feedback? Questions such as these attempt to find out if one treatment is better than the other.

Evaluation of the relative effects of treatment requires the experimental method. However, because most designs that can be used to answer the question of relative effects of two or more treatments do not necessarily rule out extraneous variables, investigators usually focus on the relative—not the absolute—effects. Within the group design strategy, the multigroup pretest– posttest design may be used. The number of groups is the same as the number of treatments that are evaluated. An extra group that does not receive treatment is needed if the absolute treatment effect also is of concern. Factorial designs such as the randomized blocks design and the completely randomized factorial design also are excellent means of evaluating the effects of multiple treatments.

The single-group time-series design with multiple treatments can also be used to determine if one treatment is more effective than the other. The within-subjects crossover design can answer the same kind of questions.

The *ABACA/ACABA* single-subject design may be used to evaluate the relative effects of two or more treatments. Also appropriate is the alternating treatments design, which may be the most frequently used single-subject strategy in assessing multiple treatment effects.

Is There an Interaction Between Treatment Components?

Many treatment procedures contain different elements. Questions regarding their independent and interactive effects often are raised. Does muscular relaxation and reinforcement for correct pitch interact in the treatment of a voice disorder? Does reinforcement for correct production and punishment for incorrect production of phonemes in articulation therapy produce a cumulative effect? Is it more effective to combine stimulus pictures and objects in language therapy? Questions such as these are about interaction. Analysis of interaction requires use of the experimental method. Selected elements of a treatment program are typically applied in isolation and in certain combinations to assess the independent and interactive effects of those elements.

Within the group design strategy, the factorial design can be used to answer questions about the interaction of treatment elements. Of the several factorial designs, the completely randomized factorial design is best suited for an analysis of interaction. In this design, the effects of more than one treatment or more than one treatment element can be studied.

In the single-subject strategy, the interactional design can help answer the same question. It is generally thought, however, that the factorial (group) interactional designs are better than the single-subject interactional design. In a factorial design, multiple treatments are not confounded because different treatments are applied to different groups of participants. But the possibility of confounding effects exists in the single-subject interactional design because it evaluates the effects of multiple treatments in the same clients.

Do Participant Variables Interact with Treatment Variables?

Interaction can exist not only between treatment variables but also between treatment and participant characteristics. The same treatment may have different effects in male and female participants, high school and college graduates, and urban and rural clients. A treatment may be more or less effective depending on the severity of the disorder treated. Such assigned variables (see Chapter 3) interact with treatment. Therefore, to establish the generality of findings, one must know who reacts in what way to the same treatment procedure. This type of research is experimental because the treatment is always an active variable.

The randomized blocks design of the group (factorial) design strategy is considered best for analyzing the interaction between the participant variables and treatment. By juxtaposing participant characteristics and treatment variables, the design can assess the interaction between these two sets of variables. Within the single-subject approach, a particular design that can help answer this kind of question is lacking; the question must be addressed through replications. In a series of single-subject designs, the investigator studies participants of different characteristics and notes possible differences in the effects of treatment. Eventually through this approach, data on interactions between participant variables and treatment may be accumulated. Many investigators consider this approach less precise than that of the factorial design.

Is One Treatment Preferred Over the Other?

Two or more treatments may be equally effective in treating a disorder, but clients may prefer one over the other. As long as the preferred method is effective, it may be better to select it over the less preferred method. In the treatment of stuttering, for example, a verbal "no" provided contingent on stuttering and the reinforcement of fluency skills may be equally effective. In this case, the participants may prefer the reinforcement procedure. A knowledge of client preference as well as objective effects of treatment can be useful in clinical practice. This kind of research requires experimental methods.

The group design strategy does not offer a direct approach to study client preference of treatment. Client preferences can be assessed indirectly by differential dropout rates when different treatments are offered and by post hoc analysis in which the participants are questioned about their preferences. However, these procedures do not permit an experimental analysis of client preferences. Within the single-subject strategy, the simultaneous treatments design offers a direct method for analyzing participant preferences. When different treatments are offered simultaneously to the same client, the client may seek one treatment more frequently than the other. This then suggests client preference. However, a preferred treatment may or may not be the most effective technique, as noted in Chapter 9.

What Components of a Treatment Package Are Most Effective?

When several treatment components are included in a package, one may wish to know which ones are more effective. This question concerns an experimental analysis of existing packages whose development has not been based on systematic research. In this case, the package is broken down into its components to find out which ones are more or less effective. Two or more components may then be evaluated in a particular study. This question is of interest regardless of potential interaction, although it is better analyzed in an interactional design. As already noted, many treatments of communicative disorders are packages of different treatment components. What is needed is a strategy to discard elements that are ineffective, improve those that are somewhat effective, and identify those that are most effective.

The factorial design of the group strategy is useful in determining the relative efficacy of treatment components. The completely randomized factorial design is especially useful. Different components are applied to different participants in a factorial arrangement. In the same process, one can also analyze the interaction between the applied components. Of the single-subject designs, the interactional design can be used for the same purposes. The design can help determine the relative and interactive effects of treatment components. Other factors being equal, the group factorial designs are a better alternative to single-subject interactional design.

Can an Effective Treatment Package Be Developed?

This question concerns the *development* of a treatment package when no effective one exists. It is generally true that multiple treatment variables are more effective than single variables. However, when treatment variables are combined without a separate analysis of their independent effects, the resulting package may contain useless elements. The total package may continue to be used because of the overall effectiveness. A better approach is to test each component in separate studies and then combine only those that have produced effects in isolation.

A treatment package cannot be developed in a single study. There is no single design to accomplish this task. The research aimed at developing treatment packages is done in two stages. In the first, the clinician performs several independent studies to isolate the effects of specific components. The components that produce effects are retained and those that do not are discarded. If it is found that a few components produce the maximum effects, those that produce less impressive effects may also be discarded. In the second stage of research, the few components that are most effective are combined into a treatment package. The independent and the interactive effects of the components of the package are then determined.

Any of the group or single-subject designs that help evaluate the effects of a treatment variable may be used in the first stage. Factorial group designs or single-subject interactional designs can be used in the second stage of research. However, for various practical reasons, single-subject designs have proved to be more useful than group designs in developing treatment packages.

What Is the Optimal Level of Treatment?

This question concerns the mechanics of arranging treatment sessions or the intensity of treatment. The question can be asked even about the most effective treatments. For example, assuming that a given treatment is effective, one can ask whether a 50-minute treatment session is more effective than a 30-minute session. Is therapy two times a week just as effective as therapy four times a week? The answers to such questions help arrange effective and economical schedules of treatment.

Questions about the optimal level of treatment are better answered within the single-subject strategy. Single-subject designs that permit parametric variations of treatment are best suited for answering questions of this kind. The same participants may be exposed to the same treatment but with variations in the durations of sessions or the weekly frequency. Such variations are counterbalanced across participants. A second choice would be the single-group time-series design with multiple temporary treatments. The multiple temporary treatments would consist of variations designed to determine the optimal level of treatment.

Can We Predict the Group Behavior?

Although I have emphasized the importance of studying individual participants in a clinical science, it is sometimes necessary to ignore the behaviors of individual participants and ask questions about behaviors of groups. For example, a classroom teacher may wish to keep a group of children relatively quiet although every child may not necessarily be quiet all the time. Small variations in individual behaviors are ignored as long as the collective behavior of the group is acceptable. The speech and language clinician treating a group of children may face a similar situation.

Analysis and prediction of group behaviors is better accomplished by the group design strategy. Most group prediction studies are not experimental, however. A pollster who predicts the winner of an election is simply measuring and predicting group behavior without trying to change that behavior. On the other hand, some questions of group behaviors involve experimentation. Scientific or professional organizations may wish not only to find out about some particular behaviors of a group of people, but also to change some of those behaviors. A speech and hearing organization, for example, may attempt to first find out how much people know about its services and then design an experimental publicity campaign to increase the amount of information people have. Of the group designs, the time-series designs with repeated measures before and after the experimental manipulations are especially helpful. Single-subject designs are not efficient in predicting group behaviors.

How Effective Is the Treatment Across Individuals?

Clients or their families often wish to know the overall success rate of treatments they seek. They ask such questions as these: How many people who stutter generally improve under treatment? What is the success rate of articulation therapy? Can patients with aphasia be helped? What percentage of the children who receive language therapy improve? How many children with early language intervention can attend regular educational programs? Such questions attempt to predict treatment effects across large numbers of participants. Differential predictions may be attempted on the basis of diagnostic categories, age levels, and such other variables. These questions are important because clinical services are supported by those who ask them.

The overall effectiveness of treatment procedures is better evaluated with group designs. Group designs with a relatively large number of treated and untreated individuals can answer these questions more effectively than single-subject designs. However, with accumulated evidence, single-subject designs can eventually answer such questions as well. A review of replicated single-subject studies can help determine the percentages of clients who improve with treatment. Nevertheless, a well-conducted group design study with a large sample can provide that information more expeditiously.

The types of questions described so far are by no means exhaustive, but they do illustrate the relation between research questions and designs. Each question is answered by different kind of data, and each design generates its own kind of data. After asking a question, the investigator must determine what kind of data will answer it and what kind of design will generate those data.

ADVANTAGES AND DISADVANTAGES OF DESIGN STRATEGIES

Throughout the book, the various advantages and disadvantages of the group and single-subject design strategies have been discussed in several contexts. Therefore, what follows is a summative evaluation of both the group and single-subject design strategies. I shall list the major advantages and disadvantages of each of these approaches.

Advantages of Group Designs

Group designs have the following advantages over single-subject designs:

1. Group designs are generally effective in assessing the distribution of dependent variables in a population.

2. Group designs offer a means of evaluating the differential distribution of variables in defined populations (normal vs. clinical groups).

3. Group designs are effective in the analysis of the relative effects of multiple treatments.

4. The group strategy offers useful methods for assessing the interaction between two or more treatment variables.

5. Group designs are the most effective in assessing the interaction between treatment and client characteristics.

6. The group strategy is especially useful in determining and predicting group behaviors.

7. The group strategy is effective in predicting treatment effects based on diagnostic categories.

8. Because group designs have well-defined structures, the investigator need not make too many decisions while implementing a study.

Some of the advantages just listed may be hard to realize in practice. However, the advantages relative to group behaviors and predictions often are realized. The designs are best suited for investigating nonclinical and nontreatment-related issues in which the behavior of individual participants is not of particular interest.

Disadvantages of Group Designs

Because of their reliance on group performance differences, the group design strategy has the following disadvantages:

1. The group strategy is generally not practical in clinical sciences that emphasize the experimental method in treatment evaluation.

2. The group strategy is weak in evaluating treatment effects on individual participants. Because it lacks logical generality, the clinician cannot extend the conclusions of a group study to individual clients.

3. Group designs are somewhat weak in empirical manipulations because of the excessive reliance on statistically significant changes in dependent variables. Instead of producing larger effects of the independent variables, the group approach seeks more powerful statistical techniques that show that smaller effects are significant.

4. The group strategy is generally inadequate in measuring dependent variables. The pretests and posttests are a poor substitute for reliable and continuous measurement of dependent variables.

5. The group strategy is weak in the analysis of individual behaviors and their controlling variables.

6. The group strategy is not productive in the development of treatment packages.

7. The group strategy is not suited for evaluating the optimal level of treatment.

8. The group strategy is not effective in assessing the individual preference of treatment procedures.

9. Group designs are not flexible. They must usually be carried to their conclusion even when things go wrong during a study.

10. The group design strategy is not conducive to replication. Because of the practical problems, group design studies are not replicated as often as single-subject studies.

Advantages of Single-Subject Designs

Single-subject designs have the following advantages over group designs:

1. Single-subject designs are better than group designs in the analysis of individual behaviors and their controlling variables.

2. Single-subject designs are more effective than group designs in the experimental assessment of the effects of single treatment variables on the behaviors of individual participants.

3. Single-subject designs can produce data that are especially applicable to individual clients. The designs are high on logical generality.

4. Single-subject designs are generally more practical than group designs. They have the potential of being replicated more easily than the group designs.

5. Single-subject designs are effective in building treatment packages.

6. Single-subject designs can help determine client preferences of treatment procedures when multiple treatments are equally effective.

7. Single-subject designs are effective in determining the optimal level of treatment.

8. Independent variables in single-subject designs typically produce larger effects on the dependent variables than group designs.

9. Single-subject designs offer more reliable and extensive measurement of the dependent variables than group designs offer because in single-subject designs the measurement is continuous.

10. Single-subject designs are more flexible and allow modifications during the course of investigations.

Disadvantages of Single-Subject Designs

Compared with group designs, single-subject designs have the following disadvantages:

1. The single-subject strategy is less effective than the group strategy in predicting group behaviors.

2. The single-subject strategy cannot make statistical statements regarding the overall effectiveness of treatment programs across large numbers of clients.

3. Single-subject designs are not efficient in evaluating the interaction between treatment variables and client characteristics.

4. Single-subject designs are not efficient in assessing the effects of multiple treatments without interference among treatments.

5. The single-subject approach is weak in its assessment of interaction between different treatment variables.

6. Single-subject designs require on-the-spot decisions at various stages of a study.

The advantages and disadvantages of all designs should be placed in a philosophical perspective, which will be done later in this chapter. Also, the advantages should be weighed against the disadvantages in the context of a particular study and its purpose.

PROBLEMS COMMON TO DESIGN STRATEGIES

Some problems are common to both the group and the single-subject strategies. It is necessary to note the common problems because they may sometimes be blamed on one or the other design strategy. Many problems are simply a part of the research process.

Intersubject and Intrasubject Variability

All research designs must handle variability in the phenomenon they observe. Generally, variability is not a creation of research strategies but a creation of nature itself. A participant's behavior varies because the factors that affect that behavior vary. Different individuals vary because they are exposed to different factors or independent variables.

However, design strategies handle this variability in different ways. In the group design strategy, this variability is typically handled statistically; in single-subject strategy, it is typically handled experimentally.

Unexpected Change in the Control Mechanisms

Though the control condition, participants, or behaviors should not change in either strategy, they sometimes do. Participants in a control group may improve without treatment. In a single-subject design, the behavior under a control condition may change; for example, a behavior in a multiple baseline may change before the treatment is applied to it.

Problems of change in the control mechanism suggest that either the conditions were not well controlled or the behaviors were correlated (i.e., the behaviors were not independent response classes). Other independent variables may have been active, or the treated and as-yet-untreated behaviors may be responses of a single class.

Generality

Generality is a common problem of research, but the proponents of group designs usually make it appear to be predominantly a problem of single-subject designs. Because group designs are supposed to draw random samples that represent the population, it is usually believed that they have generality. However, in using group experimental designs, investigators rarely can draw random samples from clinical populations. If a random sample is drawn, inferential generality to the population may be achieved, but there is still no assurance of other kinds of generality. For example, clinician generality and setting generality would not be established by a group design study even if it had an adequate random sample.

Generality is not a problem of designs; rather, all designs have to face this problem. It is a problem that requires replication. To achieve generality, both group design studies and single-subject design studies must be replicated. No strategy offers it automatically. In fact, the group strategy lacks logical generality by design and inferential generality by default. The single-subject strategy lacks inferential generality by design, but it does provide logical generality. Both strategies can demonstrate other kinds of generality only through replications.

Slow Accumulation of Scientific Evidence

Scientific data, especially experimental data, accumulate at a slow rate. The rate is slower still in clinical sciences in which the variables are many and hard to control and in which ethical restrictions are justifiably stringent. It often is thought that group designs advance the rate of data accumulation whereas single-subject designs retard it. This is not true because replication is what takes time. Whether an effect is initially demonstrated in 10 participants or 100 participants is not as critical as is generally thought because in either case, replication is required.

In behavioral research, single-subject designs have generated more experimental clinical data than have group designs. Because of their relevance to clinical work, which involves single participants or small groups of participants, single-subject designs have been used in many more treatment evaluation studies than group designs.

Though scientific data generally tend to accumulate slowly, it is possible to accelerate the pace. Among other factors, practical methods of research, better training of clinicians in research, and better support for research can make a difference.

Problems of Implementation

Many problems of research are not problems of design strategies but simply problems of implementation. Research is a complex task, the implementation of which can go wrong at any time. Participants may be hard to find and, once found, hard to retain until the end of the study. Needed instruments may be expensive, and once they are acquired, they do not seem to give notice before they break down. These and many other problems of implementing research studies are common features of research.

PHILOSOPHICAL CONSIDERATIONS IN EVALUATION

In the comparative evaluation of design strategies, one cannot ignore the philosophical considerations that created some of the differences between the group and the single-subject approaches. Many of the procedural differences grew out of different conceptual bases.

As noted elsewhere, the group design strategy is heavily influenced by the logic and procedures of statistics. Statistical reasoning treats individual variability as controllable mostly through methods of statistical analysis, not through methods of experimentation. The behavior of the individual is of interest only as it contributes to the statistically stable measure, such as the mean. Theoretically, the group design approach tries to build a science of behavior by observing many subjects in single studies.

The single-subject strategy, on the other hand, was influenced heavily by the tradition of experimentation, not by the statistical analysis of data. It treats individual differences and variability as experimentally controllable phenomena. The behavior of the individual is of primary concern. The approach considers the statistically stable mean a creation of methods of analysis; therefore, the mean is not considered an empirical value. Theoretically and practically, the single-subject approach starts with one or a few individuals, studies them, draws conclusions, and extends those conclusions only to similar individuals—if at all. This approach also tries to build a science of behavior by intensively observing many individuals across studies but few individuals in given studies.

THE INVESTIGATOR IN THE DESIGN SELECTION PROCESS

A theme of this book is that science is both a public and a personal matter. Many scientific decisions are made for objective reasons, and many others are made for personal reasons. Still others are made for practical reasons. There is nothing good or bad about these reasons; that is simply the way it is. Also, there is no other way because scientists are people, and science is what these people do.

All responsible scientists first consider what they think are the objective bases of selecting a design. The investigators first determine the nature of the question asked and what kind of data will answer it. Then a design that will produce relevant data in as clear and as practical a manner possible is selected. Once the method has been selected, scientists try to use it as precisely and thoroughly as they can.

Objective reasons are not entirely free from personal reasons, however. Personal reasons are nothing but the past training and experience of the investigator. As such, they are not necessarily subjective in the prejudicial sense of the word. An excellent design choice is as subjective as a poor choice; both are partly determined by the scientist's training and experience. Generally speaking, those who are trained in a particular tradition of research try to make the best possible decision within that tradition. Sometimes, scientists reject the tradition of research in which they were trained; in such cases, the scientists are said to "adopt a different tradition." This happens because their experience has taught them a different lesson. When scientific behavior itself becomes the subject matter of scientific analysis, these reasons will be objective in the same sense that any other behavioral phenomenon is objective.

Finally, the selection of a design is partly a matter of practical exigencies. The investigator may know very well that an elegant factorial design with multiple cells is the best design to analyze the interaction between treatment variables, but not having enough clients, he or she may settle for the less efficient single-subject interactional design. Another investigator may select a single-group treatment design because of a preference for avoiding a control group that must be denied treatment or given deferred treatment. Practical exigencies seem to play a greater role in clinical treatment research than in basic laboratory research. Availability of clients, the need to offer treatment as promptly as possible, and other ethical considerations create a host of exigencies for the clinical investigator.

FINAL CRITERION: SOUNDNESS OF DATA

In the evaluation and selection of a design, it is better to keep in perspective that, after all, a design is only a means of producing data. A method is as good as the data it generates. As pointed out by Sidman (1960), though the type and the quality of data depend upon the method used, sound data can stand by themselves. Bad methods may not produce sound data, but sound data must be accepted regardless of methodological biases one may hold.

The soundness of data must be judged in a broad context, and no objective rules are available to make this judgment. Even the original investigator's judgment regarding the importance of his or her data cannot always be trusted (Sidman, 1960). Data rejected by the investigator may be important or may prove to be important in light of evidence that comes later. Data hailed as important may be worthless or may prove to be irrelevant later. Methodological or theoretical faddishness may make poor data look good as long as that faddishness lasts. Relevant data that contradict faddish trends of the times may be considered irrelevant.

The value of given data can and must be judged regardless of the hypothesis they are supposed to support or repudiate. A set of data may not serve the purposes of an investigator, but it may still be sound. The data generated by a particular study may fail to confirm a pet hypothesis or may force the acceptance of an unfavored one. Data not sought in a study may emerge accidentally, and those sought may not emerge. None of these contingencies are important in evaluating the soundness of data.

Another consideration in the evaluation of data is the methodological soundness of studies, which can be determined regardless of theoretical or personal biases (Sidman, 1960). Data that are generated by acceptable methods of observation and experimentation must be welcomed even if the data contradict the investigator's preconceptions. Strong and unambiguous effects of independent variables demonstrated under controlled conditions must be accepted regardless of theoretical or personal points of view. Data that resolve contradictions, shed light on poorly understood phenomena, clarify relations between events, and show patterns in seemingly chaotic happenings are always important. Similarly, data that show effective treatment of disorders, methods of solving practical problems, and effective ways of studying a difficult phenomenon are valuable. As Sidman (1960) has pointed out, it is the cumulative development of a science that eventually determines the importance and soundness of data.

SUMMARY

In evaluating designs and design strategies, the clinician should consider the type of research question, applicability to clinical science, and soundness of data. Table 11.1 summarizes the major research questions and design options.

Several designs may answer the same research questions. In such cases, selection may be based on applicability and the investigator's expertise. Some designs may be more applicable than others. In clinical treatment evaluation, a strict adherence to the requirement of sampling equivalence is not practical. Therefore, the applicability of group designs in treatment

TABLE 11.1

Comparative Summary of Design Options

| Research Question | Design Options | | Comments |
	Group	Single-Subject	
What are the dependent variables?	Case study	Case study	Descriptive studies
How are the variables distributed in a population?	Uses the group method; no particular design; descriptive studies	None available; unattractive because it is nonexperimental	Descriptive and normative studies
How are the variables differentially distributed in a population?	Uses the group method; no particular design; descriptive studies	None available; unattractive because it is nonexperimental	Normal versus clinical group comparisons use this approach
What factors may have caused this effect?	Case study	Case study	Not experimental; no controls
What are the effects of an independent variable?	Pretest–posttest control group design; posttest-only control group design; within-subjects and time-series designs	*ABA* reversal or withdrawal design; *BAB* design; *ABAB* multiple baseline, and changing criterion design	Controlled design is needed; both the strategies offer designs; consider the strategic and design-specific limitations
Is a treatment associated with improvement?	One-group pretest–posttest design	*AB* design	Uncontrolled treatment evaluations
Is a treatment effective?	Pretest–posttest control group design; posttest-only group design; within-subjects and time-series designs	*ABA* reversal or withdrawal design; *BAB* design; *ABAB* multiple baseline, and changing criterion design	Controlled design is needed; both the strategies offer designs; consider the strategic and design-specific limitations
Is one treatment more effective than the other?	Multigroup pretest–posttest design; factorial designs; crossover designs; time-series designs	*ABACA/ACABA* design; alternating treatments design	Only relative effects are frequently assessed; control groups may be added; group designs are somewhat better
Is there an interaction between treatment components?	Completely randomized factorial design	Interactional design	Group strategy is better; multiple treatments interference in the single-subject design

(continues)

TABLE 11.1 *Continued.*

Research Question	Design Options		Comments
	Group	**Single-Subject**	
Do some clients benefit more than other clients from the same treatment?	Randomized blocks design	An efficent design is not available	Group strategy can isolate an interaction between assigned variables and treatment
Do clients prefer one treatment over the other?	An efficient design is not available	Simultaneous treatments design	Preference, not necessarily effectiveness, is analyzed
What are the most effective components of a treatment package?	Completely randomized factorial design	Interactional design	Relative as well as interactive effects are analyzed
Can an effective treatment package be developed?	Any controlled design to begin with, and then a factorial design	Any controlled design to begin with, and then the interactional design	Requires a two-stage evaluation of independent components and their interactions
What is the optimal level of treatment?	An efficient design is not available except for the single-group time-series design with multiple temporary treatments	Most single-subject designs; parametric variations of treatment may be introduced in successive stages of treatment	Single-subject approach is preferable because of its flexibility
How do certain groups behave?	Time-series designs with repeated measures before and after treatment	An efficient design is not available; handled through replications	Group strategy is efficient in describing and predicting group behaviors
How efficient is the treatment across clients?	Any well-controlled group design	An efficient design is not available; handled through replications	Group designs, though better in this respect, are not efficient in evaluating treatments in the first place

evaluation research is limited. When they are used in clinical research, group designs almost always involve major compromises in achieving sampling equivalence.

Group designs are more effective than single-subject designs in determining the distribution of dependent variables in samples of participants, group trends and characteristics, the differences between clinical and nonclinical groups, interaction between treatment variables, and interaction between treatment and participant variables. Group designs also are effective in predicting treatment effects based on diagnostic categories. Finally, the designs are well structured, so that the need to make on-the-spot decisions is minimal.

The disadvantages of group designs include limited applications in clinical treatment evaluation, lack of logical generality, weak empirical manipulations, inadequate measurement of dependent variables, insensitivity to individual uniqueness, and rigidity of experimental conditions. Also, group designs are not able to evaluate optimum levels of treatment or client preferences for treatment procedures when multiple procedures are equally effective. Finally, group designs are not conducive to direct or systematic replications.

The advantages of single-subject designs include their sensitivity to individual behaviors and uniqueness, appropriateness to treatment evaluations, high logical generality, practicality, replicability, reliable measurement of dependent variables, large magnitude of treatment effects, and flexibility. Also, the designs are advantageous in building treatment packages, determining client preferences for treatment procedures, and in establishing optimal levels of treatment.

The disadvantages of single-subject designs include their limited usefulness in predicting group behaviors and performance under given treatments. They are less effective than group designs in evaluating the interaction between multiple treatments or between treatment and client characteristics. Also, they require on-the-spot decisions.

Problems such as intersubject and intrasubject variability, unexpected changes in the control mechanisms, problems in achieving generality, slow accumulation of scientific data, and practical problems of implementation are common to both design strategies.

The final criterion in the selection of design strategies is the soundness of data. Procedures that produce sound data are always acceptable.

STUDY GUIDE

In answering questions 1 through 11, make sure you (a) identify the type of research, (b) specify the type of design (group or single-subject), (c) describe the basic elements of the procedure, and (d) justify the selection of the design. You must make up such needed information as the age of the participants, the kind and the severity of a disorder, and sample size.

1. Design a study in which you would investigate the potential independent variables of conductive hearing loss in a group of school-age children.

2. Suppose you wish to find out the stages in which children acquire the passive sentence forms. Design a study that would have a local but adequate sample. Use hypothetical information regarding the size of the population.

3. Compared with normally hearing persons, how frequently do adults with hearing impairment initiate conversation in a group? Design a study to answer this question.

4. Design two studies in which the effects of an independent variable are evaluated under controlled conditions. In the first study, the temporary effect of a variable on some aspect of speech, language, or hearing will be evaluated. For example, the effects of white noise or delayed auditory feedback on speech may be temporary. In the other study, the relatively permanent effect on some aspect of speech–language behavior will be evaluated. The effects of treatment or teaching procedures are of this kind.

5. You wish to find out if one teaching or treatment method is more effective than another. From your study of your specialty, select two potential treatment procedures and design a study to evaluate their relative effects to determine if one of them is more effective than the other.

6. Find a treatment procedure that contains at least two dissimilar elements. Then design a study in which you would determine the interactive effects of the two selected components. Design both a single-subject study and a group design study.

7. You suspect that the social class of your clients influences the outcome of language treatment. Design a study to investigate this possibility.

8. Find two equally effective treatment procedures for a given disorder. Then design a study in which you would determine if selected clients prefer one procedure over the other.

9. Suppose you wish to find out if one of the components of a treatment package is more effective than the other. Find a treatment package used in your field and select two of its components. Design a study to find out the relative effects of the two.

10. Design a study in which you would evaluate the optimum level of a selected treatment procedure. Let your independent variable be either the duration of treatment sessions or their weekly frequency.

11. Suppose you have repeatedly faced parents of children with language disabilities who ask you whether language therapy for these children will increase their chances of completing high school. Assuming an answer is not available, how would you design a study to find out?

12. Summarize the advantages and disadvantages of the group design strategy.

13. Summarize the advantages and disadvantages of the single-subject strategy.

14. What kinds of problems are common among all design strategies?

15. Specify why the soundness of data is an important criterion in the evaluation of design strategies.

Chapter 12

◆◆◆◆◆◆◆◆◆◆◆◆◆◆◆◆◆◆◆◆◆◆◆◆◆◆◆◆◆◆◆◆◆◆

Designs Versus Paradigms in Research

Most books and graduate courses on research concentrate on research methods. Methods, however, are only a part of research. Two other parts of research are equally important: knowledge of the subject matter and knowledge of its philosophy. It is necessary to understand what to investigate and why it is important to investigate it, as well as how to investigate it. It is not clear why, in discussions of research, the knowledge and philosophy of subject matters do not receive much attention. Many writers pay exclusive attention to the methods of research and ignore the questions of the conceptual and philosophical bases of research.

LIMITATIONS OF EXCLUSIVELY METHODOLOGICAL APPROACHES

It is important to know how research is done. The methods and procedures by which research questions are investigated constitute a large body of technical information. **Methodology** is defined as the study of how to do research and includes a discussion of the following: how to observe, measure, and record a phenomenon; how to fit research questions to research methods; how to set up conditions in such a way that a cause–effect relation is revealed; how to manipulate independent variables; and how to make sure that unwanted variables do not influence the results. Methodology tells a researcher *how* to investigate.

However, methodology does not tell a researcher *what* to investigate. A thorough study of the methods of research may still leave the investigator with nothing to investigate. Knowledge of the group and single-subject designs or of the various statistical techniques will not necessarily suggest research questions. The knowledge of research designs is useless without a worthwhile question that needs to be answered.

An important point about research methods is that they are secondary to the subject matter and its philosophy. In many ways, the nature of a subject matter and its philosophy shape methodologies. Meaningful studies can be designed only when an investigator has a critical understanding of the subject matter, its philosophy, and the concepts and methods of science and research.

RESEARCH METHODS AND SUBJECT MATTERS

It was pointed out in Chapter 3 that the basic methods of science are independent of any subject matter. Investigators can borrow methods from science as long as those methods are applicable to a given subject matter. A subject matter that successfully applies the methods of science will be regarded as a branch of science. However, the methods of science are not a closed set. The set is open, dynamic, and shaped by the nature of different disciplines that have used the basic scientific approach in studying common and unique problems. New methods are added to the set by different disciplines. Such additions of methods that do not violate the basic logic of science enrich scientific methodology.

The independence of most methods of science and subject matters does not suggest that an understanding of the methods alone will lead to significant research in given subject matters. A thorough knowledge of the subject matter is necessary before the application of research methods in answering important research questions. Theoretically, students can learn how to do research independently of their subject matters. They can later combine this information on research methods with their independently acquired knowledge of the subject matter. In practice, however, this may not be the best strategy for learning how to do research.

The way many graduate students are asked to study research methods suggests that it may not be important to understand *what* to investigate and *how* to investigate in the same context. Graduate courses on research methods, often taken in departments outside students' major discipline, offer methods independent not only of the subject matter of research but also of all philosophical concerns. Because of the highly prevalent notion that statistics and research designs are the same thing, more and more students in a variety of social, behavioral, and health-related disciplines are asked to take courses on statistics that count as courses on research designs. Students from different disciplines take these courses with the implied assumption that information on research can be acquired with no philosophical concerns relative to their subject matter. Many students, however, cannot integrate the subject matter with research methods that are offered in a content-neutral manner. They do not appreciate the philosophical issues relative to their subject matter. A knowledge of analysis of variance or a knowledge of specific group or single-subject designs does not necessarily make a student a competent researcher.

An exclusive concern with methodology leaves the student with no philosophical sophistication needed to do research. Therefore, in this chapter, I will address some of the philosophical issues that play a major role in the research process.

At the very outset, I wish to make a few points clear. An examination of philosophical issues inevitably raises questions about personal biases and views. Also, such an examination raises the question of what kinds of research (unrelated to methodology) are more or less valuable. The discussion can raise unsettling questions about a person's philosophy, which is an inclination to investigate certain kinds of questions with certain methods. Perhaps partly because of this reason, authors typically shy away from more personally colored philosophical issues and stay close to more objective methodology.

Methodological questions have relatively straightforward answers. Although different tactics can be used to investigate a certain problem, some are clearly more appropriate than others, and some are undoubtedly wrong.

However, philosophical issues are not as easily resolved. Therefore, the philosophical questions to be discussed in this chapter do not have right or wrong answers. The sole purpose of this chapter is to draw attention to a neglected aspect of research. I take certain philosophical positions, as everyone else does, and surely (and I believe appropriately) my positions will be clear in the following discussion as one of the different views.

Another point that must be made at the very beginning is that both methodology and philosophy are important. There is no suggestion here that philosophical considerations should supersede methodological considerations. The main emphasis here is on giving philosophical issues the attention they deserve. In the best tradition of research, both methodology and philosophy play a significant role. They influence each other and help each other evolve. At a more advanced stage, there is a productive interplay between the philosophy and methodology of a subject matter. I shall return to this point later.

PHILOSOPHY AS METHODOLOGY

It is appropriate to contrast philosophy with methodology, but probably a more significant factor about philosophy is that it can have very direct consequences for methodology. In many respects, the philosophy of a subject matter is also its methodology. This section explores this idea; the text then returns to the question of interplay between philosophy and methodology.

Very few, if any, disciplines have a single philosophy. Different philosophical approaches coexist in many disciplines. Therefore, disciplines are likely to have different paradigms. **Paradigms** are conceptual frameworks that include certain basic assumptions about a discipline. Such assumptions dictate the nature of questions asked and the methods used to answer them. Philosophical or paradigmatic variations within a discipline create several methodological issues. This discussion is concerned with (a) the philosophy of subject matters, (b) the philosophy of the science of speech and language, (c) the philosophical ways of handling methodological problems, and (d) the interplay between philosophy and methodology.

PHILOSOPHY OF SUBJECT MATTERS

The philosophy of a subject matter is different from the accumulated knowledge and methods of that subject matter. However, an overall **philosophy of a subject matter** is a broader view of what that subject matter has been and what it ought to be; the philosophy of a subject matter is a conceptual evaluation of the methods, questions, theories, social applications, and overall implications of that subject matter. Such a philosophy does not necessarily evaluate the empirical findings of a discipline; that is the stuff the subject matter is made of. It does not directly evaluate particular designs, methods, or modes of data analysis. Instead, the philosophy concerns itself with the way the subject matter and its methods have been conceptualized, the approaches taken to the issues of methodology, the strengths and the limitations of those concepts and methods, and the overall significance of the knowledge generated within the discipline.

When a discipline is also an applied profession, additional philosophical considerations emerge. Among the questions a clinical profession attempts to answer are these: Can the discipline solve its problems? Does it address the concerns philosophically as well as methodologically? Does the profession have a philosophy that moves it forward? Are the methods used consistent with the profession's applied objectives? Does it promote a discussion of ethical issues? In essence, the philosophy of an applied discipline asks and evaluates a generic question: Is the profession able to meet its scientific and social challenges in an efficient and responsible manner?

The philosophical concerns of the kind described here are not totally independent of the subject matter and its methodology. In fact, questions of philosophy can be answered only in the context of a particular discipline, its methods, and their outcome.

The philosophy of a subject matter is not a discussion of vague and irrelevant issues. Contrary to the popular notion, philosophy is concerned with conceptual as well as practical issues. There is nothing more practical than an evaluation of the degree to which a profession has achieved its scientific and applied objectives. Such an evaluation is a philosophical venture. A serious examination of the philosophy of a subject matter and its conceptual frameworks can suggest better ways of reconceptualizing the issues or even the entire subject matter. This may help meet the practical challenges of the profession.

When a discipline reaches a certain stage of sophistication and advanced knowledge, philosophical issues become clear and often pressing. For example, the question of life and death, certainly one of the most profound of the philosophical issues, became pressing when medical technology advanced to the stage where life (as defined in a technical and legal sense) could be sustained through artificial means. On the other hand, if individuals belonging to a discipline are sensitive to philosophical issues from the beginning, then it is possible that certain faulty concepts and methods can be avoided.

Different traditions of research within disciplines often are a product of divergent philosophical positions. Whether philosophical assumptions are made explicit or not, they have a profound influence on what sorts of phenomena are researched and how. Natural sciences are bound by some common assumptions about natural phenomena. As noted in Chapter 3, natural scientists believe that events are caused and that causal relations between events can be discovered (determinism). Scientists also believe that some form of sensory observation is necessary for a thorough study of a phenomenon (empiricism). Also, natural sciences have certain common philosophical assumptions about their methods. Most natural sciences have a commitment to experimental methodology. They have a strong tradition of experimental research. As a result, there is a large body of replicated knowledge. Natural scientists also believe that variability is mostly extrinsic and therefore subject to experimental control. This philosophical assumption may have done more than anything else to successfully control and alter the variables dealt with in natural sciences. It also shows how a philosophical assumption dictates a certain methodology.

In natural sciences, there is a long tradition of empirical research as opposed to logical speculation. This may be partly due to the philosophy of natural sciences, which drives the scientists out of their armchairs and into their laboratories. The philosophy of natural sciences insists that empirical investigation is the best method of producing knowledge: One must find out through experimentation. Speculation can serve a purpose only when it leads to experimental verification.

The philosophy of science makes a distinction between scholarship and scholasticism. **Scholarship** is the product of informed, authoritative, and evaluative awareness of the existing knowledge in a given subject matter. Scholarship is needed and valued in sciences, art, literature, and the professions. **Scholasticism,** on the other hand, is a *method* of generating knowledge that does not necessarily use observational and experimental methods; instead, it relies on authorities, traditions, ancient sources, and logic. Natural sciences have moved away from scholasticism, which is good at generating controversies but inefficient in producing empirically validated knowledge. Unfortunately, some of the lesser developed sciences have not been especially successful in rejecting scholasticism and moving on to the realm of empirically verified knowledge based on observation and experimentation.

PHILOSOPHY OF THE SCIENCE OF SPEECH AND LANGUAGE

A philosophy of the *science* of speech and language should have emerged before a philosophy of clinical intervention in speech and language disorders. However, the sequence of development within this field has been the other way around. The field started as a profession and then slowly began to move in the direction of scientific study. It is probably accurate to say that failures and inadequacies in the practice of the profession have prompted it to become more and more scientific. Therefore, it is not clear whether the profession has a dominant philosophy of the science of speech and language, and if so, what it is.

When a subject matter starts as a profession, it is very likely to borrow philosophies from relevant disciplines. Probably three major sources influenced speech–language pathology: medicine, education, and behavioral and social sciences. Most of the early clinical conceptual models were influenced by medicine. Medical concepts such as symptomatology, diagnosis and differential diagnosis, etiology, prognosis, and functional–organic distinction were all influential in speech–language pathology.

Much of the training and practice model of speech–language pathologists was influenced by schools of education. Largely because the public schools provided most of the jobs, the philosophy of education has had a large influence on the way the profession was conceptualized and the way clinicians were educated. Most speech–language pathologists were and still are asked to take several courses in the department of education with the idea that both the science and the profession of speech and language have something to gain from such courses. Possibly, this approach had some negative impact on the development of speech and language as a science.

Among the behavioral and social sciences, psychology and linguistics have had the greatest influence on speech–language pathology. The early influence was from psychology, which probably had a more favorable impact on audiology than it did on speech pathology. Experiments in sensory psychology, especially auditory sensations and perceptions, had a tremendous effect on the new science of audiology. Initially, the branch of psychology that tended to influence speech pathology was not experimental but clinical. The clinical psychology of the time was mostly Freudian in its orientation. Psychodynamics and psychodiagnosis were and have been the dominant themes of clinical psychology. These themes blended well with the medical philosophy of finding an internal cause and treating it; the only difference was that the cause in clinical psychology happened to be in the mind of the client (such as the bad self-image of a person who stutters).

Subsequently, applied behavior analysis, another kind of psychology, began to influence speech–language pathology. Techniques of behavior change began to be used in the modification of speech, language, fluency, and voice disorders. However, this influence, even today, is strictly methodological. The parent of applied behavior analysis or modification—radical behaviorism—has had very little impact on the way the behavioral principles are applied in speech–language pathology. In other words, there is some appreciation of methodology of behavior change but not of the philosophy of that change (behaviorism). Consequently, the application of behavioral technology within the field of speech and language pathology has been devoid of philosophical strengths. Behavioral methodology is often grafted onto the incongruent philosophies of cognitivism and nativism, whose major sources of influence have been linguistics and psycholinguistics.

Linguistics did not exert much influence until the entry of speech–language pathologists into the realm of language and its disorders. At the time when language clinicians began to be involved with language disorders, Chomsky's (1957) generative transformational grammar dominated linguistics. The same philosophical approach, with its purely structural orientation and a tendency toward nativism, was borrowed by speech–language pathologists. This philosophical approach encouraged speculative writing, which has been flourishing ever since. Ironically, speech–language pathologists did not lead the experimental research on the treatment of language disorders. Behavioral psychologists who did not share Chomsky's philosophy of nativism and rationalism led that research.

The observation that a philosophy either encourages or discourages certain kinds of research is clearly demonstrated in the case of language. Structurally oriented linguistics encourages normative and descriptive research. The presumed independent variables are often not susceptible to experimental manipulations. Innate structures, cognitive notions, knowledge of the universal grammar, and grammatical competence are not experimentally manipulable independent variables, though they figure importantly in linguistic theories of language. On the other hand, environmental contingencies that are supposed to control language within the behavioral philosophy encourage or even require experimental methodology. Experimental research on language and language treatment has typically been the product of behaviorism, whereas descriptive, normative, and predominantly theoretical writing has been the product of the linguistically oriented approach.

If the contemporary scene of speech–language sciences and disorders does not permit definitive statements about a philosophy, that is probably because it has not been philosophically aware as a discipline. There have been no systematic attempts at creating a unifying philosophy of speech–language research and clinical practice. The *science* in the profession has followed a certain subject-matters-are-science approach. Anatomy and physiology and acoustics are typically considered under *speech science*, whereas the study of articulation or fluency disorders is *clinical*. Offended by this approach, some who studied language simply renamed their subject matter *language science*, with very few consequences.

In treatment and applied research, eclecticism has prevailed. Within the best tradition of eclecticism, one is supposed to select what is valid from different approaches. Validity is determined on the basis of controlled, replicated evidence. In practice, however, eclecticism has meant borrowing from different sources with no regard for philosophical or paradigmatic differences. Such borrowings have been based on subjective opinions and feelings. The most distressing thing about this trend is that the prevailing approaches from which clinicians chose were also based on unsupported opinions.

When the basic study of a subject matter and its clinical activities are influenced by contradictory philosophies, that subject not only lacks a unifying philosophy but is also riddled with controversies. This has been a major problem in the study of language and, more recently, phonology. While the basic analyses of language and phonological aspects of language have been based mostly on structural properties, remedial approaches have necessarily looked elsewhere for help. Behavioral and other approaches that are not necessarily congruent with purely structural approaches have influenced remedial efforts and research. Consequently, conceptual inconsistencies and philosophical problems have resulted.

In its efforts to establish a philosophical base, a new discipline must consider several factors. Some of these factors will now be addressed.

Philosophical Aspects of Dependent Variables

It is generally true that researchers, knowing the effects and not knowing the cause, start an investigation. Therefore, much scientific discussion centers on independent variables (causes), not dependent variables (effects). Nonetheless, the neglected question of the dependent variables is important.

The question of the dependent variables is none other than the all-important question of what it is that one is trying to study. A scientific study starts with an observed effect, but the scientist may face two problems to begin with. The first problem, which is generally appreciated, is that the effect may not have been understood fully. For example, in the study of stuttering, the analogy of the six blind men trying to explore an elephant is often used to describe the problem of each investigator seeing only a part of a large effect. When the totality of an effect is not understood, descriptions, explanations, and theories of that effect will be inadequate. In the course of a causal search, more may be understood about the effect itself. Descriptions and explanations of the effect will be modified as more is learned about the nature of the effect.

The second problem is not as well appreciated as the first. A serious problem with the dependent variable can arise when its conceptualization is inadequate, is mistaken, or does not allow experimentation. It is known that a science makes progress when its dependent variables are firmly and clearly established. This means that when researchers are sure of what they are studying, they may be better able to explain it through experimental research. Obviously, experiments on vague effects may not isolate specific causes. Physical sciences have made great strides partly because of their definitive dependent variables.

The problem with the dependent variables used in speech–language sciences and pathology is basically conceptual and philosophical. Researchers in this field face methodological problems largely because of ignored conceptual and philosophical issues. Whether the dependent variables one studies are inadequate or mistaken depends upon particular points of view, but whether the variables are experimentally accessible can be better argued or illustrated.

Many controversies about language have resulted from the confusion regarding the dependent variables themselves. The grammatical, semantic, and pragmatic so-called "revolutions" in linguistics that have affected speech–language pathologists are mostly a debate about the dependent variables. The single most critical question for these controversies is this: What is language? As the answers have differed, so have the dependent variables. Is language the innate knowledge of the rules of universal grammar, as Chomsky claimed? Is language simply grammar, as is also claimed by the generative linguists? Is language semantic notions, as is claimed by generative semanticists? Is language pragmatic structures or notions or rules? Is language the use of those pragmatic rules? Is language cognitive structures? Is language an unobservable mental system, or is it the observable production of whatever it is supposed to be? Is language a type of behavior? Is it similar to other kinds of behaviors, or is it special? These are only a sampling of questions asked in the study of language, and as can be seen, they are not about the *causes* of language but the *effects* being studied. In essence, researchers have been wondering about the dependent variables themselves.

The way a dependent variable is conceptualized can make it more or less susceptible to an analysis of cause–effect relations. The philosophy of the dependent variable will determine to a large extent what kinds of methods will be used to study it and, in turn, what kinds of knowledge this study will generate.

When the effects are supposed to lie in a realm not accessible to observation, the causes also tend to be hypothesized to exist within that unobservable realm. If the dependent variable is a mental system, then its independent variable is typically thought to exist within the same mental domain. It need not necessarily be that way, but those who postulate internal effects also tend to explain them on the basis of internal causes; unfortunately, neither internal effects nor internal causes are observable, and science requires that both the effect and the cause be observable. However, on a temporary basis, scientists can tolerate the idea of causes that have been postulated but not yet demonstrated. There is then an expectation that such a demonstration is forthcoming. On the other hand, scientists may not have much patience with effects that are not observed and that perhaps cannot be observed. In such cases, scientists do not see anything to be explained. Mental rules, cognitive structures, innate systems, and such other internal dependent (or independent) variables fall into this category.

The same situation exists in phonology. The real dependent variables, it is argued, are not the production of particular phonemes, but the knowledge of the speech sound system. Phonological rules, which are extracted from behavioral regularities, are considered the essence of phonological behaviors. The dependent variables are once again unobservable.

The question of the dependent variable also has plagued the study of stuttering. The multitudinous definitions of stuttering reflect nothing but a controversy (or confusion) about the dependent variable. Stuttering is variously defined as role conflict, avoidance behavior, prosodic defect, phonatory problem, laryngeal aberration, incoordination between neuromotor systems, auditory perceptual defect, production of certain kinds of dysfluencies, or production of all kinds of dysfluencies at a certain frequency level, just to name a few. When investigators within a discipline do not agree on the nature of the effect, there can be little agreement on its causes.

In a clinical discipline, controversies concerning the dependent variables are carried into treatment. Such controversies make it difficult to conduct research on treatment effects. When certain treatment effects on controversial dependent variables are evaluated, the clinician does not know which dependent variables change under what treatment conditions. Such treatment evaluation studies also are not easily replicated.

Empirical specification of a dependent variable is essential for successful treatment of a disorder by different clinicians. If clinicians are researching and treating different dependent variables, there can be very little unambiguous communication between them. In the case of stuttering, for example, the clinician who corrects the prosodic defect may not be doing the same thing as the one who reduces the avoidance behaviors. Success rates of treatment procedures also vary tremendously, not necessarily because people who stutter are heterogeneous, but simply because different dependent variables are targeted.

From the standpoint of the philosophy of science (not that of a subject matter), the dependent variables must at least be observable in some empirical sense. Effects that do not generate empirical consequences cannot be observed or explained. Scientists, like everyone else, do not try to solve problems that do not exist. Unobservable dependent variables are a luxury especially for the clinician who must stay close to empirical data. Dependent variables in language, speech, fluency, and voice must be empirically real. There is no assurance that such variables as the rules of universal grammar and knowledge of phonological systems are not simply inferred entities. There is not even assurance that grammatical categories, semantic notions, and pragmatic rules are separate and independent behaviors in the sense that they are empirically real.

Questionable dependent variables pose another danger to the researcher and the clinician. It is easy to confuse those dependent variables with independent variables. Is knowledge of the rules of universal grammar a dependent variable or an independent variable? In other words, is it part of the language or is it the cause of language? It can be either, depending on whose work one is reading. In the Chomsky-type theory, knowledge of the rules is sometimes the dependent variable and at other times the independent variable. Similar confusion exists in phonological and pragmatic analyses.

Sometimes a confusion between dependent and independent variables can exist even when a given variable is clearly dependent. This problem exists in stuttering research concerned with various neurophysiological activities of people who stutter. For example, is the slow phonatory reaction time in people who stutter a dependent variable or an independent variable? In other words, when people who stutter take more time to say what they are asked to say, do clinicians observe a part of stuttering or do they observe a cause of stuttering? Is the observed excessive tension in the laryngeal muscle during stuttering a part of stuttering, an effect of stuttering, or the cause of stuttering?

It is not suggested here that all researchers should agree on certain dependent variables so they can make collective progress. Such a prescriptive suggestion is not acceptable to scientists because it is likely to inhibit creativity. What is suggested here is that researchers pay attention to some fundamental philosophical issues when considering, advocating, and researching certain dependent variables. At the least, investigators, in formulating their dependent variables, must address questions such as these: Are the dependent variables observable? Do they have empirical validity? Do they have more than speculative substance to them? Do they encourage experimental research? Clearly, these questions do not stem from a particular view of the subject matter, but rather from the philosophy of science itself.

Philosophy of Measurement

It was noted briefly in Chapter 6 that measurement philosophies are a part of the subject matter. Such philosophies influence the kinds of research done in a discipline. The point is that the philosophy of measurement is itself a part of methodology used in many investigations and that those philosophies are intricately connected with the conceptualizations of the dependent as well as the independent variables.

The two interrelated issues relative to the philosophy of measurement are what is measured and how it is measured. Both dependent and independent variables are measured in research, but it is the measurement of the dependent variable that can pose significant problems. It is obvious that the measurement of any variable depends on the way it is conceptualized. In the case of dependent variables, some can be measured directly, others only indirectly, and some not at all.

Social and psychological sciences have devised a variety of indirect measures of their dependent variables, largely because of the prevailing tendency to hypothesize dependent variables that are not directly observable and hence not measurable. Elaborately developed rating scales; personality inventories; and interest, attitude, and opinion questionnaires illustrate a complex set of measures analyzed through an equally complex set of statistical techniques. Unfortunately, the scientific return on such complex activities is usually poor because the nature of the dependent variable thus measured is not at all clear. It is one thing to measure the number of times a college student visits the library over a period of time, and an entirely different thing to measure what the student says or indicates on a questionnaire about the same behavior. The dependent variable, in this case the frequency with which he or she visits the library, is perfectly observable, although not without some inconvenience on the part of the researcher. The shortcut often taken is to simply ask persons about a particular behavior and treat their verbal statements as the measure of the dependent variable.

In communicative disorders, indirect measures have been used frequently. Instead of stuttering being measured directly, it may be measured through a rating scale. Experts may be asked to judge whether a person's stuttering is mild, moderate, or severe. Different judges' ratings may be averaged to derive a single rating on a given client. The rate of speech has sometimes been used as a measure, not of rate itself but of stuttering, on the assumption that slower rate is indicative of stuttering. If one wonders why stuttering could not be measured directly, the answer lies in the way stuttering was conceptualized. Evidently, to some investigators, stuttering is not a dependent variable that can be observed and measured in *real numbers.* When stuttering is conceptualized in terms of bad self-image, it is difficult to count it in mathematical units. Some indirect number systems that give the impression it is being measured will have to be devised.

It is probably better to have dependent variables that permit at least indirect measures than to have those that do not permit any measurement at all. Many of the variables that figure in the linguistic analysis of language and phonology can hardly be measured. It is not clear how one measures the knowledge of the grammatical or phonological rule system. In such cases, observable behaviors are measured and their patterns established. Patterns of correct and incorrect responses are thought to reflect the underlying knowledge systems. Such knowledge systems are then thought to have been measured indirectly. In this case, measurement is by inference, which is a highly questionable scientific practice indeed.

It appears as though the philosophy of the subject matter of speech and language pathology considers direct measures of behaviors either not adequate or not valid. The prevailing practice of measurement by inference in communicative disorders suggests that somehow counting the production of various language responses in numbers and percentages is either unimportant, invalid, or both. There is probably a prevailing opinion that directly observable dependent variables are superficial and that in-the-head, inferred variables are complex and scientifically more valuable.

In summary, one can measure only what one thinks it is important to measure, and what one thinks is important is a matter of one's philosophy of the subject matter. Once again, it is possible to think of some conditions of measurement purely from the philosophy of science. It is preferable to measure the dependent variable as directly as possible. It is also preferable to measure the variable in mathematically valid units (numbers) and not with a simulated system of numbers with nonmathematical definitions (see Chapter 6 for details). It is certainly best to avoid measurement by inference when the inevitable effect is unchecked speculation.

Locus of the Independent Variables

How independent variables are conceptualized is another philosophical matter that profoundly affects the methods of research and research reporting. It may be recalled that to establish cause–effect relations, the experimenter manipulates independent variables under controlled conditions. The cause of a certain event may be discovered accidentally, in which case the influence of prior conceptualization may not have played a critical role. In fact, prior conceptualization can sometimes delay accidental discoveries by making the scientist less observant of unsuspected relations. In any case, the following two questions are considered in this section: What are independent variables? Where are they located within the operating philosophy of a given discipline?

Systematic thinking about the nature of causes and the philosophy of causation has a long history because this is the stuff science is made of. As noted in Chapter 3, most dependent variables have a chain of causes, which can be analyzed at different levels. A patient's aphasic speech problem may have been caused by brain damage, but the brain damage also is an effect of some other cause such as a head injury or a stroke. The head injury and stroke have their respective causes, and so forth. In this chain of events, a particular event and its cause may be the focus of analysis at a given time, but it is important to remember that there is a larger picture of more interrelated events.

In the case of communicative behaviors and their disorders, causes are complex and perhaps involve multiple chains of events. But more important, the causes are often historical. By the time a clinician sees a child who has a language disorder or any other disorder of communication, the independent variables will already have occurred. That is why a retrospective search for causes through the method of case history is commonly employed in clinical sciences. As noted in Chapter 5, such ex post facto studies are done with the hope of uncovering past causes of current effects.

Uncovering the past causes of current effects has many pitfalls. One can never be sure that the event identified as the cause in a historical record was indeed the cause of the effect under study. Because the experimenter is not able to manipulate the suspected independent variable under controlled conditions, the cause–effect relation remains correlative and somewhat speculative.

The search for a cause that is still in the system has been prompted by the medical model. A virus or a bacterium or a lesion may be found in the body while the disease is still current. In this sense, the past cause is still active and observable, and in many cases that cause can be removed, killed, or neutralized. In the case of communicative and other behavior disorders, causes that are in the system are not encountered frequently. Even when they are, they are confounded with events in the life of the client. Such factors as a cleft palate, mental retardation, and brain damage are often suggested as the causes of certain communicative disorders. These causes are comparable to the causes found in medical diagnoses. While this may be true to a certain extent, the resulting effect is not entirely the product of those causes. In most cases, environmental events interact with those causes and produce a more complex effect on communication. This point is illustrated by the intact need for speech modification even when a cleft is surgically repaired. People with similar organic conditions may have vastly different behaviors or behavior potentials.

The nature of the independent variables in communicative disorders is complex because some of them are *relations between events*. Such relations are transitory. They have occurred in the past, and they often produce effects that accumulate over time. In this process, many variables come together to produce the eventual, magnified effect (called a disorder) that the clinician sees all at once and often after a lapse of time. If one suspects a certain pattern of parent–child interaction as the cause of stuttering in young children, then those interactions are simultaneously transitory, historical, cumulative, and interactive. Tracking such cause–effect relations is one of the most challenging tasks clinicians face.

The *locus of the independent variables* is an issue that has not received much direct attention, but it has been debated in an indirect manner. The questions, phrased in nontechnical terms, are these: Where are the independent variables located? Where do we look for them? Some look for them in the genetic mechanism of individuals, others in the dynamics of the neurophysiological systems of speech production. Still other investigators look for the causes in the environmental events that may have produced the effects under study. At a more complex level of analysis, interaction between some of these variables may be the target of study.

The philosophy of the locus of the independent variable that one adopts has a significant impact upon his or her methods of research. Of course, the philosophy has an initial impact on the kinds of causes looked for: genetic, neurophysiological, environmental, interactive, and so on. The kinds of causes thought of will influence the methods used to track them down.

If the causes looked for are within the *genetic and neurophysiological mechanisms*, then the methods are mostly nonexperimental. Genetic studies of human behaviors and disorders are retrospective, and they make the best effort at reconstructing the events so that a pattern emerges. The patterns may suggest different possibilities of inheritance or potential genetic mechanisms at work. Investigations of neurophysiological mechanisms examine existing structural variables and functional (working) dynamics. Such investigations compare the structures and dynamics found in individuals with a given effect against those without the effect. In other words, the method is mostly that of standard-group comparison. Observed structural and dynamic differences may then be related to the existing effect in one population and its absence in the other. People who stutter, for example, may be found to be slower than people who do not in their muscular or vocal reaction times. The two groups may be different in their reactions to certain central auditory stimulus materials.

When independent variables have an **internal locus,** analysis concerns what happens internally when an observable response is made. For example, when it is proposed that some fault in the phonatory or auditory system is responsible for stuttering, the fault, which is the independent variable, will not have been observed. It will have been inferred from a dependent variable (responses that are different from those of people who do not stutter).

Similar problems exist with such proposed independent variables as grammatical competence, knowledge of the rules of grammar or phonology, cognitive structures, and pragmatic rules or notions. These independent variables do not allow direct experimentation, and, therefore, they have to be inferred from dependent variables (client responses of one kind or another). This comment does not necessarily question the validity of those inferred independent variables. A knowledge of phonological rules may indeed underlie articulatory productions, both normal and deviant. But the method used to analyze that knowledge has its limitations, which are not often appreciated.

Independent variables that have external loci can be investigated with experimental methods. Those independent variables can be controlled by the investigator. Opportunities for direct experimentation in themselves do not validate the proposed independent variables, but they are opportunities for self-correction. Various environmental reinforcement, punishment, and other kinds of contingencies are more susceptible to experimental analysis than are genetic or neurophysiological independent variables. Indeed, most of the experimental research in speech–language pathology consists of independent variables of external locus. Controlled treatment research in articulation, language, fluency, and voice disorders have necessarily manipulated independent variables in the form of various stimuli and response consequences.

The question of the locus of the independent variables is also related to the issue of variability discussed in Chapter 7. The assumption of intrinsic variability is the same as the assumption of internal locus of independent variables, and the assumption of extrinsic variability is the same as that of the external locus of independent variables. These philosophical positions have similar methodological implications. The notions of intrinsic variability and internal locus of independent variables are hard to adapt to the experimental methodology.

PHILOSOPHICAL WAYS OF HANDLING METHODOLOGICAL PROBLEMS

Generally, and often appropriately, investigators think of methodological solutions to methodological problems. However, there are philosophical solutions to methodological problems. An investigator should at least be aware of such solutions, even if he or she rejects them after due consideration. Methodological problems can be handled philosophically. A few illustrations will serve to make this point.

When I say that a methodological problem is handled philosophically, I do not mean that somehow the need to design a procedure is bypassed. I mean only that the problem is approached from a different philosophical, rather than methodological, perspective. Instead of adding another procedural component to the methodology, the investigator reconceptualizes either the dependent or the independent variable or some aspect of the experimental control. The new perspective may lead to new methods.

Intersubject Variability

As noted in Chapter 7, intersubject variability poses a significant methodological problem in most animal and human research. This problem is handled with relative ease in animals by controlling their genetic as well as environmental history. Obviously, such tight control cannot be achieved with human participants. Therefore, human intersubject variability must be handled differently.

Intersubject variability can be handled either methodologically or philosophically. Statisticians have historically offered methodological solutions to the problem of intersubject variability. When a given sample of participants shows unacceptable amounts of intersubject variability, the investigator is advised to increase the sample size. The assumption is that the greater the number of participants, the higher the chances of neutralizing the effects of variability, because the opposing directions of variability within large groups may cancel each other.

A related methodological solution to intersubject variability is the use of statistical procedures of analysis. Bypassing the variability within the group, one can analyze the results through such techniques as the analysis of variance and still be able to draw some conclusions regarding the effect of independent variables on dependent variables. To be sure, within-group variability affects the analysis, but having more participants will make it possible to tease out the effects in spite of background variability.

There are two philosophical ways of handling intersubject variability. First, variability is not treated as an unwanted or interfering problem. Within this philosophy, intersubject variability is not a problem that needs bypassing techniques. This position also holds that statistical methods of handling variability are not effective. Those methods leave variability untouched and in fact magnify it by increasing the number of participants. Variability, on the other hand, is thought of as a matter of exerting greater control over the extraneous variables that are responsible for that variability. Instead of leaving the variability intact and finding methods of analysis that would still show the effects of independent variables, the investigator may take extra steps to control the conditions of the experiment so that the variability across (and within) participants is reduced. Behavioral research has shown that variability is often the result of poorly controlled experimental conditions or weak independent variables.

Second, variability itself may be the subject of experimental analysis. Within this philosophical view, questions about why individuals differ are considered worthy of research. This approach may need new methods, but only after such a philosophical shift.

Integrity of Dependent Variables

The kinds of dependent variables selected for study are often a matter of the philosophy of a given subject matter. A problem that has plagued investigators in psychological and social research is the reactivity of the dependent variable (see Chapter 7). Reactive dependent variables are those that change simply because they are measured. Such changes then confound the effects of the independent variables. Because the dependent variables must be measured before the independent variable is introduced, reactivity can pose significant problems.

It was noted in Chapter 8 that Solomon (1949) had devised a methodological solution to the methodological problem of measurement effects on dependent variables. His four-group design, considered one of the most complex and ideal of the group designs, makes it possible to identify the presence and the magnitude of reactivity. He simply increased the number of groups in a design so that the effect of the independent variable could be tested with and without pretesting. This is an excellent illustration of methodological handling of a methodological problem.

A philosophical approach to the same problem would prompt serious thinking about the integrity of the dependent variable under study. Perhaps the dependent variables must be reconceptualized. Possibly, attitudes and opinions that are notoriously reactive are not solid dependent variables. Such unctuous dependent variables may suggest that at best they are indirect measures of whatever is measured. Perhaps there is a more direct way of measuring what the reactive variable is supposed to measure. Such a philosophical approach asks some basic questions: What is it that we wish to change? What is the true dependent variable? Is it a person's response to a questionnaire, or is it the actual behavior under some specified conditions? Can we measure the behavior more directly than by accepting an indirect measure of it from what the person says about it?

A reconceptualization of *attitudes*, for example, would show that they are a surrogate for real behaviors and that the only practical reason to measure them is the difficulty in measuring those real behaviors. However, it is not impossible to measure the real behaviors for which the attitudes are a surrogate. A philosophical shift, then, would suggest that instead of a four-group design to handle reactivity, one might measure dependent variables that have a greater degree of integrity.

Reconceptualization of dependent variables is perhaps the most important philosophical method of handling a methodological problem. The very first question an investigator should ask about a research problem is the integrity of the dependent variable. It should be reliably and validly measurable. When there is no reasonable assurance of this, the investigator must consider other dependent variables. Generally speaking, if a dependent variable has to be measured only indirectly and without its actual occurrence, then a reconceptualization should be considered. Such dependent variables are abundant in speech–language pathology.

Magnitude of Change in the Dependent Variable

How much of an effect the independent variable should produce to suggest a cause–effect relation is a significant problem in research. The problem is compounded by intersubject and intrasubject variability. Under an experimental condition, the dependent variable must change more than it typically does on its own. How much more should it change has always been a difficult question, for which the traditional answer has been methodological.

The methodological approach is to use statistical methods of analysis that, depending on the sample size, require relatively small amounts of change in the dependent variable. Statistical significance is a measure of the effect of the independent variable over and beyond chance variations in the dependent variable. An important factor related to statistical significance is the sample size. When the other variables are held constant, the larger the sample size, the smaller the magnitude of change (in the dependent variable) needed to conclude that the manipulated variable was indeed responsible for the change. In essence, to show an effect, the methodological approach recommends that a large number of participants be used. Taking this recommendation seriously, social scientists have produced increasingly smaller effects in their experiments with increasingly larger numbers of participants.

A philosophical approach may not accept a methodological shortcut to this problem. Accordingly, there is no substitute for producing a large enough change needed to show that the independent variable did produce a change. Therefore, the only acceptable solution is to make the changes large enough to convince an observer without help from levels of statistical significance. This philosophy has gained additional strength in clinical sciences, where the effect of treatment procedures must be large enough to make a difference in the life of the clients. Statistical significance may or may not mean much in this respect. So the philosophical solution, which of course is no solution at all from the critics' standpoint, is to produce large effects after all.

INTERPLAY BETWEEN PHILOSOPHY AND METHODOLOGY

Under consideration so far has been how philosophical positions can influence methodological problems. However, methodology also has philosophical implications. Different methods shape different philosophies. Methods limited to naturalistic observations lead to different philosophies than do those that involve experimentation. For example, pure normative research is likely to shape a philosophy of language that is very different from the philosophy that would emerge from experimental analysis of the language acquisition process. Investigators who merely observe language and those who affect it by experimentation give different answers to questions regarding what language is and how and why is it acquired. In a more advanced stage of scientific research, there is a lively interplay between philosophy and methodology.

Although it was suggested earlier that philosophy can help resolve some of the methodological problems, it is not necessary to have a firm philosophy of the subject matter before one ventures into research. Also, in the beginning stage of a discipline, a commitment to a philosophy of a subject matter can be premature and can limit the kinds of questions asked or methods tried. In the absence of a philosophy of the subject matter, empirical scientists should adopt the philosophy of science. The basic philosophy of science can often be a better guide than premature philosophies of a subject matter. The philosophy of science also can suggest more fruitful questions for research than can existing nonexperimental data, speculative theories, untested clinical procedures, or personal philosophies, which are often no more than pet notions.

In the context of behavior science, Skinner (1956) has stated that when he started his research career, he had no particular physiological, mentalistic, or conceptual model of behavior. He was committed to the methods and philosophy of the natural sciences. Behaviorism, which is the philosophy of his kind of behavior science, evolved as data evolved. As the philosophy evolved and began to be applied to various behavior disorders, new methods evolved. Some of the experimental designs, including the multiple baseline design and the changing criterion design, were developed or modified in the applied contexts. However, in this endeavor, the applied researchers were guided by the philosophy of behaviorism.

A long tradition of research helps accumulate replicated data on the important questions pertaining to a given field of study. Whether this research is done with the philosophy of the subject matter or within the philosophy of science may not be crucial. Once an experimentally valid data base is created, philosophical implications begin to emerge. Those implications then guide further research. From this point on, methodology and philosophy influence each other.

When a given philosophy is not yet capable of suggesting appropriate methods, one should again follow the lead of the basic methods of science. Whenever possible, the experimental methodology should be preferred, since this method can pay larger dividends than any other. Cumulative experimental research can help shape a more useful philosophy of the subject matter and take both the subject matter and its philosophy to a level of development where new methods can be derived from that philosophy. Perhaps speech–language sciences and disorders will soon reach this level.

SUMMARY

- Researchers who exclusively consider methods to advance their discipline ignore another valuable factor that shapes research and knowledge: the philosophy of a subject matter.

- A philosophy of a subject matter
  - Asks questions about the value, usefulness, practicality, and overall implications of a subject matter and its methods
  - Can suggest *what* to research while methodology only can suggest *how* to do research
  - Can be a source of methodological innovations

- The philosophy of speech and language is still being developed. Some of the issues it needs to consider include the following:
  - Definition of dependent variables
  - Philosophy of methods of measurement
  - Locus of the independent variables

- There are philosophical ways of handling methodological problems. The following variables typically are handled methodologically, but they also can be handled—sometimes more appropriately—philosophically:
  - Intersubject variability
  - Integrity of dependent variables
  - Magnitude of change in the dependent variables

- A discipline makes progress because of an interplay between philosophy and methodology.

STUDY GUIDE

1. In addition to a knowledge of methodology, what are the two other parts of research that an investigator must be familiar with?

2. What are the limitations of a pure methodological approach to research?

3. Why should you be concerned with the philosophical issues relative to research?

4. How is a philosophy of a subject matter different from its accumulated knowledge and methods?

5. What are some of the philosophical concerns of an applied (clinical) discipline?

6. What discipline seems to have had an early influence on the training of speech–language pathologists?

7. What are the two behavioral and social sciences that had an influence on the development of the field of communicative disorders?

8. Specify the importance of dependent variables in developing a philosophical base for research.

9. What are some of the problems associated with many of the dependent variables used in speech—language pathology? Give examples.

10. Specify the relation between the way a dependent variable is conceptualized and the method of measurement used to measure that variable. Give an example.

11. What is meant by the locus of independent variables? How are the loci of such variables related to research methodology?

12. Which kind of locus is more susceptible to experimental methodology? Why? Illustrate your answer.

13. How is intersubject variability handled methodologically? How is it handled philosophically?

14. What is meant by integrity of dependent variables?

15. What is a methodological approach to handling the issue of the magnitude of the effects of independent variables? What is a philosophical approach?

PART III

◆◆◆◆◆◆◆◆◆◆◆◆◆◆◆◆◆◆◆◆◆◆◆◆◆

Doing, Reporting, and Evaluating Research

Chapter 13

◆◆◆◆◆◆◆◆◆◆◆◆◆◆◆◆◆◆◆◆◆◆◆◆◆◆◆◆◆◆◆◆◆

How To Formulate Research Questions

One would think that it should be possible to tell a beginning graduate student how to do research and the student in turn should be able to follow the suggestions and complete a study. Unfortunately, telling someone how to do research is not easy and the effects are not always predictable. Therefore, I realize the potential pitfalls in writing this and the other chapters in this final section of the book. Nonetheless, it is possible to offer a few suggestions that may help in the pursuit of knowledge.

Most graduate seminars on research methods and designs require the students to write a research proposal. Students are typically expected to suggest a research question and describe an appropriate method for investigating it. A majority of students probably do not find this to be an easy assignment. The very first question they face is simple but often debilitating: Where do I start? Students will also quickly find out that answering one question will only make them qualified to face other questions.

As described in Chapter 2, research generally does not follow a fixed pattern that can be described. The formative process of research is a set of ever-changing contingencies. Therefore, the researcher should train himself or herself to become more sensitive to the changing contingencies in the process of research and keep learning in that process. In the beginning, this learning is difficult and full of uncertainties; that is, the difficulties faced by graduate students in writing a research proposal are both natural and inevitable.

Uncertainties in the research process are never totally resolved, no matter how experienced the investigator. Therefore, students should hope to do their best, start the work as early as possible, and believe that research can be fun.

In this chapter, the emphasis will be on formulating research questions. Once a research question is formulated, the investigator thinks of the best method of studying it. The information on methods of study is the essence of many previous chapters. Therefore, the issue of selecting methods will be addressed only briefly in this chapter.

HOW TO FORMULATE RESEARCH QUESTIONS

The first problem the student faces is how to find a topic of research. This is essentially the problem of finding research questions. Research questions are sometimes literally found in some sources, and at other times they are formulated. On the one hand, a research paper, a textbook, a review article, or another researcher may suggest a problem that needs to be investigated. In this case, the student literally finds a research question. On the other hand, the student's own scholarship may prompt a new question that needs to be answered. In this case, the student will have thought of an original idea, and the resulting question is a self-formulated one.

As long as the question is considered worthy of investigation, either a found or a formulated research question is acceptable. Nevertheless, it is best for students to learn the process of formulating research questions. The best way to learn to be independent researchers is to know how to formulate research questions based on critical scholarship.

Research questions identify gaps in the knowledge about a phenomenon. When those questions are validly answered with methods of science, the gaps in knowledge are filled. Questions that are researched may produce new information or verify the reliability and validity of known information. Research that produces new information is original, and that which verifies the results of earlier studies is replicative. Both kinds of research are valuable. However, to learn more about the research process, the student should think of a question that has either not been answered or not been answered appropriately. An exercise of this kind will teach the student more about research than will an attempt to replicate a well-done study. In any case, the student needs to start looking for a problem to investigate, and there are several places to look.

Formulating research questions may be relatively easy or difficult depending on the degree of knowledge and scholarship the student has in his or her field of study. Knowledge itself does not guarantee that research questions will be found, however. The student should read the literature critically, taking note of the kinds of research done and the methods used. The student should judge how well the research has been done. The student should come to understand what is still not known.

At this point, it may be appropriate to give the student the bad news: No amount of "how to" suggestions will replace careful and scholarly review of the literature. But even before doing that, there are a few things the student should do. What follows is a series of interrelated steps the student should take to formulate a research problem and plan for an investigation.

Identify a Broad Area of Research

The first thing to do is find a broad area of investigation or a general topic that is of interest. In communicative disorders, the student may consider such areas as cleft palate, dysarthria, language acquisition, phonological disorders, treatment of stuttering, types of aphasia, or maintenance of treatment targets. It is better to select an area that is personally interesting; after all, the student will be spending much time on it.

Once an area or topic has been selected, the student should read or re-read the basic information covering it. It is often useful to read what is written on that topic in a recently published standard textbook. Even research that produces advanced information requires a command of the elementary information. For example, a student wishing to do a piece of research on language acquisition should have a good grasp of the basic textbook information on this subject. A student who goes directly to theoretical writings, more advanced books, or journal articles without a good grasp of the basic information will waste time.

Identify the Current Trends

The researcher should then proceed to find the current trends on the topic. The research done in recent years must be carefully reviewed. There are no specific guidelines on what is recent and what is not; it depends on the amount and the chronology of research on a given topic of investigation. Some topics have both a long history and a high level of current research activity. Other topics have a long history but a low level of current research activity. Still other topics have a recent history with a high density of studies. Finally, there are recent topics with few studies. No recent trend can be fully understood without a historical background, however. Therefore, it is essential to know the classic studies and theories before reading recent research papers. Students should not refrain from reading sources that may be hundreds of years old with the fear that the sources my be dated. Classic, scholarly information is never dated, even if there is disagreement about it.

Generally speaking, in most empirical research with no compelling reason to go back, 7 to 10 years of research may be considered current or recent. This guideline, however, may be more often violated than followed, and for good reasons. For instance, to gain a good historical understanding of a specific topic, one may need to go back more than 10 years. Other topics may be of very recent origin. In any case, there are many ways of finding the current trends, and the student must use most if not all of them. The basic task, however, is to search the literature to find both a general topic of interest and its recent trends. A thorough and systematic literature search is essential in finding possible topics for research.

Several sources help identify the current trends in research. Most likely, scientific and professional journals are a good starting point.

Journals

The student must find the major journals that publish research articles on the selected topic. Journals published by one's own professional organization (such as the American Speech-Language-Hearing Association) are usually excellent sources because they are most likely to publish articles of immediate relevance. To achieve a broader understanding of the context and issues involved, the student may expand this search and read articles in national and international journals, related professional organizations, research institutes, and private publishing houses. For instance, journals published in many branches of medicine, psychology, linguistics, education, special education, education of the deaf, biology, and acoustics may provide information from different perspectives that might suggest research questions.

Depending on the general area of investigation being considered, the student will have to concentrate upon certain kinds of journals. In the case of most topics in communicative disorders, various national and international journals in the discipline will be the primary source of information. If the general area of investigation is the normal acquisition of speech and language, journals in linguistics and psychology are likely to have relevant articles. If the research topic is treatment of various behavioral disorders, including communicative disorders, various journals of applied behavior analysis and behavior modification may be searched. Researching diagnosis and treatment of communicative disorders may require a search of medical and educational journals.

Most journals are published quarterly. Some medical journals are published more frequently; some are published weekly. Typically, the final issue of a volume contains an annual index. Most journals have an author index, a subject index, and a title index. As an initial step, it is best to look into the final issues of selected volumes and go through the indexes to find the articles of interest.

Printed Abstracts

Another method of literature search is to use the printed abstracts, which help investigators make a quick review of recent research. Most abstracts publish brief and nonevaluative summaries of research published in various sources, both national and international. Some specialized abstracts include such unpublished research as doctoral dissertations and master's theses.

The American Psychological Association (APA) publishes *Psychological Abstracts*, which can be useful in literature search. They are a monthly publication of nonevaluative summaries of the world's literature on psychology and related subject matters, often abstracting speech and hearing related articles. Articles are classified according to subject–topic areas. Of particular interest to students in communicative disorders are the subtopics *Speech and Language* under *Communication Systems* and *Speech Therapy* under *Treatment and Prevention*.

Another major abstract service is offered by the University Microfilms International (UMI). UMI publishes *Dissertation Abstracts International*, a monthly publication of doctoral dissertations and master's theses accepted in North American universities. Each monthly edition has two sections, bound separately. Section A abstracts dissertations and theses submitted in the humanities and social sciences; it includes such relevant fields as communication, education, language, and linguistics. Section B of each issue is devoted to natural sciences and engineering including biological sciences, health sciences, and psychology.

Another publication of the University Microfilms International is the *Comprehensive Dissertation Index*. This may be especially useful to students because it lists dissertation and thesis research under the heading *Speech Pathology*. Research on audition is included under this heading.

When the general topic of interest is medically related, the *Cumulated Index Medicus* may be useful. It is a bibliography of the literature on biological and medical sciences. Many articles related to communicative disorders may be abstracted in this index. This is an annual publication of the National Library of Medicine (National Institutes of Health, U.S. Department of Health and Human Services).

Finally, *Linguistics and Language Behavior Abstracts*, published quarterly by Sociological Abstracts, Inc., can be useful in searching literature on a variety of subjects including audiology, speech pathology, laryngology, neurology, otology, linguistics, and applied linguistics. It was originally published under the title *Language and Language Behavior Abstracts*.

Aggregated Databases

An efficient method of information retrieval is to use one of the several computerized data search services available on the Internet. They are known as aggregated databases. Students and faculty may gain access to database services free of charge if they go through their university library's Web site. University libraries subscribe to many database services and offer the information free of charge to students and faculty.

Most database services provide only abstracts of articles, but they may provide a bibliography of published research. There are a few databases that provide full texts of some, not all, articles. Practically all databases are interactive; that is, a student can first ask the system to list articles on a general topic and then narrow the field down to a specific area of investigation. Most entries may be printed outright. Students can request the full text of articles through the library. Within a few days, the library will obtain a copy of the article for the student. In some cases, there may be a photocopy charge although in most cases, the copies arrive free of charge.

Most students now have the skill to navigate through the Internet and the specific databases to get the information they need. University libraries offer workshops and other forms of assistance to students who need to learn the basics of database search. Information specialists in the library may also offer individual assistance upon request. It is best for the student to learn advanced database search skills as early as possible.

Most computerized services save time, although the specificity of information on speech and hearing publications may be variable. Students with Internet connections can search the databases of the world from their own home. Nonetheless, the student must plan the search well and make sure the terms to be used in the search are specific and are known to be a part of the database. A random search may yield a few good results but may also frustrate the student. Also, because it takes time to obtain articles through interlibrary loan program, it is important for the student to submit requests for full texts of articles as soon as possible.

Several specific databases are especially useful to students in speech and hearing sciences and special education. For instance, ERIC (Educational Resources Information Center) is a vast computerized database service devoted to research in education. Many articles of relevance to speech–language pathologists are available on ERIC. Exceptional Child Education Resources is a related service, and it can be combined with ERIC in the process of information retrieval. If the topic of interest is related to special or regular education, ERIC is the most valuable source for the student in communicative disorders.

Another vast database is PsycINFO, maintained by the American Psychological Association. This well-known database offers millions of articles abstracted from around the world. Although the number of journals abstracted varies from time to time, a recent check of the PsycINFO Web site revealed more than 1,800 journals being abstracted. PsycINFO does not provide full texts of articles; however, another database, known as PsycARTICLES, also maintained by the American Psychological Association, does that for a fee. It may also be available through universities free of charge.

Research publications in medicine, nursing, and health sciences are computerized by MEDLINE, which includes most of the printed information found in *Cumulated Index Medicus*. The original MEDLINE program was not especially helpful to students in communicative disorders. In recent years, the specificity with which research studies in communicative disorders are entered has been increased with additional terms and topic entries. It is possible to obtain a list of articles on specific topics such as language disorders or speech disorders, or, more specifically, stuttering or cleft palate. The system can also search for articles whose titles or abstracts contain specific terms such as *Dysfluency* or *Presbycusis*. The system can print out a bibliography as well as abstracts of articles.

MEDLINE's search engine is called PubMed, which can be accessed directly or through MEDLINE. MEDLINE usually gives only the abstracts, but its affiliated program, MEDLINE (SilverPlatter) provides many full-text articles. Another useful database is LexisNexis, which provides abstracts of articles in medicine and health-related disciplines. In addition, Elsevier Science Direct can give abstracts of most medical and scientific articles and in some cases, full texts. Again, students can access all of these databases through their university libraries.

Any computerized data search helps the student in identifying articles published in various sources. In some cases, the number of available articles may be few, but in many cases, the number may be overwhelming. Therefore, the student must narrow the search, be more selective, obtain the most essential articles, and read them thoroughly and critically.

In reading journal articles on the topic, the student should take note of the kinds of studies that are repeated. In a given period of time, several persons may have published on a particular topic, and the questions researched may be the same or similar. Should the student find this to have happened during the last few years, a recent trend may have been identified. In such cases, it is also necessary to find out why similar studies were repeated. It is possible that a controversy about the first one or two studies stimulated people with different views. This may have led to studies designed to produce contrary evidence. If this is the case, the research information will be controversial, and the student may find it relatively easy to find a problem, because controversies are an excellent source of research questions.

Other Sources

Review articles are especially good sources for research questions. In a review article, the author will have surveyed most of the published information on the topic and made a critical analysis of what is known and with what degree of generality, and what kinds of research need to be done. The author will have pointed out the good and the bad about the research attempts in a particular area of investigation. A good review article points out both the methodological strengths and weaknesses of the past studies. Frequently, a well-written review article identifies research questions for future investigations. One of those questions may be quite appropriately selected.

Studies that are described as exploratory or preliminary may also be a source of research questions. These labels are sometimes an excuse for poorly designed studies, but when they are not, they may contain seeds of new studies. Even when they are methodologically inadequate, the student with a good knowledge of designs can improve upon them if the basic idea is sound. Good exploratory studies suggest emerging trends in the field. They often suggest the topics of the future.

Descriptive studies can also be a source of new experimental investigations. Some of the original investigators of descriptive studies suggest further experimental studies on the issue. Many descriptive studies, however, do not have any hints of experimental studies. In such cases, the student is alone in going beyond the investigator's descriptions to think of experimental questions.

The student should not ignore scholarly exchanges between authors as a source of research questions. Some journals publish such exchanges, sometimes called *Letters to the Editor*, which typically are critical responses to published research followed by the author's rebuttal. Some of these exchanges can fail to illuminate the issues at hand because of a personal and subjective tone, but several of them can suggest questions for further research. Journals also may publish critical commentaries on previously published articles as regular papers. Some journals publish special issues devoted to scholarly exchange between experts.

Additional sources of information can be found in books. After having reviewed the basic information and some journal articles, the student may be ready to read some specialized books. Books on recent advances are occasionally published in every field, and most contain critical reviews and summaries of recent research information. Such books can serve the student well by giving both a current overview and suggestions on potential research questions.

Books on controversies in selected clinical or theoretical issues can be helpful to students and more advanced researchers. Books on controversies are edited by an expert, and the chapter authors are experts who are generally known for their contrasting views. Students should not shy away from controversial issues because, as suggested earlier, they are a good source of research problems.

Finally, the workshops, symposia, seminars, and presentations at professional meetings and conventions are expected to give the most recent information on a variety of topics and issues. The quality of presentations at such gatherings varies tremendously, however. With a critical approach, the student can find many research questions. A significant advantage of professional meetings is the opportunity to meet researchers who have done exceptional research in the selected area. Through these meetings, the student researcher can often get expert advice. Such advice, however, can be sought at any time during the planning and implementation of a study by contacting experts, who are usually happy to advise interested students.

Identify the Classic Questions

Many graduate students and professionals find it attractive to do research on topics of recent interest, often resulting in an overemphasis on identifying current trends in the search for a research question. Furthermore, research on current topics is generally more easily published than research exploring unknown, unappreciated, or unpopular areas and views.

Nothing is wrong with researching currently popular topics, but a potential problem must be avoided: Current trends of research are not necessarily the most creative or worthwhile. Research and theory also have their fashionable trends or *zeitgeist*. For instance, the semantic analysis of language, the distinctive feature analysis of articulation, and the phonatory reaction time of people who stutter have had their heyday, only to be overshadowed by newer trends. Therefore, one should be aware that some highly regarded current trends may be nothing more than a passing fancy, and such trends are not the only ones that generate original research. Indeed, researchers should not be discouraged from asking old, unusual, novel, or unpopular questions. All problems without solutions are of current interest. Any question whose answer has a potential for producing new knowledge or replicating old knowledge is worthy of investigation.

A significant question, posed long ago, may be still unanswered, perhaps because past methods were inadequate and unproductive. Therefore, investigations on that question may have dwindled; a student could investigate new and more productive methods to study the old but unresolved question. In some cases, theoretical or conceptual advances in the field may suggest new ways of looking at old problems. In such cases, it is appropriate to renew an old line of investigation.

The basic experimental questions of causality are timeless. For example, clinical research questions concerning the effects of treatment procedures and refinement of those procedures are never out of date. In fact, new trends have a tendency to emerge in the theoretical explanation of phenomena, but some of these theoretical trends may prove unproductive. When one is interested in the basic experimental and empirical analysis of phenomena, most of the procedures are well established, and the questions of causality are classic, simplifying the selection of a topic and methods for studying that topic.

Concentrate on a Specific Area of Research

After the preliminary information-related research on a general topic, such as language acquisition or the treatment of phonological disorders, the student should narrow the problem down to a more specific area of investigation. In language acquisition, for example, one might think of morphological acquisition. Even more specifically, the acquisition of the irregular morphemes, adjectives, or some specific sets of semantic or pragmatic notions may be considered. The research done so far should guide the student in this regard; obviously, the student would not select a research question that has been overly and perhaps quite adequately researched. The initial survey of the literature should have indicated that the selected problem or some aspect of it still needs to be investigated.

When the student has selected a specific area, more reading is needed. The student must go back to the journals and carefully read reports of major studies on the specific area being considered. This reading is more critical and analytical than the first pass. The student should make a critical analysis of theoretical and conceptual information, pay particular attention to methods. Indeed, detailed notes should be taken of the methods and procedures of the studies because the student may use some of those methods and because the student may wish to avoid the methodological deficiencies of past studies.

Formulate a Specific Research Question

A critical reading of a particular area should lead to a more specific research problem. The student should know that the journey from a general topic to a particular research problem can be long and frustrating. One may have a desire to do some research on language treatment, but a specific research question may not emerge for some time.

At this point, it may be useful to write a general description of the research problem. Once again, the student should recheck the major sources to make sure that the problem either (a) has not been researched, (b) has not been researched in the manner being considered, or (c) has been researched but with room for significant methodological improvement. A difficult problem a majority of students face at this point is confirming that the study as planned has not been done. Students often find themselves discarding their pet ideas one by one because previous investigators were ahead of them.

Writing research questions takes some skill and practice. Research questions should be as direct as possible and as technical as necessary. Furthermore, they are typically about some objective phenomenon, perhaps asking whether the phenomenon exists and if so investigating its descriptors.

Research questions can also ask whether a certain variable (such as a treatment) has an effect, and whether two or more variables interact. Purely descriptive research involves somewhat simpler questions than experimental research. For example, "How many phonemes are produced by 2-year-old children?" is a relatively simple descriptive question. On the other hand, the question of whether two or more phonological treatment components have certain independent and interactive effects, and if so to what extent, is experimental in nature and therefore more complex.

A variety of research questions were described in Chapter 11. The kind of research question formulated for a particular investigation depends on the type of research contemplated. Normative and standard-group comparison research mostly involve questions that evoke descriptions. Ex post facto, experimental, and correlative research ask questions of relation between two or more variables. In fact, specifying the variables of a study is probably the most crucial step involved in planning the study.

Specify the Variables in Technical Language

The student will find that a serious attempt to specify the variables to be investigated will force clearer thinking about the entire research plan. The student must try to answer several questions: What are my dependent variables? How many dependent variables do I have? What are my independent variables? How do I control my independent variables? What kind of relation is to be studied: cause–effect relations, correlative relations, or additive and interactive relations? Direct answers to questions such as these will help the student to clarify the research problem and design appropriate methods.

The dependent and independent variables must be clearly separated in studies that include both of them. The typical dependent variables in communicative disorders include various kinds of speech, language, and hearing behaviors and their disorders. In a particular study, a specific aspect of these behaviors constitutes a dependent variable. In other words, although *language* can be described as a dependent variable, one needs to specify a particular aspect of it, for example, the production of the plural morpheme at the word level. Stuttering can be a dependent variable, but it is better to specify exactly what will be measured to document the occurrence of that disorder. In essence, the dependent variable must be described in *measurable* terms.

An independent variable, being the manipulated or suspected cause of the dependent variable, should be described in equally specific language; after all, this is the variable whose effects are determined in experimental studies. While reading the literature, the student should pay particular attention to the way different investigators have described dependent and independent variables. Often, students will find themselves confused about the status of the variables in their study. The student should know the definitions and characteristics of different kinds of variables (see Chapter 3).

The operational specification of variables also involves considerations of measurement. As discussed in Chapter 6, variables can be measured in different ways, some more suitable to given problems than others. The student should always think in terms of more objective, more direct, and more discrete types of measures of the behaviors under study. Sometimes, it may be found that the problem is very intriguing, but the variables involved cannot be measured easily.

After specifying their variables, some investigators formulate their hypotheses. A research investigation does not require a hypothesis, but if one is preferred, it must be written clearly so that it specifies the variables to be investigated. See Chapter 3 for additional information on hypotheses.

Talk to Someone

Talking to someone about a research problem can be a great help. The person the student talks to need not be an expert on the subject. In the process of talking, the student may find that he or she has not thought through the research question or some methodological aspect of the contemplated research. The student may also find gaps in his or her understanding of some theoretical concepts involved in the study. Such deficiencies in the understanding of the research topic or the procedure will force more homework or clearer thinking. This step can be taken at the very beginning and repeated at every stage of the investigation.

Talking to an expert, however, can have additional advantages. The expert can help the student avoid false starts or dead-end projects. In talking with the expert, the student may find out that a particular study has or has not been done. The expert may also pose gentle and supportive challenges so that the student attains greater clarity in thinking. The student may gain more confidence in the idea being considered, and under the best possible conditions, the exchange may inspire and motivate the student to go ahead with the project.

Evaluate the Significance of the Research Questions

In the process of selecting a research problem, the student must judge whether it will be a valuable study. The question to be researched must be of some scientific, theoretical, or applied significance. Some of the most common questions asked in evaluating the significance of research questions include the following: Is the research meaningful? Is it likely to contribute new knowledge or to expand on the existing knowledge? Does it help solve a problem? Does it have the potential to explain an event hitherto unexplained? Does the research show a new method of studying a difficult problem? Does it improve clinical techniques? Does it produce an effect unobserved so far? Does it help detect an effect that has been suspected but not observed? These are some of the many questions one can ask in evaluating the significance of research questions.

To judge that a given piece of research is valuable, one need not seek an affirmative answer to all the questions just posed. A single affirmative answer may be sufficient to justify a study. Evaluation of the significance of research problems and questions is one of the most difficult tasks in the research process. This important issue will be discussed in Chapter 15.

Think of the Methods

It is generally assumed that the researcher thinks of the methods only after having decided upon the problem. In practice, however, such a sequence is seldom realized. Methods must be considered even during the process of selecting a problem or rejecting others. If the investigator cannot think of a procedure for researching a particular question, that question may have to be rejected or postponed for future consideration. In fact, one way to screen out poor research ideas is to realize their methodological impracticality.

Other practical considerations assume importance in the process of problem selection. The student must consider the availability of participants, special equipment, and laboratory facilities. For example, if it is known that laryngectomy patients are not being served in a particular clinic, questions about the effectiveness of a certain laryngectomy treatment procedure may not be practical unless the student is willing to go elsewhere. If a particular research idea needs expensive biofeedback equipment that the department does not have, perhaps some other problem must be found. Similarly, if the research idea requires a specially constructed acoustic laboratory that does not exist, then that idea may have to be rejected.

When a research question is sound, a lack of available methods (not physical instruments) should only signal a challenge to one's scientific ingenuity. The idea need not be rejected, but it may not be implemented immediately. It may take some time before an appropriate method is devised to study the problem. Meanwhile the graduate student needs a practical problem for the thesis or some specific assignment so that he or she can graduate within a reasonable period of time. Sometimes, even a seasoned researcher is likely to move on to something that can be done more easily than the project that takes extra time, effort, and thinking.

Questions that are too broad (What causes language disorders?) or too vague (How do children acquire language?) do not lend themselves to methodological planning. As soon as the student begins to consider how a piece of research can be implemented, the problem itself begins to be seen in a different light. In essence, methodological considerations force problem specificity. Therefore, it is a good idea to think about the problem and the methods in an interwoven fashion. However, once a specific problem has been found, the investigator can spend more time working out the details of methods.

One of the first methodological considerations is the participants of the study. The student must decide on the number of participants and their characteristics. Clinical or nonclinical participants and their social, personal, health, and other relevant characteristics must be considered. The age and gender of the participants should also be decided. The clinical and nonclinical participants must be described in terms of the criteria used in separating them. If patients with aphasia are going to be used in the study, how are they going to be diagnosed? Who are not aphasic? Who will make the judgments? By what means? How and where are they going to be found? By what criteria are they finally going to be included in the study? These are the questions of participant selection procedures or criteria. There are both inclusion and exclusion criteria—they specify the characteristics that will admit individuals to the study as well as those that will exclude individuals from it.

Whether one wishes to use a large random sample or a small group of homogeneous participants is also an important question. In most clinical studies, available participants are used with a few restrictions. For example, an investigation concerned with language disorders may exclude those with neurological handicaps or hearing impairment. Certain syndromes or special conditions that complicate language problems may be excluded. A relatively narrow age range may be specified as acceptable. With some such restrictions, the participants may be selected on the basis of availability.

A difficult aspect of planning for a study is determining the kinds of instruments that will be used in it. The term *instruments* includes all the kinds of equipment or apparatus that will be used in the study. The type of instruments needed for a study depends mostly on the nature of the dependent variables and the kind of measures selected for the study (see Chapter 6 for details).

The stimulus materials to be used in the study also are part of the instruments. Questions designed to evoke responses, modeling, and the specific target behaviors, and instructions to be given the participants, also should be prepared beforehand.

Another important aspect of the procedure is the overall plan and the specific design of the study. The selected design may be of the single-subject or group variety. The design typically dictates the number and sequence of the conditions of the study. These conditions, such as the pretest, experiment, and posttest, must be specified. As noted in Chapter 11, the selection of a design depends on the nature of the research question asked.

Finally, the student must have some idea of the kinds of data the study will generate and how they will be analyzed. The method of analysis is mostly determined by the design and the kinds of data. Studies of group designs generate data that are appropriately handled by statistical methods of analysis, whereas single-subject design studies generate data that can be evaluated visually and quantitatively, but not with statistical methods.

When statistical methods of data analysis are used, the student must understand the limitations and appropriateness of the tests to be used. Each statistic is based on certain assumptions, such as the normal or nonnormal distribution of the dependent variable being measured and the methods of measurements used (continuous, categorical, etc.). The data for which the selected statistic is applied should not violate those assumptions. Most students need to consult an expert in statistics before selecting statistical techniques of analysis.

The foregoing is by no means an exhaustive survey of questions that must be addressed in planning a research study. The list can, however, promote the understanding of some major steps that must be taken in developing a research study.

PREPARATION OF THESES AND DISSERTATIONS

In a majority of graduate programs in communicative disorders, a master's thesis is optional; however, a few programs may require a thesis from all candidates for the master's degree. A dissertation is always required of doctoral candidates.

In formulating questions for a thesis or dissertation, the student follows the same steps as described earlier. However, theses and dissertations require a more careful and thorough literature search than that needed for a class project. It is expected that a student planning a thesis or dissertation has a good background in the field, and therefore the search can be more specific and goal directed from the beginning.

An initial step in the preparation of a thesis, however, is to find a faculty advisor who is willing to direct the research. Unlike class projects and research assignments, theses and dissertations need close supervision from the advisor. In completing an original study for a thesis or dissertation, the student works closely with the faculty advisor.

It is in the best interest of the student to find a faculty advisor who is an expert in the particular area selected for investigation. In this way, the student can be sure of getting expert advice and help in the conduct of the research study. Generally speaking, the student and the advisor will spend much time discussing potential research problems. When a problem is finally selected, it is the student's responsibility to make sure that current information on the topic has been thoroughly researched. The design and the procedures of the study are then discussed with the advisor and finalized.

Most theses and dissertations are evaluated by a committee of three to five members. The advisor serves as chair of the committee. The student, in consultation with the advisor, selects members for the committee. Depending on the research problem being investigated, the student may select a committee member from outside the department. Psychologists, statisticians, linguists, and medical and other professionals may be selected.

Once the committee is formed, the student must write a detailed proposal of the study and submit it for approval. Usually, an oral presentation is also made. During this oral presentation, the student briefly reviews the literature and justifies the study and its procedures. The committee's task is to ensure that the student understands all aspects of the proposed research and that the methods and procedures are appropriate. If necessary, the committee may suggest changes in the methods of the proposed study.

After obtaining the approval of the committee, the student must submit the proposal to an institutional review board (IRB), which reviews the proposal from the standpoint of human participant or animal subject protection. An IRB's task is to determine whether the study poses any risks to the participants, and if so, what steps must be taken to minimize them. Chapter 16 offers discussion of the ethical issues involved in the conduct of research, along with human participant and animal subject protection procedures.

The student can begin the actual investigation only after the thesis or dissertation committee and the IRB approve the study. When the study is completed, it is written according to the guidelines established by the student's department and the graduate school of the university. Most departments of communicative disorders use the guidelines specified in the *Publication Manual of the American Psychological Association* (APA, 2001). The student should consult the most recent edition of the APA Manual or other accepted sources.

Once again, the student works very closely with the advisor (the committee chair) in writing the thesis or dissertation. Most students revise the thesis or dissertation several times before the advisor accepts it tentatively. Finally, when the advisor considers it appropriate, an oral examination is scheduled. The entire committee once again meets to judge the appropriateness of the thesis or dissertation for the degree being sought.

During the oral examination, the student describes the study and its results and conclusions and also relates the findings to previous research and theories. In essence, the student defends his or her work during this oral examination. Approval is granted when the committee is satisfied with the thesis or dissertation and its defense. Following this approval, any changes and corrections the committee suggests are incorporated, and the final copy of the thesis or dissertation is submitted to the graduate school. If it is deemed appropriate, the graduate school then accepts the document on behalf of the university.

Completing a thesis or dissertation can be extremely time consuming. It takes hard work and typically involves extra expense. However, it is a worthwhile aspect of graduate education. It is the only opportunity for students to do a piece of original research evaluated and approved by a team of experts in the field. There is no better way to learn about research than completing a thesis or dissertation. Well-planned and well-conducted theses or dissertations meet standards of publication.

SUMMARY _____

Research questions are those that when answered, fill gaps in knowledge. The first step in conducting research is to formulate a research question. The following steps may be taken to formulate research questions:

- Identify a broad area of research. Consider what general topics interest you.

- Identify the current trends of research on the selected topic. In finding the current trends, study the following sources:
  — Journals in the major field and in related fields
  — Printed abstracts
  — Computerized database services
  — Books
  — Symposia, seminars, conventions, and other presentations

- Identify the classic questions that still need to be answered.

- Concentrate on a specific area of research.

- Formulate a specific research question.

- Specify the variables in technical language.

- Talk to people.

- Evaluate the significance of the research questions.

- Think of the methods.

In preparing theses and dissertations, follow the guidelines of your department and the instructions of your advisor.

STUDY GUIDE _____

1. What are research questions? Where do you find them?

2. What are the nine steps you should take to formulate research questions?

3. Describe how the process of formulating a research question proceeds from a review of a broad area of research to a narrowly specified research question.

4. Describe the usefulness of a published review article in your search for a research question.

5. What are the main sources of information on the current trends?

6. What is meant by "classic research questions"? Why are they important?

7. Why is it necessary to specify the variables of a research question in technical language? Give an illustration by writing a research question that specifies its variables in technical language.

8. What are the advantages and disadvantages of talking to experts and laypersons?

9. What are some of the questions you would ask in determining the significance of research questions? Are the answers to those questions always clear and objective? Why or why not?

10. Specify why methodological impracticality is one of the early considerations in the selection of research problems.

11. Formulate a research question that would be considered "classic" in its import. Specify the variables in technical language. Write a brief justification of the research the question would lead to.

12. Formulate a research question that would reflect a recent trend in your subject matter. What makes it recent? What are your variables? Justify your study.

Chapter 14

◆◆◆◆◆◆◆◆◆◆◆◆◆◆◆◆◆◆◆◆◆◆◆◆◆◆◆◆◆◆◆◆◆◆◆

How To Write Research Reports

Those who do research should write. The completion of an investigation is followed by writing the report and submitting it for publication. Besides research articles, scientists and professionals also write integrative articles, critical reviews, philosophical essays, books, manuals, many types of clinical reports, and a variety of other kinds of reports.

Most universities require adequate writing skills of their graduate as well as undergraduate students. Students who wish to complete a thesis as part of the requirement for graduate degrees are especially concerned with writing skills.

This chapter is concerned with writing in general and with writing research reports in particular. I shall describe five aspects of scientific and professional writing: (a) the format of a research article, (b) writing without bias, (c) some principles of good writing, (d) conceptual considerations, and (e) style.

FORMAT OF SCIENTIFIC REPORTS

Each professional and scientific community has an accepted format for reporting scientific studies. These formats encourage a relatively uniform way of writing scientific articles. Editors of journals and books and professional organizations impose uniform formats. Such writing formats are helpful for several reasons. First, they make the job of editorial evaluation manageable. If different authors were to report their studies in vastly different formats, the process of editorial evaluation would be complicated by the problems inherent to the organization of data. Second, the mechanical aspect of printing differently reported material in a single publication such as a journal can be unnecessarily complicated. Third, a uniform reporting format is desirable for readers as well. Readers of particular journals find it easy to understand and evaluate reports written in a uniform format.

The prescriptive formats are especially required of articles submitted for publication in scientific and professional journals. Books, manuals, and other kinds of written materials are not as strictly controlled by such formats. Therefore, this section will focus on journal article formats.

A widely used format for journal articles is that of the American Psychological Association (APA). As early as 1929, a group of anthropological and psychological journal editors were concerned about a standard format of reporting scientific studies. The first edition of the *Publication Manual of the American Psychological Association* was published in 1944. The current version (5th ed., 2001, hereafter, APA Manual) has gained wide acceptance. Even many nonpsychological journals, including those of the American Speech-Language-Hearing Association (ASHA), use the APA format. Furthermore, most graduate programs require their students to write papers, theses, and dissertations according to an accepted format; in many behavioral and related disciplines, the APA format is the most frequently used.

The most common forms of journal articles include research reports or articles, review articles, and theoretical articles. Journals also may publish book reviews, commentaries, and other forms of papers. An original research study typically is written in the form of a report or an article. Reports have sections arranged in a fairly rigid format: *introduction, method, results, discussion,* and *references.*

A **review article** makes a critical assessment of published research in an area of investigation. Review articles are both integrative and evaluative. They point out research advances and summarize the state of the art. They highlight methodological and conceptual problems of past investigations and suggest questions for future research. The format of a review article is more flexible than that of a report because the article is organized according to the issues raised and data evaluated.

A **theoretical article** either presents a new theory or critically examines existing theories in an area of investigation. Theoretical articles, too, have flexible formats dictated by the nature and number of issues and theories.

Many journals also publish scholarly exchanges among authors. In some journals, such exchanges are published in the form of letters to the editor. The letters often are critical evaluations of articles published in recent issues of the same journal. The author of the original article usually writes a rebuttal. These exchanges do not have a fixed format, and they generally do not have subheadings.

Theses, projects, and **dissertations** have a fixed format, but academic departments and universities often have their own variations of a general format. The formats of these documents contain certain unique aspects, such as an approval page, a table of contents, and a copyright authorization page. However, the body of the text, references, figures, tables, and appendixes may be prepared according to one of the widely accepted publication styles, such as that of the APA.

A **research proposal** typically is not published. Research proposals are made to various government and private agencies that financially support research. Each agency has its own guidelines and formats within which the proposals should be prepared. Those who seek funds should strictly follow these formats and guidelines. Also, to demonstrate their knowledge of research methods and scientific writing style, graduate students taking seminars on research methods may be required to write a research proposal.

Writing a **technical report** on a piece of empirical research is the prototype of scientific writing. An investigator who can write an acceptable report generally can write other kinds of articles and proposals, with necessary modifications. Sections such as *introduction, review of literature,* and *discussion* are common to most types of scientific writing, so the goal here is to write a technical report of an empirical investigation according to the APA format. The topics to be discussed will follow the order required by the publication style.

Title Page

The title page contains the title of the article, the author's name and affiliation, and a running head. The title of an article should be brief and to the point. Long, wordy titles do not easily signal the essence of a paper and thus may fail to draw reader attention. It is best for the title to specify the experimental variables that were investigated. For example, the title *The Effect of Time-out on Stuttering* specifies both the dependent and the independent variable studied. The title is also direct, brief, and self-explanatory. The APA Manual recommends 10 to 12 words for a title.

The author's name is written on a separate line, starting with the first name, the middle initial, and last name. Words such as by or from are not added to the author's name. Titles and degrees also are omitted.

The name of the institution where the study was conducted is written on a separate line below the author's name. Typically, the name of the department in which the study was done is omitted. When the author is not affiliated with an institution, the author's city and state are specified below his or her name.

When the author has moved since the completion of the study, the new affiliation and the mailing address are written on a separate page under "author notes," and placed after the references. A journal, however, may print this information as a footnote on the first page.

An abbreviated version of the title is printed flush left at the top of each page, preceded by the term, *running head*. A still shorter version of the title is printed as a page header, followed by the page number. The page header and the page number are printed right-justified. The APA Manual limits the running head to 50 characters, including punctuation marks and spaces between words.

Abstract

Almost all kinds of scientific articles require an abstract, which is written on a separate page. A good abstract will attract the reader to the whole article whereas a bad one may turn the reader away. Therefore, it is important to write an abstract with an attractive style. The APA Manual requires the abstract to be accurate, self-contained, concise and specific, nonevaluative, and coherent and readable. It should highlight the problem investigated, the methods, the procedures, the results, and the main conclusions. An abstract may contain abbreviations with explanations (except in the case of standard, literal abbreviations such as *vs.*). To save space, it is written in active voice (but in the third person, without the personal pronouns *I* or *we*). All numbers except those that start a sentence should be written in digits. Quotations are typically avoided in abstracts. The APA Manual limits all abstracts to 120 words; however, theses and dissertations generally have longer abstracts.

Introduction

The text of the paper starts with an introductory section without a heading. This initial section of a paper introduces the reader to (a) the general area of investigation, (b) the general findings of past investigations, (c) the specific topic of the current investigation, (d) selected studies that have dealt with the topic in the past, (e) the problems and limitations of past studies, (f) some of the questions that remain to be answered, and (g) the specific problem or research questions investigated in the present study.

The opening sentence introduces the reader to the broad area of which the present investigation is a part. In most cases, the problem of the study is not stated at the outset. The reader is prepared for the problem by an initial description of the general area and the findings of the past studies. For example, if the investigation to be reported is about a particular language treatment procedure designed to teach specific morphological features, the introductory section may first make a few statements about research on language treatment in general, and some of the relevant studies and their results may be summarized or cited. The writer then introduces the specific topic that helps focus on the investigation. In the example, the research on teaching morphological features would be highlighted. Past studies that are especially relevant to the topic investigated may then be reviewed in some detail. Methods and procedures of selected studies on teaching morphological features would be reviewed. This review would be concerned mostly with the conceptual and methodological limitations of the past studies. The review would also point out the questions that are still in need of further research. Finally, the author brings the problem investigated into sharper focus. The introduction may end with a formal statement of the research problem or problems.

A well-written introduction moves from the general to the particular. The initial general framework helps the reader place the investigation in a proper theoretical, conceptual, and methodological perspective. With each additional paragraph, the writer takes the reader closer to the particular research question investigated. Meanwhile, the author also reviews the past studies in such a way as to justify the present investigation; a smoothly written introduction does not need a separate section called *rationale* or *justification*. The entire introductory section should make clear to the reader the need for the study and the reasoning behind it.

A critical part of the introduction is the review of the past studies. A well-written review justifies the study and sets the stage for it. The review may be critical, because in many cases, a study is undertaken because of the limitations of past studies. In some cases, the same question may have been researched, but inadequately. In other cases, a new method the author has used may be expected to prove more effective than previous methods in studying a phenomenon. In still other instances, the problem may not have been conceptualized at all in the manner of the investigation to be reported. Therefore, a critical analysis of the past research often justifies an investigation.

The critical review should be fair and objective. Its tone should not be judgmental, emotional, or polemical. Nevertheless, it should be direct. The limitations of past studies should be stated honestly and unambiguously; that is, the literature review should not be an exercise in diplomacy. Some investigators can write critical reviews more tactfully than others, but tact should never conceal valid criticisms that help advance the cause of knowledge.

The introduction to a direct or systematic replicative study does not involve much critical assessment of past studies and their methodologies. Direct replication studies need very brief introductions, mainly to justify the need for replication. Systematic replication studies do this and also describe the specific ways in which the present study is different from the original study.

The review of literature should point out the logical or empirical relation between the past studies and the present research. It should show how the study is built upon the past evidence and methodology. It is good to remember that a vast majority of research questions are hinted at or directly suggested by past studies. Knowledge is both continuous and evolving; utterly original studies are often the stuff the junior scientist's dreams are made of. Therefore, the past studies are not criticized to show that the present study is so original that it bears no relation to other studies or present knowledge. Instead, the review should show how the present study is conceptually and methodologically related to the past research while also pointing out its innovative aspects.

Toward the end of the introduction, the research question is formally stated. Hypotheses, if proposed, may be stated at this point. The research questions and hypotheses should be written in direct, clear, and terse language.

Method

The second section of a research article describes the method of the study. The method is described in detail so that a reader can evaluate its appropriateness to investigate the research questions. The description should be specific enough to permit a replication of the study by other investigators.

The method section of an empirical study has at least three subsections: *participants*, *apparatus* or *materials*, and the *procedure*. Additional headings may be used when necessary. For example, clinical treatment studies may describe the *pretreatment measures* or *baselines*, *treatment procedures*, and *probe* or other *posttreatment procedures* under separate headings. Reports of multiple experiments are also likely to have additional subsections.

Participants

The participant characteristics, number, and selection procedures are de-scribed in this subsection. Studies in communicative disorders describe the participants' age, gender, health, geographical location, family background, and communicative behaviors. In most cases, studies provide detailed in-formation on the participants' speech, language, voice, fluency, and hearing. Other relevant characteristics may be described.

The number of participants initially selected and the number who eventually completed the study should be specified. In a group design, the number of participants assigned to different groups also should be described.

The participant selection procedure should be described in detail. Was it a random sample? Were the participants selected simply because they happened to be available? Was the investigator trying to achieve a sample representative of the population? Were they clinical participants seeking professional services? Were there criteria by which potential participants were excluded from the study? How were the participants screened? These are some of the questions that are answered in describing the participant se-lection procedure.

Apparatus

In this section, the physical setting in which the study was carried out and the equipment and materials used are described. Institutions or places where the data were collected are described. In a treatment study, the clinic name and the room dimensions where the sessions were held also are described.

Instruments and materials that are commonly used in the discipline need not be described in detail. Their name, model number, and the manu-facturer should be specified, however. Instruments include standardized tests whose full names are given with references. Custom-made or rarely used instruments should be described in detail. If needed, drawings, photo-graphs, and additional descriptions may be given in an appendix.

Procedure

It should be noted that *procedure* is a subheading under *method*. Procedure refers to certain specific aspects of the method, which is a more general term. Details on how the study was implemented are given in the procedure section. The experimental design is described in this section although some-times it might take a separate heading. A commonly used experimental de-sign is simply mentioned by name, but an uncommon design may be de-scribed in greater detail. The design should be referenced by a book or an article that describes it.

Instructions given to the participants, how the variables were measured and manipulated, and the time schedules followed in completing the study are also described. How groups of participants were treated differently or how the separate conditions of an experiment differed from each other should be specified. Finally, how the reliability of the data was established should be described.

It is not possible here to specify everything that should be included under *procedure*. It is the author's responsibility to report all steps taken to complete a study. There should be a valid reason if something done in the study is not reported. The author can use the criterion of replicability in determining whether procedures were described in full. If by reading the article, another investigator can replicate the study, then the descriptions are adequate.

Results

This section opens with a brief statement of the problem investigated and the general findings of the study. An overview of the results is followed by a detailed presentation of the findings in quantitative and qualitative terms, and in graphic and tabular format.

In the results section, the findings are simply reported without interpretations and evaluations. Quantitative data may be presented concisely in tables. The changes noted in the dependent variables across experimental conditions are better represented graphically. Group design studies do not report individual data, but single-subject designs do. Tables and graphs should supplement, not duplicate, the text. Statistical tests are always reported in terms of their value, the probability level (significance level), and degrees of freedom when appropriate. The meaning of the obtained statistical value is also briefly stated.

The results section may have subheadings (e.g., Experiment 1, Experiment 2). It may also have subsections in which different kinds of data are reported (e.g., Treatment 1, Treatment 2). In organizing the results of a study, the student should consult the APA Manual and several exemplary articles published in the professional journal to which the author plans to submit the paper for publication.

Discussion

In the discussion section, the author points out the meaning and significance of the results. The section opens with a brief statement of the problem and the results of the study and proceeds to discuss the theoretical and applied implications of the findings. The results of the study are related to the findings of previous investigations. In this section, the problems and limitations of the study also may be pointed out, along with suggestions for further research.

A well-written discussion places the results of the study in the larger context of past research on the issue at hand. Ideally, a discussion is an integrative essay on the topic investigated, but it is written in light of the data generated by the study. The similarities between present and past findings are highlighted, as are the differences. When the results are consistent with past findings, the discussion will give a coherent, possibly advanced, picture of the phenomenon investigated. When the results contradict previous findings, the author may discuss possible reasons. Methodological problems and differences typically explain such contradictions.

The discussion should answer the research questions posed in the introductory section. The author should try to answer them as directly as possible. The answers may be positive or negative, but they should be stated clearly. Possibly, the author may say that the results failed to answer the questions. In any case, vagueness and hedging should be avoided. It is possible, though, that the results of a study do not support a strong and direct answer. In such cases, some authors prefer to be vague and tentative. Even then, a direct statement that the results were ambiguous is preferable to vagueness that leaves the reader confused.

Hypotheses, when proposed by the author, are supported or refuted in the discussion section. Clarity and directness are important here, too. Some authors may be reluctant to admit that their hypotheses were not supported by data, and the discussion may therefore be vague or distorted. There may be reasons to suspect the results, however. If so, the reasons may be clearly stated, along with better tests of the hypotheses. Even then, the author should state unambiguously that the results obtained did not support the hypotheses.

A common problem in many discussions is a labored effort to explain the results, especially when the results are unexpected from a particular view. Excessive speculation is the result. Such speculations are typically so far removed from the results that the discussion and the results seem almost disconnected. Why the results were the way they were is an interesting question, but it should not lead to unnecessary speculation. The best approach is to describe implications that are close to data. Obviously, data that cannot be explained need further study. Speculation will not explain them unless it is verified by additional experiments.

Single-Subject Studies and Multiple Experiments

Discussion of single-subject studies and those of multiple experiments is handled differently. In a single-subject study, a common discussion section is appropriate as long as the research questions and methods were common across the participants. However, sometimes a single-subject study may involve more than one experiment, each with single or multiple participants. The questions researched with various participants may be different though closely related. Such may be the case within a group study as well, and then it is better to write the discussion separately for each experiment. In this case, brief discussion follows the results of each experiment. However, at the end, a general discussion of the experiments taken as a whole is also needed. Different experiments are a part of a single study mainly because they are related in some conceptual and methodological manner; therefore, a common discussion is needed to suggest the significance of the results and their interrelation.

References

Within the body of a paper, references support statements the author makes about past investigations and the views of other authors. The authors and their works cited in the text are listed under the references. The reference list is placed after the discussion section.

The citations in the text and the reference list should match perfectly. There should be no citation in the text that is omitted from the reference list, and there should be no reference that is not cited in the text.

A reference list should not be confused with a bibliography. A reference list contains only those studies that are cited in an article. Studies not mentioned in the text, no matter how relevant, are not included in a reference list. A bibliography, on the other hand, is a comprehensive list of published studies on a particular topic or area of investigation. One can prepare a bibliography without writing an article, but a reference list is always a part of an article.

The APA Manual specifies the rules for citing references and arranging a reference list. The reader should consult the current edition of the manual for details.

Appendix

The use of appendixes increases the production cost of journals and books. Therefore, they should be included only when necessary. Appendixes provide information that cannot be integrated with the text. For example, a new test protocol, detailed description of a new equipment, and drawings of certain stimulus materials may be provided in an appendix.

Appendixes are used more frequently in dissertations, theses, and projects than in research articles. Raw data on individuals or groups of participants, instructions, papers relative to human participant protection, and details of statistical analyses may be placed in appendixes.

Following the APA Format

Authors in communicative disorders, including student writers in most educational and clinical programs, are expected to follow the APA format. The APA Manual should be studied carefully in preparing manuscripts. To begin with, the manual gives a brief description of the content and organization of manuscripts. In subsequent chapters, it gives comprehensive guidelines on the format of research articles. There are guidelines on punctuation, spelling, capitalization, use of italics, abbreviations, the arrangement of headings and subheadings, quotations, the use of numbers, the metric system, preparation of tables and figures, the reporting of statistical and mathematical formulas, footnotes and notes, reference citations, and reference lists. In addition, the manual also gives detailed instructions on how to type a manuscript.

The APA Manual will not be summarized here. Every author should have a copy for constant reference. In their preparation of reports, projects, and scientific articles, students need to refer repeatedly to the manual. Once the paper is written, the student should make sure that it conforms to the format. It is the author's responsibility to prepare the manuscript according to the manual.

Prescriptive formats are not intended to discourage interesting and unique writing styles. When a scientific article is boring, it is not because of the rigidity of the format, but because of a lack of style on the part of the author. Within an acceptable format, one can write with an interesting individual style. A mistaken assumption is that scientific writing should be devoid of individual style and that research reports should be necessarily monotonous and uninteresting.

This misconception is due to a confusion between lack of style and objectivity in scientific reporting. Scientific writing can have an attractive style while retaining objectivity. However, scientific writing style does have certain characteristics that may not be found in literary writings. Some of these differences will be discussed in later sections.

WRITING WITHOUT BIAS

Scientific writing is objective in that it is free from bias. It avoids words and expressions that unfavorably reflect on individuals and groups. Stereotypic and prejudicial expressions about genders, individuals, and ethnic groups are found often in everyday language. Inadvertently, they may be used by persons who do not necessarily share the implied sexism or racism. Nevertheless, such expressions are offensive and, therefore, inappropriate in everyday usage as well as in scientific writing. In their pursuit of knowledge, scientists are committed to fair treatment of individuals and groups of persons and must not use language that implies bias.

Among the biases that can creep into writing, racism and sexism are probably the most common. Racist expressions in describing participants and in exploring the meaning of research findings should be avoided. If it is necessary to identify participants as belonging to particular ethnic or cultural groups, terms that are nonevaluative should be used. The best practice is to select the terms the groups use to refer to themselves in formal writings and discussions.

Such expressions as *culturally deprived* or *disadvantaged* have a pseudoscientific connotation, but they are also biased. They imply that one culture is the standard against which other cultures are evaluated. For example, in communicative disorders, the expression *standard English* is often contrasted with *Black English;* this expression implies that the language spoken by one group is the standard by which the language spoken by the other group is judged. Another mistake made by many writers is to describe foreign languages they know very little about as *dialects.*

Many expressions that imply sexism are a part of long-established traditions of language usage, and therefore, they may not be easily recognized as sexist. One of the most inappropriately used personal pronouns is *he.* It is often used to refer to any child, student, customer, or client. Indiscriminate use of male personal pronouns may imply that all executives, doctors, nurses, firefighters, engineers, supervisors, department heads, garbage collectors, or professors are male. Another frequently misused pronoun that implies sexism is *man.* It is *man* who searches for knowledge, achieves great things, provides the work force. It is *mankind* that experiences great problems or solves those problems. In cases such as these, other terms, including *human beings, people, persons, humanity,* and *humankind* are appropriate. (See Hegde [2003] for additional examples.)

Besides implying bias, indiscriminate use of certain words may create ambiguity. The word *men,* for example, cannot be used to refer to people of both genders; *men* can only refer to male persons. In other words, a term should be chosen for its particular relevance, not because of habitual usage. This will help writers avoid both bias and ambiguity.

The APA Manual has additional guidelines for describing clinical populations and research participants. According to these guidelines, in descriptions of people with disabilities, "person-first" language must be used; for example, the phrase *a person who stutters* is preferable to the term *stutterer.* Furthermore, in reporting empirical studies, the classic term *subject* should be replaced with *participant* because the latter suggests that participants play an active role. The APA Manual contains guidelines on writing without bias and ambiguity (see Chapter 2 in the 5th edition). The American Speech-Language-Hearing Association has adopted similar guidelines. The student should consult the current APA Manual for details.

GOOD WRITING: SOME PRINCIPLES

A format of research articles, such as the one discussed earlier, may not necessarily ensure good writing. Scientific writing should be good writing, and it also should adhere to an accepted format. Good writing involves an understanding of both structural principles and conceptual considerations.

Structural Principles

Grammar specifies the structural principles of language. The term *grammar* includes the morphological as well as the syntactical aspects of language. In addition, one also should consider punctuation. Minimally, good writing is grammatically correct. It is not possible to specify all the rules of grammar here; the student should consult a good source on grammar. Many books on writing include basic information on grammar and correct usage. The student should have one or two such books for permanent reference (Baker, 1981; Bates, 1980; Hargis, 1984; Hegde, 2003; Kane, 1988; Kirszner & Mandell, 1992; McWhorter, 1993; Streng, 1972; Turabian, 1996; Zinsser, 1990).

Grammar and usage are two closely related but separate matters. Grammar is a collection of finite and fixed rules, whereas usage is a matter of change and diversity. Grammatical rules are not empirical, but usage always is. How people talk and write and what kinds of changes they thus force in their language are a matter of usage. Scholars are concerned with usage for several reasons. In some cases, popular usage may violate the rules of grammar. In other cases, popular usage may be grammatically correct but not effective, direct, clear, or concise. Generally, popular usage forces changes in language mostly at the level of vocabulary, syntax, idiom, and expression. These changes may promote or hinder direct communication in writing or speaking. Therefore, the writer should be aware of the past and present usage of language.

There are excellent books on the contemporary usage of the English language. Although to write correctly, one needs books on grammar, to write more creatively and effectively, one needs books on usage and writing that go beyond the basics of grammar. The writer should consult the current editions of such excellent sources as *Modern American Usage* by Follett (1998), the *New Oxford Guide to Writing* by Kane (1988), and the *Harper Dictionary of Contemporary Usage* by Morris and Morris (1985). *The Elements of Style* by Strunk and White (1979) is a classic, and every writer should have a copy of this book. Written with a great sense of humor, *A Civil Tongue* by Newman (1976) is a delightful book on the contemporary misuse of American English. Some of these books are periodically revised.

Though it is not the purpose here to review rules of grammar, it is necessary to point out a few common problems that should be avoided in writing research papers. There also are some guidelines that are not a matter of correct or incorrect grammar but rather of preference.

Sentence Structure

By definition, a sentence is grammatical: It is correct and complete. Therefore, the writer should avoid sentence fragments that result from a lack of certain grammatical features or inappropriate punctuation.

Missing grammatical features create sentence fragments of the following kind:

> ⮚ **Incorrect:** The group was scheduled to come to the laboratory on Monday. But got there on Tuesday. (The subject is missing from the second sentence, making it a fragment.)

> ⮚ **Revised:** The group was scheduled to come to the laboratory on Monday but got there on Tuesday.

> ⮚ **Incorrect:** The author finally found the participants. In the Psychology 10 class. (The fragment has no verb.)

> ⮚ **Revised:** The author finally found the participants in the Psychology 10 class.

Many problems arise when punctuation marks are used to break strings of words at inappropriate junctures. For example, a subordinate clause, which needs an independent clause, should not be punctuated as a sentence:

> ⮚ **Incorrect:** The testing was completed in two sessions. Because the instrument broke down. (The subordinate clause is punctuated as a sentence.)

> ⮚ **Revised:** The testing was completed in two sessions because the instrument broke down.

Similar problems arise when a prepositional phrase, a verbal phrase, an absolute phrase, an appositive, a compound sentence, or an incomplete clause is punctuated as a sentence. None of these can stand alone as sentences. An example of each illustrates these problems:

> ⮚ **Incorrect:** The dysfluency rate decreased dramatically. In the final two sessions. (The prepositional phrase is punctuated as a sentence.)

> ⮚ **Revised:** The dysfluency rate decreased dramatically in the final two sessions.

> ⮚ **Incorrect:** The experiment had 50 participants. Divided into two groups. (The participial phrase, a type of verbal phrase, is punctuated as a sentence.)

⮑ **Revised:** The experiment had 50 participants. They were divided into two groups.

⮑ **Incorrect:** The participants were eight men. Their speech characterizing severe stuttering. (The absolute phrase is punctuated as a sentence.)

⮑ **Revised:** The participants were eight men. Their speech was characterized by severe stuttering.

⮑ **Incorrect:** The participants were tested in a sound-treated room. A room that was especially built for the experiment. (The appositive is punctuated as a sentence.)

⮑ **Revised:** The participants were tested in a sound-treated room, a room that was especially built for the experiment.

⮑ **Incorrect:** Many patients with aphasia have word-finding problems. And may also find it difficult to remember names. (The second part of the compound sentence is punctuated as a separate sentence.)

⮑ **Revised:** Many patients with aphasia have word-finding problems and may also find it difficult to remember names.

⮑ **Incorrect:** Regulated breathing, a highly researched technique known for its effectiveness with young children who stutter, which is developed by Azrin and associates. (The subject, regulated breathing, has no predicate.)

⮑ **Revised:** Regulated breathing, a highly researched technique known for its effectiveness with young children who stutter, was developed by Azrin and associates.

Many grammatically incorrect sentences can be rewritten in different ways because the same idea can be expressed in different forms. Therefore, the revised versions of incorrect sentences that are given here are only illustrative.

Generally, the longer the sentence, the easier it is to make a mistake in its structure and the harder it is to find the missing element or confusing feature. Shorter, simpler sentences are preferable because they reveal their problems somewhat easily. Such sentences also are easy to understand. However, many times transition words (e.g., *but, so, or*) that show relations between thoughts and sentences prevent ambiguity and keep the text from seeming fragmented.

Verbs

It is preferable to use verbs in their active voice. Active voice is more direct and emphatic than passive voice. Active voice is also brief.

> ⮑ **Passive:** The children were brought to the clinic by their mothers.

> ⮑ **Revised:** The mothers brought their children to the clinic.

However, passive voice may be preferable when the agent of an action is unimportant or unknown:

> ⮑ **Correct:** An increased prevalence of stuttering in the female population was reported in the literature.

Most scientific papers are written in the past tense. Reports of empirical studies review past studies and describe a completed study. Therefore, the review, the methods, and the results are reported in the past tense:

> ⮑ **Correct:** Smith (1985) reported similar findings.

> ⮑ **Correct:** Ten adults who stutter were selected.

> ⮑ **Correct:** The scores of male and female participants were the same.

When reporting something that began in the past and continues into the present, the present perfect tense is used:

> ⮑ **Incorrect:** Since the invention of the tape recorder, nearly all audiologists used it.

> ⮑ **Revised:** Since the invention of the tape recorder, nearly all audiologists have used it.

> ⮑ **Incorrect:** Over the years, many scientists replicated Piaget's results.

> ⮑ **Revised:** Over the years, many scientists have replicated Piaget's results.

It is preferable to write the discussion section in the present tense:

> ⮑ **Correct:** The data suggest a need for further research.

> ⮑ **Correct:** The result shows that it is better to use both the treatment procedures.

> ⊋ **Correct:** One conclusion of the study is that reduced rate of speech affects the frequency of dysfluencies.

Agreement

Agreement between various elements of a sentence is one of the critical tests of grammatically correct sentences. Mistakes often are made in this case. Subjects and verbs must agree in number and person, whereas pronouns and their antecedents must agree in number, person, and gender. See Hegde (2003) for more examples.

Singular subjects take singular verbs and plural subjects take plural verbs:

> ⊋ **Correct:** The result is questionable.

> ⊋ **Correct:** The results are reliable.

In simple and direct sentences, it is easy to see a mistake in subject–verb agreement that may be less conspicuous in complex sentences. Mistakes are likely when intervening phrases are included in a sentence:

> ⊋ **Incorrect:** This result, also reported by many past investigators, are not consistent with the theory.

> ⊋ **Revised:** This result, also reported by many past investigators, is not consistent with the theory.

> ⊋ **Incorrect:** These techniques, when used appropriately by a competent clinician, is known to be effective.

> ⊋ **Revised:** These techniques, when used appropriately by a competent clinician, are known to be effective.

Intervening phrases such as *as well as, along with, in addition to, including,* and *together with* do not change the number of the subject:

> ⊋ **Incorrect:** The accuracy of phoneme productions as well as the rate of correct responses increase during treatment.

> ⊋ **Revised:** The accuracy of phoneme productions as well as the rate of correct responses increases during treatment.

> ⊋ **Incorrect:** Error scores, along with the correct score, was used in the analysis.

> ⊋ **Revised:** Error scores, along with the correct score, were used in the analysis.

Generally, compound subjects joined by *and* have plural verbs (e.g., Mother *and* child *were* interviewed together). Exceptions are when an expression, though containing *and*, suggests a single concept or individual:

> ⊇ **Correct:** Who says country *and* western *is* dead?

> ⊇ **Correct:** The president *and* chief executive officer *is* Mr. Smith.

Additionally, a singular verb is used when *each* or *every* precedes a compound subject joined by *and:*

> ⊇ **Correct:** *Each* test and measurement procedure *was* pilot-tested.

> ⊇ **Correct:** *Every* child and adult *goes* through the same procedure.

When two subjects are linked by *or, either/or,* or *neither/nor,* the verb should be plural if both subjects are plural and singular if both subjects are singular:

> ⊇ **Correct:** *Either* verbal praise or informative feedback *is* combined with modeling.

> ⊇ **Correct:** *Either* verbal reinforcers or tokens *are* combined with modeling.

However, when a singular and a plural subject are linked by *neither/nor, either/or,* or *not only/but also,* the verb form is determined by the subject that is nearer to it:

> ⊇ **Incorrect:** Neither the treatments nor the *result are* replicable.

> ⊇ **Revised:** Neither the treatments nor the *result is* replicable.

> ⊇ **Revised:** Neither the treatment nor the *results are* replicable.

> ⊇ **Incorrect:** Not only the instruments but also the *procedure are* described.

> ⊇ **Revised:** Not only the instruments but also the *procedure is* described.

> ⊇ **Revised:** Not only the instrument but also the *procedures are* described.

A few indefinite pronouns (*both, many, several, few, others*) are always plural and therefore take plural verbs.

> ⊇ **Correct:** Both of us are busy.

> ⊇ **Correct:** Only a few were interested.

Most other indefinite pronouns (*another, anyone, everyone, each, either, neither, anything, everything, something,* and *somebody*) are singular and therefore take a singular verb:

> ⊇ **Correct:** Anyone is acceptable, providing the participant selection criteria are met.

> ⊇ **Correct:** Something was missing in that procedure.

> ⊇ **Correct:** Everything is fine.

> ⊇ **Correct:** Either of them is acceptable.

However, some indefinite pronouns such as *some, all, none, any, more,* and *most* can be singular or plural. The verb form is singular or plural depending on the noun the pronoun refers to:

> ⊇ **Correct:** None of the *participants were* pretested.

> ⊇ **Correct:** None of the *techniques were* correct.

> ⊇ **Correct:** Some of this *effect is* understandable.

> ⊇ **Correct:** Some of the *techniques are* useless.

Collective nouns also take singular or plural verbs. A collective noun that refers to a single unit takes a singular verb; one that refers to individuals or elements of that unit takes a plural verb:

> ⊇ **Singular:** The *group was* tested in a single session.

> ⊇ **Singular:** The *number* of participants *was* small.

> ⊇ **Plural:** The *members* of the control group *were* tested separately.

> ⊇ **Plural:** A number of *participants were* absent.

As a general rule, *the number* is singular, *a number* is plural. But phrases that refer to fixed quantities (*majority, three quarters*) are collective nouns:

> ⊇ **Singular:** *The majority was* against the idea.

> ⊇ **Plural:** *A majority* of people *were* against the idea.

> ⊇ **Singular:** *Three quarters* of the amount *is* withheld.

> ⊇ **Plural:** *Three quarters of those* completing the treatment *improve* significantly.

Some subjects that are typically in the plural form still take singular verbs:

❯ **Correct:** The *news is* bad.

❯ **Correct:** *Statistics is* but one method of data analysis.

❯ **Correct:** *Economics is* not an exact science.

❯ **Correct:** *Politics does* not thrill me.

However, when words like *statistics* refer not to a *set* of techniques but to certain *data*, a plural verb is appropriate:

❯ **Correct:** The *statistics show* that the treatment of aphasia is successful.

Certain nouns have unusual plural forms and should not be used with singular verbs:

❯ **Plural:** The baseline *data were* recorded on a separate sheet.

❯ **Singular:** The *datum* is as solid as it can be.

❯ **Plural:** Similar *phenomena were* observed by several scientists.

❯ **Singular:** The same *phenomenon was* reported by other scientists.

❯ **Plural:** The *loci* of stuttering *were* studied by Brown.

❯ **Singular:** The *locus* of response control *was* shifted.

❯ **Singular:** The *thesis was* completed on time.

❯ **Plural:** The *theses were* too long.

In popular writing, *data* may be treated as singular. The singular form, *datum*, is rarely used for this reason. In scientific writing, however, *data* is always plural. A few other words have dual plural forms, though one of them may be preferred. For example, *appendices* and *appendixes* are the two plural forms of *appendix*, but *appendixes* is the preferred form. Similarly, both *indices* and *indexes* are acceptable plural forms of *index*, but *indexes* is preferred.

In using a linking verb, it is important to make sure that the verb agrees with its subject. A typical mistake is to make the verbs agree with the subject complement.

❯ **Incorrect:** The problem were the instruments.

❯ **Revised:** The problem was the instruments.

Correct Use of Modifiers

Modifiers connect ideas while adding information. In a sentence, the word or phrase to which a modifier refers should be clear. A *misplaced modifier* (an adjective or an adverb) refers to a wrong word or phrase in a sentence. A *dangling modifier* does not modify any word or phrase in a sentence.

Misplaced modifiers confuse the reader by not specifying which word or group of words is being modified (Hegde, 2003). This is more likely to happen when the words that are modified and the modifiers are too far apart.

> **Incorrect:** The author and her assistants tested the hearing of all participants using the procedure described earlier. (Who used the procedure?)

> **Revised:** The author and her assistants, using the procedure described earlier, tested the hearing of all participants.

> **Revised:** Using the procedure described earlier, the author and her assistants tested the hearing of all participants.

> **Incorrect:** Distant and mysterious, he stared at the sky. (Who or what is distant and mysterious?)

> **Revised:** He stared at the sky, distant and mysterious. (The sky is distant and mysterious.)

Generally, it is better to place modifiers immediately before or after the words or phrases that are modified. Certain modifiers (*only, hardly, simply*) should be placed before the words they modify. Different placements will change the meaning of sentences:

> **Incorrect:** The past studies *only offer* limited solutions to this problem.

> **Revised:** The past studies *offer only* limited solutions to this problem.

> **Incorrect:** The male participants scored a mean of 23.9, but the female participants scored *only a mean* of 14.6.

> **Revised:** The male participants scored a mean of 23.9, but the female participants scored a *mean of only 14.6*.

> **Incorrect:** The implications *are simply* not clear.

> **Revised:** The implications *simply are* not clear.

⮕ **Incorrect:** The results *hardly are* impressive.

⮕ **Revised:** The results *are hardly* impressive.

Sentences with dangling modifiers should be rewritten to include words or phrases that are indeed modified:

⮕ **Incorrect:** Several additional effects are observed *using this technique*. (The modifier has no reference in the sentence.)

⮕ **Revised:** Several additional effects are observed in *clients* using this technique.

⮕ **Revised:** Several additional effects are observed when *therapists* use this technique.

⮕ **Incorrect:** Using the standard procedure, the participants were screened for hearing problems by the experimenter.

⮕ **Revised:** Using the standard procedure, the experimenter screened the participants for hearing problems. (The experimenter, not the participants, used the standard procedure.)

⮕ **Incorrect:** Consistent with past studies, Johnson and Williams (1985) found that their female participants performed better than the male participants.

⮕ **Revised:** Johnson and Williams (1985) found that their female participants performed better than the male participants. This result is consistent with that of past studies. (The result, not Johnson and Williams, is consistent with past studies.)

Parallel Forms

Sentences expressing parallel ideas can be especially troublesome. Parallel ideas should be expressed in the same grammatical form: words, phrases, clauses, or sentences (Hegde, 2003). Parallel forms are used for emphasis, clarity, and variety. Such forms help maintain continuity of ideas. When used judiciously, parallel forms add force to writing. They also facilitate conciseness. Many parallel forms require a careful use of coordinating conjunctions: *and, but, or,* and *nor.*

⮕ **Correct:** The author studied books, charts, and tables.

⮕ **Correct:** The clients found the procedure complex but useful.

⮞ **Correct:** The experimental participants were either adults or children.

⮞ **Correct:** The responses were neither correct nor adequate.

Parallel forms are necessary in expressing paired ideas:

⮞ **Correct:** His comment was brief but forceful.

⮞ **Correct:** Stuttering is aversive, but silence is painful.

⮞ **Correct:** The research was concerned with immediate generalization and subsequent maintenance.

⮞ **Correct:** The more patients you treat, the more you learn.

⮞ **Correct:** The treatment phase was over; the maintenance phase was beginning.

Parallel forms also can help highlight contrast or opposition between paired elements in a sentence:

⮞ **Correct:** It is better to treat stuttering children than to merely counsel the parents.

⮞ **Correct:** Establishing target behaviors is easier than making them last.

Several mistakes result in faulty parallelism. A common mistake is to write the different terms of a parallel construction in different terms:

⮞ **Incorrect:** Many people who stutter have suffered because their therapists lacked adequate training, supervised experience, and *the therapists' knowledge of stuttering has been limited.* (The final element in the list is not parallel.)

⮞ **Revised:** Many people who stutter have suffered because their therapists lacked training, supervised experience, and *scientific knowledge of stuttering.* (Parallelism is restored.)

Another mistake is a failure to repeat a parallel element in a series that signals the parallelism. The result is a broken pattern. Such sentences should be revised to restore parallelism:

⮞ **Incorrect:** Persons with communicative disabilities have difficulty talking, reading, and *self-confidence.* (The final element is not parallel with the previous elements.)

⮞ **Revised:** Persons with communicative disabilities have difficulty *talking*, *reading*, and *maintaining* self-confidence. (All three elements are parallel.)

➜ **Incorrect:** Some of the side effects of punishment are aggression, emotionality, and the *client may also learn to punish others.* (The last element causes mixed construction.)

➜ **Revised:** Some of the side effects of punishment are *aggression, emotionality,* and *imitative punishment.* (Parallelism is restored.)

➜ **Incorrect:** Differential reinforcement helps maintenance by *not* allowing a rapid extinction, increasing the response strength, and improving the chances for generalization. (*Not* does not apply to all the elements in the series.)

➜ **Revised:** Differential reinforcement helps maintenance by not allowing a rapid extinction, by increasing the response strength, *and* by improving the chances of generalization. (The preposition *by* is repeated to prevent confusion between the elements in the series.)

➜ **Incorrect:** Regulated breathing, developed by Azrin and associates (1975), *which* was researched by many other investigators, is known to be effective.

➜ **Revised:** Regulated breathing, *which* was developed by Azrin and associates (1975), and *which* was researched by many other investigators, is known to be effective.

Shifts Within and Between Sentences

Sentences and paragraphs must be consistent in tense, voice, mood, person, and number. Wrong or unnecessary shifts in them confuse the reader:

➜ **Incorrect:** The therapist *told* the client that she would not take him to outside situations unless he *maintains* fluency in the clinic. (There is a shift in the tense.)

➜ **Revised:** The therapist *told* the client that she would not take him to outside situations unless he *maintained* fluency in the clinic.

➜ **Incorrect:** The clinician *was* well trained. She *knows* how to treat a variety of communicative disorders. Nevertheless, she *had* difficulty treating this particular client. (There is a shift in tense between the sentences.)

➜ **Revised:** The clinician *was* well trained. She *knew* how to treat a variety of communicative disorders. Nevertheless, she *had* difficulty in treating this particular client.

⇒ **Incorrect:** Van Riper first *developed* cancellation and later pull-outs *were* also developed. (There is a shift from the active to the passive voice. Who developed pull-outs?)

⇒ **Revised:** Van Riper first *developed* cancellation and later *developed* pull-outs.

⇒ **Incorrect:** It is important that a client *possess* a tape recorder and *uses* it regularly to record speech. (There is a shift from subjunctive to indicative mood.)

⇒ **Revised:** It is important that a client *possess* a tape recorder and *use* it regularly to record speech.

⇒ **Incorrect:** When *one* is reviewing the literature, *you* find that not many studies have been done on the issue. (There is a shift from second to third person.)

⇒ **Revised:** When *one* is reviewing the literature, *one* finds that not many studies have been done on the issue. ("A review of the literature shows that not many studies have been done on the issue" is probably preferable to either sentence.)

⇒ **Incorrect:** If a *client* does not attend at least 90% of the treatment sessions, *they* will not show significant improvement. (There is a shift in number.)

⇒ **Revised:** If a *client* does not attend at least 90% of the treatment sessions, *he* or *she* will not show significant improvement.

Punctuation

The student writer should consult a good source such as *The Holt Handbook* (Kirszner & Mandell, 1992) for a complete discussion of punctuation and mechanics. The APA Manual and other sources (Hegde, 2003) cover the basic information on the correct use of the period, the comma, the semicolon, the colon, the dash, quotation marks, parentheses, and brackets. The student should learn to correctly use these elements of punctuation.

Other Structural Matters

The student should be familiar with other structural matters the APA Manual specifies. It has sections on capitalization, italics, abbreviations, headings and series within a manuscript, quotations, numbers, metrication, tables, figures, reference citation, reference lists, and so on. In writing scientific papers, the student should adhere to the recommendations made in the manual.

Conceptual Considerations

A mastery of the principles of grammar, punctuation, and related matters will help the writer organize a piece of writing. Those principles are matters of structure necessary for correct and acceptable expressions. However, a mastery of those principles may not necessarily assure concise, adequate, clear, and coherent writing. In spite of a good command of the structural principles, a writer may find it difficult to write well. Such a difficulty typically is the result of conceptual, rather than structural, problems.

While most principles that govern matters of structure may be specified, conceptual matters can be discussed only in general terms. There are no finite and explicit rules that dictate conciseness, comprehensiveness, clarity, and coherence. These parameters of writing are often judged by a reader's response to a piece of writing. The writing is not concise if unnecessary words and expressions distract readers. The writing is not adequate if readers think that some information is missing. The writing is not clear if readers are not sure what is said. Finally, the writing is not coherent if readers become confused. Good writing is effective. Therefore, good writing is often judged by its effects on the reader.

Knowledge of the Readership

A knowledge of the readership can help one write effectively. A main difficulty of writing is that the author knows what he or she wishes to say even without writing it out, but the reader does not know. Therefore, even if his or her writing is deficient, the author will have no difficulty understanding it. Unfortunately, what is perfectly clear to the author may be ambiguous to the reader.

The writer should read his or her writing from the viewpoint of the reader. The writer should judge whether a reader *without* the knowledge of what is being said can understand the material. This skill in reading one's own writing from the viewpoint of a naive reader is important for all writers.

The author should know the educational level of the readership. The extent of a readership's technical sophistication will determine the overall writing style, the number of examples given, and the amount of elaboration. Successful writers always know who their audience is and adjust their writing accordingly.

Concise Writing

Many first drafts are too long. Therefore, conciseness should be the main target for the second draft. If new sentences should be added, the writer should see whether a comparable number of sentences can be deleted. Long papers tend to be wordy, clumsy, redundant, and indirect. The writer can usually cut the number of words, phrases, and sentences to make a piece more readable. It is best to read what you have written with the assumption that the length as well as the number of sentences can be cut.

The writer should examine every sentence and judge whether it is necessary and whether it can be shortened. The meaning of a sentence should be understood by the reader at the first reading. A sentence that must be reread to be understood is probably too long, clumsy, or ambiguous. Shortening it may help achieve effective as well as concise communication. Some experts suggest that the average sentence length should be 20 or fewer words (Bates, 1982). Most readers prefer shorter to longer sentences. Therefore, other factors being equal, the author is more likely to hold the reader's attention with shorter sentences than with longer ones.

Neither the sentence length nor the type should be monotonously uniform, however. There should be a balance between shorter and longer sentences. Also, not all long sentences are necessarily difficult to understand; some longer sentences can be made more readable by breaking them up with chunking devices such as semicolons and dashes. Other longer sentences can be clear and direct without such devices. Longer sentences are sometimes necessary to express a complex concept. Also, when longer sentences are used sparingly and mixed with shorter ones, the reading becomes less monotonous.

Simple, active, declarative sentences are typically short and direct, but they can be dull, too. Therefore, an interesting piece of writing usually has a mixture of different types of sentences. Some sentence types, such as those using the passive voice, generally tend to be longer than other types. A shorter sentence type should be preferred as long as it is just as effective as the longer type.

Writing is not concise when it is redundant and wordy. Saying the same thing in different ways is sometimes necessary in teaching a difficult concept. However, when it seems necessary, the writer should check whether the clarity of the first statement can be improved. If a statement can be tightened up, a subsequent redundant statement can be avoided.

A typical redundancy is a result of saying the same thing in both positive and negative ways:

> The female participants generally performed better on the experimental task, and the male participants' performance was inferior to that of the female participants.

The second clause says in negative terms what the first clause says in positive terms. One of them is unnecessary, and most experts prefer the positive sentence forms.

Some of the warning signs of potentially redundant statements are phrases such as *in other words, to put it differently, to repeat,* and *to reiterate.* What follows such phrases or clauses can be redundant, although in some kinds of writing (such as in textbooks), such repetition serves a teaching purpose.

Some redundancy in talking and writing is necessary to facilitate a proper understanding of complex materials. In scientific articles and books, summaries and abstracts repeat what has been elaborated in the body of the text. Readers are better able to focus on the text when they are given the gist of the material at the very beginning. A summary at the end may help readers remember the main points of the text; such devices that reinforce a reader's understanding are not redundant.

Wordiness results when words that do not add any meaning at all are used in a sentence (Hegde, 2003). Needless words and phrases and circumlocution cause wordiness. The result is an unnecessarily long sentence:

> **Wordy:** It seemed to the author that it is important to consider many factors in selecting a specific design for the study.

> **Revised:** Many factors were considered in selecting a design for the study.

In many cases, phrases such as *who were (are)*, *which were (are)*, *that is*, and *there were (are)* can be eliminated:

> **Wordy:** Eighteen persons *who were* living in rural areas were participants.

> **Revised:** Eighteen persons living in rural areas were participants.

> **Wordy:** Two instruments, *which were* in good calibration, were used in the study.

> **Revised:** Two instruments in good calibration were used in the study.

> **Wordy:** The study *that is* well known was done by Smith (1980).

> **Revised:** The Smith (1980) study is well known. Or, Smith's 1980 study is well known.

> **Wordy:** *There were* several factors that prompted the selection of only the male participants.

> **Revised:** Several factors prompted the selection of only the male participants.

Many standard phrases often used to initiate sentences can also be eliminated:

> **Wordy:** As far as the results are concerned, they appear reliable.

> **Revised:** The results appear reliable.

> **Wordy:** *For all intents and purposes*, the two treatment techniques are similar.

> **Revised:** The two treatment techniques are similar.

> **Wordy:** *With reference to* the Smith (1980) study, the methods were appropriate.

> **Revised:** The methods of the Smith (1980) study were appropriate. Or, Smith's (1980) methods were appropriate.

> **Wordy:** *In terms of its effects*, the treatment was good.

> **Revised:** The treatment was effective.

Many words used as fillers are known as *utility* words (Kirszner & Mandell, 1992). Often, they are unnecessary:

> **Wordy:** It was *actually* a good study, but it did not produce worthwhile data.

> **Revised:** It was a good study, but it did not produce worthwhile data.

> **Wordy:** The deteriorating response *situation* was a problem.

> **Revised:** Response deterioration was a problem.

Certain needlessly wordy, though popular, phrases should be replaced with single words or shorter phrases:

due to the fact that	because
in spite of the fact that	though
on account of the fact that	because
at the present time	now
at this point in time	now
until such time as	until
used for the purposes of	used to (for)
the question as to whether	whether
have the ability to	be able to
hands on experience	experience
in the event that	if
by means of	by

See Hegde (2003) for additional examples of wordiness and means of revising them.

Certain other, longer, phrases include words with overlapping meanings. Such phrases can be reduced to single words or shorter phrases:

future prospects	prospects
advance planning	planning
absolutely incomplete	incomplete
exactly identical	identical
repeat again	repeat
each and every	each *or* every
totally unique	unique
uniquely one of a kind	one of a kind (*or* unique)
reality as it is	reality
solid (*or* actual *or* true) facts	facts
famous and well known	*either* famous *or* well known
goals and objectives	goals *or* objectives
three different kinds	three kinds

See Hegde (2003) for additional examples of redundant writing and means of correcting them.

Although concise writing is a virtue, writing that is too concise can pose problems for the reader. Depending on the readership, some elaboration is necessary; that is, sometimes the same thing needs to be said differently. Examples duplicate what is said otherwise, but they are essential in any kind of writing. Therefore, conciseness should not supersede the purpose of effective communication. The final criterion is economical as well as effective communication.

Conciseness is an issue of degree, and different types of writing require various degrees of conciseness. Journal articles are written for specialists with technical knowledge and therefore are concise. Books are written for readers with different levels of formal and informal education and, therefore, have a greater range of style than journal articles. Theses, dissertations, term papers, and other pieces of writing that are expected to demonstrate a writer's knowledge of an area are more comprehensive than concise. Details are expected in these writings so that the knowledge of the writer can be evaluated. Though the instructor who evaluates the writing "knows what the student is talking about," the student should still furnish the details necessary for an evaluation.

Adequate Writing

Most books on writing do not emphasize adequacy. The typical mistake made by an established writer is to write too much rather than too little;

therefore, books on writing tend to emphasize conciseness. On the other hand, beginning writers, especially student writers, tend to write too little rather than too much. Essay answers at the undergraduate and graduate levels are often overly restricted, and important information is often missing in such restricted writings. The first drafts of theses and projects tend to omit necessary details, so many graduate students are asked to expand their first drafts to include various details.

Inadequate writing is as problematic as excessive writing. In scientific reports, theses, and essay examinations, the writing should be adequate. These pieces of writing are evaluated by other individuals. Those who read essay answers should judge whether the student knows the information requested. Inadequate answers are taken to represent inadequate knowledge. Students often complain that, although they knew the material, they did not write all they knew; however, it is the students' *writing*, not their knowledge, that the instructor has access to. Therefore, answers should be adequate.

Scientific reports, including theses and dissertations, also are evaluated by other individuals. This evaluation is done to find out, among other things, if the procedures used were appropriate to answer the research questions and whether the results were reliable. To make this evaluation, the reader should have sufficient details about the procedures, results, and methods of analysis. The reader also should have enough background information. An adequate overview of past research should be available in a report. Omission of significant details makes it difficult to evaluate the significance of a study.

Inadequate writing is one of the main reasons why certain scientific reports cannot be replicated. Insufficient information on the types of participants used, experimental manipulations, independent and dependent variables, and control procedures can make replication difficult for other investigators.

Clear Writing

Clear writing is important in both science and everyday life. When there is no clarity, there is no communication. Much worse, there may be serious misunderstanding. Clear writing cannot be achieved by doing just one thing right. Several factors contribute to clarity. To write clearly, the author should avoid ambiguity, euphemism, jargon, clichés, colloquial expressions, and dead metaphors and similes. At the same time, the author should use the right words and exercise care in the use of abstract versus concrete words and figures of speech.

Ambiguity results from many structural problems of the kind discussed in some of the previous sections. For example, misplaced and dangling modifiers, faulty parallelism, inappropriate shifts within and between sentences, and wrong punctuation can make the meaning of sentences unclear. Structural accuracy, combined with directness and simplicity, will reduce ambiguity.

Unclear writing also may result from words and phrases that, for many reasons, do not convey the precise meaning to the reader. Euphemisms, clichés, colloquial expressions, and ineffective figures of speech are some the reasons for this lack of precision.

Avoid Euphemisms. Euphemisms are neutral or positive-sounding expressions that replace expressions with negative connotations. Several euphemistic expressions have become a part of everyday language. Children with mental retardation are *exceptional children*, poor people are *disadvantaged*, and older persons are *senior citizens*. Failing students are not dismissed but *counseled out*, and a student is not asked to retake an examination but is *given another opportunity to demonstrate knowledge*. Such euphemistic expressions hamper clarity.

Technical-sounding euphemisms can distort meaning in scientific reports. Instead of saying that some speech clinicians do not like to treat people who stutter because of lack of training, one may say that the treatment of stuttering is negatively affected by some clinicians' unfavorable attitude toward people who stutter. It is difficult to determine the meaning of this sentence, but it could possibly be that *the negatively affected treatment* is ineffective treatment, and *the clinicians' unfavorable attitude* may be a euphemistic reference to clinicians' inadequate training or incompetence. Intellectual honesty is an important aspect of scientific writing. Euphemism is anything but intellectual honesty and therefore has no place in scientific writing.

Avoid Jargon. *Jargon* is defined as the technical or specialized terms of a particular discipline as well as useless and incomprehensible vocabulary. Scientific reports cannot be written without technical terms. Technical terms are often preferable to lay terms because of the latter's imprecise and varied connotations. Therefore, jargon, in the sense of technical and specialized terms, cannot be altogether avoided in scientific writing. However, when a scientist or a professional writes for the general public, extra care should be taken in the selection of words. Technical words should be used most sparingly and with enough explanation in everyday language.

Technical words should be used only when necessary, however. A nontechnical word may be preferred to a technical word if it conveys the same meaning with the same precision. For example, if the word *language* will do, there is no sense in using *linguistic competence*. Of course, there may be a reason to prefer *linguistic competence* over *language*. In essence, the use of every technical word should be justified.

The most debilitating form of jargon is pseudotechnical gibberish. Its sole purpose is to obscure the message and presumably impress the naive audience. Careful writers avoid this kind of jargon. Sometimes, acceptable jargon in one field may be befuddling nonsense that gives an air of pseudotechnicality in a different field. Speech–language pathology is full of this kind of borrowed and grafted jargon: *input, output, end gate, information processing, governor, filter, comparator,* and so on. Most of it is borrowed from engineering and computer science. The relevance of such jargon for speech–language pathology is mostly presumed and theoretical. In fact, unless there is a scientific justification, jargon borrowed from other disciplines should not be used. It makes very little technical sense to say, *"The child seems to have processed the linguistic input as a single unit,"* when all that the child did was to point to the right picture when requested to do so.

Avoid Clichés. Standard phrases give brevity and clarity to writing. Minimal use of phrases such as *wear and tear* and *at its best* is acceptable. However, overuse of clichés (standard expressions that have become dull because of overuse) obscures writing. A writer who uses too many standard phrases lacks creativity in his or her use of language. Besides, many overused standard phrases have lost their precise meaning. As a result, the writing becomes vague. For example, a clinician who writes, "This technique is not my cup of tea," is not saying anything clearly. The statement possibly means, among other things, that the technique is ineffective or that the clinician simply does not know how to use it. Or, when a clinician writes about the *dashed hopes of parents whose children have language disabilities*, one does not know whom to blame for the dashed hopes.

Avoid Colloquial Expressions. With few exceptions, technical writing should not contain colloquial expressions. Colloquial expressions may not be appropriate in formal writing of any kind. In a scientific report, *the author feels that* is too loose and colloquial. The author's feelings are probably irrelevant in the context. *Feels that* should be replaced by *thinks that* or *believes that*. Similarly, *language* should be preferred to *tongue*, and *stomach* to *tummy*. Other kinds of colloquialism to be avoided include contractions (*isn't*, *won't*), abbreviations such as *TV*, *phone*, and *exam*, and phrases such as *sort of*, *you know*, *get across*, and *come up with*. An extreme form of colloquialism is called *slang* (e.g., *spaced out*, *uptight*, *for sure*, *rad*). They have no place in scientific writing unless this form of speech is itself the matter of investigation.

Avoid Dead Metaphors and Similes. These are expressions that were once colorful and effective but now are cliché. Expressions such as *dead as a door nail*, *a shot in the arm*, *off the beaten path*, *sit on the fence*, and *beyond a shadow of doubt* are best avoided in scientific writing. They are probably not useful in any kind of writing. In exploring the meaning and implications of scientific data, direct and nonmetaphorical use of language is essential.

Use the Right Words. Words with exact meaning should be selected over those that are too broad or vague in their meaning. In scientific writing, technical words offer more precise meaning than their counterparts used in everyday language. For example, in the behavioral science literature, *reinforcer* is a technical term that should not be used interchangably with *reward* or *award*.

Sometimes, when none of the everyday words serve the scientific purpose, a scientist may create new words to suggest a specific event or process. Such neologism is acceptable in scientific writing. However, neologisms of bureaucracy (including educational, scientific, and professional bureaucracy), the advertising industry, and business can only obscure the meaning of a message. Many neologistic adverbs and verbs have been created by adding -*wise* and -*ize* to nouns, and although many such expressions eventually become standard usage, a careful writer will not rush to use them. For instance, words such as *inferiorize, therapize, rigidize, gradewise, economywise,* and *timewise,* even if they are commonly used, are better avoided. Another set of words has been created by adding the prefix *de-* to certain words resulting in such creations as *decriminalize,* and *dehumanize.* Neologisms of this kind should be left out of scientific writing.

The careful writer should be aware of subtle distinctions in meanings of words. Many pairs of words are mistakenly used interchangeably. For example, in the following pairs of words, the meaning of each word is different: *disinterested* and *uninterested, alternate* and *alternative, anticipate* and *expect, continual* and *continuous, farther* and *further, imply* and *infer, stationary* and *stationery, economic* and *economical, historic* and *historical, affect* and *effect.* A dictionary or a thesaurus can help distinguish the meanings of these and other commonly confused words. (See Hegde [2003] for additional examples of commonly confused or misused words.)

Use of Abstract and Concrete Words. Abstract words refer to concepts and relations between concepts. Abstract words do not stimulate the senses because they do not always refer to sensory experiences. Concrete words refer to things and events that stimulate the senses. Such words help recall sensory images of all kinds. Therefore, concrete words are more direct and easy to understand. To be understood, abstract words require a certain level of conceptual understanding of the subject matter.

A general rule is that concrete words are preferable to abstract words. By generating sensory images, concrete words help the reader understand experiences the author has written about. Concrete words are especially useful in literary essays, journalistic reports, stories, and novels. These kinds of writings conjure up vivid images and sensations. Poetry, on the other hand, consists of many abstract words. That is why a serious poem is more difficult to understand than a novel or a short story: Undefined, abstract words lead to different interpretations. By not defining the abstract words used, the poet creates multiple meanings, which make a small poem a complex piece of writing.

Abstract words, however, are useful in scientific writing. Scientific reports are typically about events and their relations, and many of these relations are abstract. But, unlike the poet, the scientist defines the abstract words precisely so that multiple meanings are not suggested. Many abstract words are found in the literature review and discussion sections of a scientific report. However, even in scientific reports, concrete words should be used in describing persons, things, and events. Participants should be described in specific terms (*12-year-old boys*) rather than in general terms (*young people*). Similarly, instruments, procedures, and results should be described in concrete terms.

Sparing Use of Figures of Speech. Figures of speech, including similes and metaphors, also help make the writing vivid to the reader. Similes suggest a similarity between two essentially unlike items (a new house is *like* a black hole; it sucks in all your money). Metaphors equate two dissimilar things (*all the world's a stage*). Analogies describe a new concept in terms of a familiar concept (*the nervous system is like a telephone network*). Personification attributes human qualities to inanimate entities (*the dark clouds were mean and ferocious*).

Overuse of figures of speech can hinder direct and technical communication. Once again, they are more appropriately used in literary writings than in scientific reports. An exception is scientific writing meant for the general public, in which figures of speech can help readers understand complex ideas.

Some forms of figures of speech extend beyond single sentences. For example, *analogical reasoning* can be considered a figurative approach to thinking about a subject matter in terms of another subject matter. Descriptions of the nervous system and its functioning that use computer language or the language of industry illustrate this approach.

Coherent Writing

One writing problem often shown by student writers is incoherent writing. An essay or a review paper may lack a structure, an orderly progression of ideas and concepts, or smooth transitions from sentence to sentence, paragraph to paragraph, and section to section.

Some planning and thinking can improve the coherence of writing. The different sections of a paper and the contents of each section or topic should be determined first. Next, the sequence of these sections should be determined. Even though sections and contents of most scientific reports are relatively fixed, subheadings under these major sections vary. Therefore, some planning is needed to make scientific reports coherent and easy to understand. The sequences of sections, headings, and subheadings of articles with more flexible formats should be carefully thought out.

When sections and their contents are planned, an orderly progression of ideas can be achieved by using transitions between units of writing. The paragraph is the most important of these units. Each section or topic contains several paragraphs, and smooth transitions between them are important in good writing.

A single concept or a brief topic gives a paragraph its unity. For example, the age, socioeconomic status, and the occupational level of the participants in a study may be described in a single paragraph. How the participants were selected may be described in a different paragraph because of a change in the idea or topic. If the selection criterion can be expressed in a single sentence, it may be a part of a larger paragraph. The basic rule is that a paragraph should have conceptual unity. Therefore, the beginning of a new paragraph suggests a transition to a new idea, topic, or subtopic.

Paragraphs should not be too long, nor should they (except rarely) consist of single sentences. Readers find lengthy paragraphs formidable, but a succession of very brief paragraphs can make the writing fragmented. A single-sentence paragraph is generally inappropriate, but it is acceptable on occasion; for example, single-sentence paragraphs can make a point emphatically or can highlight a transition to a new topic.

The first sentence in a paragraph usually suggests the topic or concept to be described in it (Hegde, 2003). If the paragraph continues with the same idea described in the previous paragraph, then a transitional sentence, which makes a reference to the previous paragraph, is needed. To achieve a smooth transition, a paragraph should begin as well as end appropriately. If the same general idea is to be discussed in several paragraphs, the end of each paragraph should be linked to the beginning of the next paragraph. Such linking can often be achieved by a common word or a phrase that is repeated in the final sentence of the previous paragraph and the first sentence of the new paragraph.

There are also many kinds of paragraphs; perhaps the most important are those that introduce or conclude a section or topic. Some topics should be introduced slowly, preparing the reader with a few sentences; other topics can be introduced without much background information. Each section or topic should begin with an introductory paragraph. The need for paragraphs that suggest conclusion is somewhat varied; they are needed at the end of major sections and topics but may not be needed at the end of subtopics. Complex and lengthy discussions almost always need paragraphs that give a summary.

So far, concise, adequate, clear, and coherent writing has been discussed. These qualities of writing require a competent conceptual handling of the subject of writing. The final point about writing is the matter of style.

WRITING STYLE

In this chapter, the term *style* is not used in the same sense as a format of writing. Format refers more to the organization and mechanics of writing than to style. A format (such as APA), grammar (structural matters), and conceptual considerations are all necessary to write well. But a style of writing is a different matter; it is the most individualistic of the aspects of writing. The style, not the knowledge of grammar and other writing principles, distinguishes one great writer from another. The style, among other qualities, separates Walt Whitman from Robert Frost, James Joyce from

Saul Bellow, and Maya Angelou from Arundhathi Roy. There are good styles and bad styles, but more important, each outstanding writer has his or her own unique style.

Grammatical correctness does not necessarily assure a unique style. A piece of writing may be structurally flawless but boring because of a lack of style. A style is a writer's creative use of language. It is the distinguishing pattern of words that a writer creates to produce a unique effect on the reader. Literary writers pay close attention to style. How a story is told is at least as important as what that story is about. Scientific writers, on the other hand, generally tend to pay less attention to style. They concentrate more on technical, correct, clear, concise, and adequate writing. The meaning of a poem can be intentionally obscure, but the poem may still be hailed as important; obscure scientific articles generally remain obscure. Scientific writers restrict the reader response to particular meanings of words, whereas a poet or a novelist, as noted earlier, intentionally broadens the reader response by using words with multiple meanings and then by not defining them. Nevertheless, style is important in scientific writing. There is nothing wrong with the creative use of language in scientific writing when the author does not violate the principles of effective and accurate communication. In fact, a creative writing style can enhance scientific communication.

Some scientific writing may be unreadable because of the authors' dull style. Bold and novel use of language within the limits of scientific communication can improve the readability of most research papers. An excessive concern with structure and format makes scientific papers extremely formal and boring to read. Surely, a breezy and informal style is not appropriate for scientific discussions, but within the limits of seriousness, one can write with lucidity, style, and beauty.

Writing with a creative style that conforms to the rules of scientific and technical communication is one of the most difficult challenges writers in sciences and professions face. A lack of serious interest in good literature among many scientists and professionals may be one reason why most scientific writing lacks unique style; a study of good literature, ideally started early in life, would help scientists improve their writing style. Such a study should focus on great writers of contrasting styles.

WRITING AND REVISING

Writing correctly and with a good style is a matter of writing frequently and revising as often as necessary. Like any other skill, good writing requires practice; very few writers manage to write very little yet extremely well. Most writers have to write, write, and write before they achieve a certain ease and style of writing.

The art of revising is very important for a writer. The writer is the first reader and, therefore, the first critic of a piece of writing. The writer also begins as a mild critic of his or her own writing, but should learn to be a strong critic of that writing, at least privately and in the process of revising.

Revisions and self-editing eventually refine a piece of writing. Self-editing requires a critical reading of one's own writing. Most writers, especially student writers, make the mistake of not having enough time to revise a piece before it is submitted for publication or evaluation, yet many problems of writing can be avoided simply by allowing enough time to make revisions of the first draft.

Even the most established writers revise their manuscripts several times. Often, the final manuscript is vastly different from the original draft. It is best to wait a few days after the original writing before attempting revisions. A few good books on writing and comments from friends and colleagues can usually help in the revision process. Suggestions from persons not familiar with the subject matter can help improve the readability and clarity of technical papers, and suggestions from colleagues and experts can help a writer improve scientific accuracy.

SUMMARY

- Scientific and professional writers should follow an accepted format of writing. The format of the American Psychological Association (APA) is widely used and is accepted by the American Speech-Language-Hearing Association.

- Most scientific reports use the following structure:
    — Title page
    — Abstract
    — Untitled introduction
    — Method
    — Results
    — Discussion
    — References
    — Appendix

- All writing should be free from gender, racial, ethnic, cultural, and other kinds of bias. The writers should follow established guidelines on writing without bias.

- Good writing requires that the author follow established structural principles.

- Good writing also requires the following:
    — Knowledge of the readership
    — Concise writing

— Adequate writing

— Clear writing

— Coherent writing

- Authors should develop a unique writing style and reserve time to rewrite and revise everything they write.

STUDY GUIDE

1. Go to your department or university library and select a thesis prepared in your subject matter. Make a complete outline of the format of that thesis. Note the differences between the format of a research article published in a journal and the thesis.

2. Survey a few journals in your subject matter and select (a) an article, (b) a report of an empirical study, and (c) a set of exchanges between two or more authors. Make an outline of these publications, retaining only the major headings. Note the similarities and differences in the formats of those three types of publications.

3. What are the characteristics of a good abstract? What is its usefulness in published papers?

4. Select a report of an empirical study from one of the journals you normally read. After having read the article, write an abstract of that report. Do not use the author's abstract. Later, compare your abstract with that of the author. Can you improve your version or the author's? If so, rewrite one or both.

5. Describe the seven factors that a well-written introduction addresses. Find a published article whose introduction is well written because it includes those seven factors. Also, find an introduction that you think is not well written. Justify your selection.

6. What are the standard subheadings of the method section of a published empirical report prepared according to the APA Manual?

7. What does the discussion section of a technical paper contain?

8. Select (a) two journal articles, one written by a single author and the other written by three or more authors; (b) one book edited by a single author; (c) one book written by a single author; (d) one book written by three authors; (e) a chapter published in an edited book; and (f) a thesis. Following the APA guidelines, prepare a reference list of these publications.

9. Distinguish between a reference list and a bibliography.

10. Select a paper you have written and critically evaluate the writing in terms of the common structural mistakes. Make sure the paper selected was not edited by someone else. Can you find faults with your own writing? Rewrite your paper to make it more effective and readable.

11. What are the conceptual considerations of good writing? What aspect of good writing seems to give you the most difficulty? How can you gain control over that aspect of your writing?

12. What six factors should a writer avoid to write clearly?

13. Give an example of the following missteps: (a) euphemism, (b) jargon, (c) cliché, (d) colloquial expression, and (e) dead metaphor or simile.

14. What are figures of speech? Give examples. What is their place in scientific writing?

15. What is meant by the "style" of writing? Should scientific writings have a style? Justify your answer.

16. Select a literary essay written by a famous writer and an article published in one of the American Speech-Language-Hearing Association journals. Compare and contrast them in terms of the use of metaphors and similes, the writing style, the use of language, and the general format.

17. Write a two-page essay on your professional objectives. Put it aside for several days or a week. Then reread it and critically evaluate your writing. Rewrite your essay to make it more attractive. Have someone read and criticize it for you.

18. Find a well-written scientific article published in a scientific or professional journal. Why is it such a good article? What aspects of that article would you like to emulate in your own writing?

19. Identify two or three outstanding contemporary American writers of fiction, poetry, or essays. Select those known to have received critical acclaim (not necessarily those on the bestseller list). Read at least one book by each of the selected authors.

Chapter 15

◆◆◆◆◆◆◆◆◆◆◆◆◆◆◆◆◆◆◆◆◆◆◆◆◆◆◆◆◆◆◆◆◆◆◆◆◆◆

How To Evaluate Research Reports

Evaluating research is an important task of scientists and professionals. Sometimes it is assumed that professionals who do not do research need not be concerned with its evaluation. This is a mistake because professionals are consumers of research. Professionals must determine the usefulness of research information they wish to use in their clinical practice. Because not all research studies are equally valid or reliable, a critical clinician is a better consumer of research.

PROFESSIONALS AS CONSUMERS OF RESEARCH

Clinical practice and research can influence each other when clinicians understand and evaluate research and when researchers understand and investigate clinical issues. It is the duty of clinicians to understand and evaluate clinically relevant research. Clinicians who can do this have a good chance of influencing the course of research so that the researchers will generate clinically useful data.

Clinicians who are not in touch with research are likely to perpetuate the use of less effective or ineffective assessment and treatment procedures. Such clinicians may also be the permanent victims of faddish changes in theory and practice. Acceptance of new research and theories regardless of their scientific merit can lead to an abandonment of proven procedures. A questionable promise of a "new and revolutionary" approach may discourage attempts at refining existing, satisfactory techniques. Such efforts are more economical than those needed to develop new techniques.

Uncritical clinicians are more likely to perceive only the popular or forcefully promoted techniques. Those clinicians may not perceive the subtle, significant, and cumulative scientific progress in their subject matter. Clinicians who cannot appreciate research may be unable to contribute to their body of knowledge.

UNDERSTANDING AND EVALUATING RESEARCH

To evaluate research, one must first understand it. Many students who read research reports find it difficult to understand them; there are many sources of this difficulty, and different students may find certain sources especially debilitating.

The first source of difficulty is lack of knowledge of the subject matter or of the particular issue of a report. A grasp of the technical vocabulary and the necessary theoretical concepts is essential for understanding research. A piece of research can be evaluated only in the broader conceptual and empirical context in which it was done. Therefore, scientists capable in one field cannot necessarily fully evaluate research in another field.

The second source of difficulty is lack of knowledge of the methods of investigation. The student needs to be familiar with the basic concepts of science, such as control, causality, and causal and other kinds of analysis. The student should understand the logic and the conditions of experimental manipulations. Knowledge of the methods of analysis, especially those of statistics, is essential in understanding many research reports.

The third source of difficulty may be lack of technical understanding of various aspects of research. Journal articles are typically written for technically competent audiences. Because of space limitations and production costs, journal articles are rarely self-explanatory. Many concepts, procedures, design aspects, and theoretical backgrounds are mentioned only briefly on the assumption that readers are familiar with them. If the student is not already familiar with such elements, other sources should be consulted.

The fourth source of difficulty is lack of experience in reading research articles. Like doing good research, evaluating research well takes experience. Students usually find that as they read more reports, the reports are easier to understand.

Students who understand research reports cannot necessarily evaluate them, however. Students may make satisfactory reports on journal articles; summarize the studies adequately; and understand the rationale, methods, results, and conclusions of particular studies. Nevertheless, students may find it difficult to evaluate the reliability and validity of the studies they seem to understand.

Students may uncritically accept the conclusions of methodologically defective studies perhaps because they do not perceive logical inconsistencies, faulty designs, questionable methods of analysis, and conclusions that the data do not warrant. Many instructors find that students need instruction and practice in evaluating research reports, and often students benefit from instructors' modeled evaluations. Some clinicians who try to read, understand, and evaluate research studies also experience similar problems.

EVALUATION OF RESEARCH

As pointed out by Sidman (1960), research studies are evaluated for the scientific importance of the data, their reliability, and their generality. These three evaluation objectives can be accomplished by a critical analysis of the conceptual background of a study, the research questions asked, the methods used, the procedures of analysis, and the manner in which the conclusions were drawn. This critical analysis also tries to place the study in the overall context of its subject matter.

Scientific studies can be subjected to two kinds of evaluation. I call the first the *internal consistency evaluation*, and the second, *the external relevance evaluation*. I shall first describe these two types of evaluations and then, in the form of an outline, offer specific suggestions for evaluating research studies.

Internal Consistency Evaluation

The internal consistency evaluation is done within the confines of the study itself. The external relevance evaluation, on the other hand, is done to judge a study's importance in enhancing the knowledge within the subject matter. Before a study's relevance to the subject matter is determined, an internal consistency evaluation should be completed.

The **internal consistency evaluation** is concerned with the integrity of the structure of the study. This evaluation judges the study on its own terms. It is concerned with consistency in its purpose, methods, results, and conclusions. An important task in this evaluation is to determine whether the effects produced in a study were indeed due to the experimental manipulations (internal validity). Reliability of the results is also considered in the internal consistency evaluation.

The purpose of an investigation is an important criterion of internal consistency evaluation. A study is internally consistent only in relation to its purpose. In judging the adequacy of the methods used, one cannot use absolute criteria. The methods of a study are adequate or inadequate to answer the particular questions of that study. As I have noted elsewhere, a design may be adequate to answer one type of question but inadequate to answer another type. A method of analysis may be correct for one kind of data but incorrect for another. Therefore, what the experimenter tried to accomplish in the study is an important basis for judging its internal consistency.

The type of question asked determines the experimental design. If the question is one of interaction between two or more variables, a factorial group or a single-subject interactional design should be used. A simple two-group design or an *ABA* design will not answer that question. When the purpose is to find a causal relation between two variables, a correlational method is not appropriate; but when the purpose is to find out if two variables covary, that correlational method is appropriate.

In most cases, methodological errors threaten the internal consistency of a study. In addition to selecting a wrong design to answer the research questions, the investigator can make other mistakes; for example, the participant selection procedure may be inappropriate. When a heterogeneous set of participants is needed or intended, the investigator may select a small number of available participants. When homogeneous participants are needed, the selected participants may be heterogeneous. Participants may be matched only on some of the relevant variables. The selection criteria may be too stringent or too lenient. As a result, participants who are appropriate for the study may be rejected and those who are not may be selected.

Mistakes in measuring the dependent variables, choosing instrumentation, arranging the experimental conditions, manipulating the independent variables, and most important, building effective control procedures into the experiment can also hamper internal consistency. The pretest measures or the baselines of the dependent variables may not be reliable. The method of measurement may not be accurate. When a direct measure (frequency) of the response is required to answer the questions, only indirect measures (questionnaire responses) may have been obtained. The reliability of the instruments used in measurement may have been questionable or unknown.

Experimental conditions are a part of the design. Once the right design is selected, the required conditions should be arranged accordingly. Unfortunately, even after the right design has been selected, mistakes may be made in arranging the experimental conditions. For example, in a single-subject interactional design, more than one treatment variable may be changed across experimental conditions. The results then cannot be interpreted because of the confounding effects of multiple treatments.

Effective manipulation of the independent variables is necessary to achieve the goals of most experimental studies. Weak manipulation of the selected independent variable may fail to produce an appreciable effect. For example, a treatment variable applied only briefly may not provide an answer if the question is concerned with long-term effects. When an everyday experimental schedule is required, a twice-weekly schedule may be ineffective. The intensity of the independent variable may also be weak. The verbal "no," for example, may be delivered in a weak, unsure, soft voice. An investigation on the effects of masking noise on stuttering may use only a 30-dB masking noise, which may be less than what is required to produce an effect.

The reader may recall from Chapter 7 that appropriate controls are necessary to establish the internal validity of an experiment. Internal validity assures that the changes observed in the dependent variable are indeed due to the manipulations of the independent variables. Internal validity can be achieved by various means, including a no-treatment control group, multiple baselines, reversal of treatment, and withdrawal of treatment. In the group design studies, mistakes in achieving equivalent groups are common. Was a population accessible for sampling? Were both random selection and random assignment of participants used? Was the matching done on all relevant variables? When answers to questions such as these are negative, control procedures of a study are not adequate.

In single-subject designs, the baselines may be too brief, unstable, or improving. Some of the baselines in a multiple baseline design may show changes without treatment. When the treatment is withdrawn, the effects observed earlier may not dissipate. These and other problems question the adequacy of control procedures and hence the internal consistency of a single-subject study.

Faulty analysis of results is another problem that thwarts the internal consistency of research studies. In group design studies, inappropriate statistics may be used in data analysis. For example, parametric statistical techniques may be used when the data warrant nonparametric statistics. In case of a pretest–posttest control group design, the pretest and posttest means of the experimental group may be compared with a *t* test and the corresponding means of the control group may be tested with another *t* test. Chapter 8 points out that this is an incorrect method of analysis.

In single-subject design studies, comparisons of nonadjacent experimental conditions may be made to demonstrate experimental effects. For example, an investigator who administers reinforcement for a desirable behavior in one condition may compare reinforcement and punishment for an undesirable behavior administered in another condition when these two conditions are separated by a baseline. This is a wrong procedure because in the evaluation of multiple treatment effects, only adjacent conditions can be compared.

Finally, mistakes are made in drawing conclusions from research studies. When faulty methods of analysis are used, wrong conclusions are inevitable. The most common of these mistakes is to draw conclusions that are not consistent with the results. The results may show weak experimental effects, but the author may conclude that the effects were strong. Much worse, experimental effects may be inferred when there were none. In the statistical approach, this mistake is known as a Type I error in which a null hypothesis is rejected when it should have been retained; in other words, a nonexistent treatment effect is asserted. On the other hand, an effect may be denied when there was one. In statistical analysis, this is known as a Type II error in which the null is retained when it should have been rejected; to put it differently, treatment was judged to be ineffective when in fact it was effective.

Many other mistakes are possible in the interpretation of data. Subtle distortions in data are thought to result from authors' convictions that are not supported by the data. Some investigators have greater faith in their own convictions than in demonstrated empirical relations. In such cases, authors may try too hard to explain-away conflicting results.

The effects of wrong statistical analyses and misinterpretations of results need not totally invalidate a study, however. As long as the report describes the results separately and completely, the methods of analyses and the author's conclusions can be separated from those results. The evaluator can come to his or her independent conclusions. A clear separation between the results and the author's conclusions is an important aspect of internal consistency evaluation. Beginning students often cannot make this distinction. They tend to equate "the study showed that" with "the author concluded that." Obviously, those who cannot distinguish the results from the wrong conclusions of a study will be misled by the author.

The reliability of the results of a study is often judged on the basis of the internal consistency evaluation. Though the author has reported acceptable intersubject and intrasubject reliability measures, serious mistakes in the implementation of a study are grounds for questioning the reliability of the results. There is no assurance that if the procedures are properly implemented, the same results would be observed.

When internal consistency questions have been satisfactorily answered, external relevance evaluation becomes important. However, should the internal consistency evaluation reveal serious problems with the study, the evaluation of external relevance is a moot issue. Unreliable results of invalid experimental operations never have external relevance.

External Relevance Evaluation

The **external relevance evaluation** determines the data's importance to the subject matter. The experimental data of a given study may be reliable and internally consistent, but their significance to the subject matter may still be limited. Do the data advance the cause of understanding the phenomenon? This is the question of external relevance evaluation.

Compared with the internal consistency evaluation, the external relevance evaluation is more global. This global evaluation is done at different levels or within different contexts. The importance of data is evaluated by placing them in the larger context of research on the phenomenon addressed by the study. In turn, the particular phenomenon is also placed in the context of the larger subject matter of which it is a part. The contexts in which the data are placed for evaluation may be multiple and ever-increasing in scope. Data are placed first in the smaller context of the research questions asked by the study, then in the larger context of the topic of investigation, then in the still larger context of the subject, and finally in the context of the total subject matter. The number of contexts in which the data are evaluated depends on the scope of the questions investigated and the scope of the subject matter.

The multiple contexts of ever-increasing scope that are used in evaluating the importance of a research study can be illustrated with an example. Suppose that a study asks the question whether the known normative sequence of morphological acquisition can be altered by experimental teaching. Taking young children, the investigator teaches selected grammatical morphemes ahead of the developmental schedule and in a reversed order. The author concludes that it is possible to teach morphemes ahead of, and in a sequence other than, the normative sequence.

In making the external relevance evaluation of this study, the student first places the data in the context of studies on language acquisition. What kinds of studies have been done in the past? What is the significance of this study? Does this study use an approach that is different from the approaches of the past studies? Does it say anything new about the language acquisition process?

The significance of the study is evaluated next in the larger context of the analysis of language, not just language development. Does it offer a way of analyzing language behavior? Does the experimental method contribute anything new toward an understanding of language behavior in general? What kinds of theoretical statements do the results support?

In the third and still larger context, the significance of the data can be evaluated by judging their relevance to the treatment of language disorders. Are the data related to the clinical treatment of language disorders? Do they shed light on the selection of target behaviors? Do the results have implications for sequencing target behaviors in clinical treatment?

Finally, the study may be placed in the context of communicative behaviors and disorders in general. Does it have implications for studying normal communicative behaviors? Does it suggest that similar methods of analysis can be used in studying phonological or other norm-based behaviors? Possibly, the study can be placed in the still broader context of analysis of developmentally based behaviors of all kinds.

Another concern of external relevance evaluation is the *generality* of data. An internally consistent study may or may not have external generality. However, as noted in Chapter 7, no single study can assure all kinds of generality because generality is a function of replication. Therefore, an evaluation of generality attempts to determine the potential for replication. The main question to be answered is whether the study is described in sufficient detail to make replications possible. The research questions, procedures, designs, and experimental variables should be described operationally. The study then can be replicated by other investigators in other settings using different participants. A report that does not describe its procedures (including the dependent and independent variables) in sufficient detail is evaluated negatively from the standpoint of generality.

The external relevance evaluation is the more difficult of the two evaluations because it involves a value judgment. This evaluation asks simple questions that are difficult to answer: Is this study important, valuable, and relevant to the field of investigation? Does it make a significant contribution to the subject matter? These questions are difficult to answer for several reasons. First, students need to have broad scholarship in the subject matter to judge the overall significance of a study. Second, individual evaluators almost always judge the importance of scientific data from the standpoint of their personal perspectives. This is necessarily so because scientists who evaluate the scientific significance of their colleagues' data do not have a common set of criteria. What is an important criterion for one evaluator may be trivial to another evaluator. After a thorough discussion of the evaluation of scientific importance of data, Sidman (1960, p. 41) said, "If science is to use the importance of data as a criterion for accepting or rejecting an experiment, it should have a set of rules within which the scientist can operate when he has to make his evaluation. Do such rules actually exist? The answer is no."

Lack of objective rules and the subjective nature of evaluation of the external relevance of data suggest that evaluators should be careful in rejecting any experimental data as unimportant. Negative evaluation of the external relevance of a study often is made on the basis of one's own theoretical biases and convictions arising from personal experiences. If the results are not consistent with such biases and convictions, a negative judgment may be rendered. However, this can be a bad practice, because the value of certain experimental data can be independent of theoretical viewpoints and personal biases. This is true of the biases and convictions of both the evaluator and the original investigator. If it appears that the methods and procedures of a study were appropriate, the data whose significance is not clear should be afforded the benefit of doubt. The original investigator may have rejected such data because they did not support his or her preconceived ideas. An evaluator may think that the data are trivial because of narrow views. In such cases, the best course of action is to reserve judgment. Sound experimental data survive negative judgments of fellow scientists.

The difficulties involved in making external evaluations should not discourage one from trying, however. For both scientific and professional reasons, one should judge the importance of the studies one reads. One should try to make the best possible judgment yet remain open to a different judgment. An uncritical acceptance of everything—perhaps desirable for personal reasons—is not helpful in advancing the science of a subject matter. Uncritical acceptance of scientific literature can be detrimental to the professional's integrity and to the progress of clients under treatment.

What follows is an integrated outline for making a summative evaluation of research studies. It includes questions of both internal consistency evaluation and external relevance evaluation.

EVALUATION OF RESEARCH REPORTS: AN OUTLINE

Before using this outline, the student should make sure that he or she is familiar with the subject matter and the concepts that serve as background to the study being evaluated. Also, the student should understand the general methods of the study, its research design, the concept of experimental control, internal and external validity, methods of statistical analysis, and statistical significance.

In evaluating published research studies, the student should try to answer the following questions:

   I. **Significance of the Problem Investigated (External Relevance)**

      A. Was the problem investigated significant?

      B. Does the problem concern an important area of investigation?

      C. Does the problem advance understanding of the issues involved?

      D. Does the problem have basic implications, applied implications, or both?

  II. **Introduction and Literature Review (Internal Consistency)**

      A. Was the introduction section clear and complete?

      B. Did the introduction help focus on the problem investigated?

C. Is the literature review sufficient in detail to justify the study?

D. Was the review objective, impartial, and appropriately critical?

E. Did the review give a historical perspective if one was required to understand the investigation?

F. Did the review point out the strengths and limitations of previous studies?

G. Did the introduction place the research questions in the context of previous investigations?

H. Overall, did this section make it clear why the study was made?

III. Statement of the Problem

A. Was the problem stated clearly?

B. Did the problem statement specify the variables in operational terms?

C. Was the problem statement clear enough to permit a replication?

D. If hypotheses were made, were they stated clearly?

E. If there were no hypotheses, did the author specify the research questions?

IV. Method

A. Were the methods described clearly and adequately?

B. Could one replicate the methods?

C. What type of study was it? (See Chapters 4 and 5)

   1. A normative study?

   2. A standard group comparison study?

   3. An epidemiological study?

   4. A sample survey?

   5. An uncontrolled unreplicated case study?

   6. An uncontrolled directly replicated case study?

   7. An uncontrolled systematically replicated case study?

   8. A controlled unreplicated study?

   9. A controlled directly replicated study?

   10. A controlled systematically replicated study?

D. What was the design of the study?

   1. A randomized two-group design? If so, what kind?

   2. A randomized multigroup design? If so, what kind?

   3. A factorial design? If so, what kind?

4. A time-series design? If so, what kind?

5. Any other kind of group design? If so, what kind?

6. An *ABA* or *ABAB* design? If so, what kind?

7. A multiple baseline design? If so, what kind?

8. The interactional design?

9. The alternating treatments design?

10. The changing criterion design?

11. Any other kind of single-subject design? If so, what kind?

12. Was the design appropriate for answering the research questions?

13. Was the selected design used correctly?

14. Were the experimental conditions arranged logically?

15. Did the design include adequate controls?

16. Did the control procedures rule out the sources of internal invalidity to a satisfactory degree?

E. Who were the participants?

1. Did the author give a full description of the participants?

2. Did the author specify the number of participants and their selection and exclusion criteria?

3. Was the selection procedure adequate for the purpose and design of the study?

4. How were the participants divided into experimental and control groups?

5. Were the participants matched, and if so, on what variables?

6. In a group design study, did the author use both random selection and random assignment?

7. In a single-subject or small group study, were the participants homogeneous or heterogeneous? In either case, were the individual participants described in sufficient detail?

8. In a clinical study, did the author describe the disorder, its history, and measured severity of the selected participants?

F. What kinds of instruments did the author use?

1. Did the author describe the instruments and give their make and model numbers?

2. Was information provided on reliability of the instruments used?

3. Were there sufficient descriptions of the functioning of complex and new instruments used in the study?

4. Were the instruments selected appropriate for the purposes of the study?

G. Were the procedures described adequately?

1. In a treatment study, did the author describe all the treatment steps (independent variables)?

2. Is the description of treatment detailed enough to permit replication?

3. How were the independent variables manipulated?

4. What was the frequency and duration of treatment sessions?

5. What kind of probes or follow-ups were conducted?

6. What was the involvement of the family members, teachers, and others?

7. Was the treatment or teaching extended to nonclinical settings? If so, how?

H. What were the dependent variables?

1. Were the variables described in operational terms?

2. How were the variables measured?

3. How were the pretests and baselines established?

4. Were the pretreatment measures reliable?

5. Did the experimenter establish reliability and validity of the dependent variable measures? By what procedures?

6. Were the reliability indexes satisfactory?

I. How were the participants instructed?

J. What were the stimulus materials?

V. Results

A. What were the results of the study? Were they described objectively and without evaluations and interpretations?

B. In a single-subject design study, did the author describe the results of individual participants separately?

1. Were the single-subject results visually represented?

2. Were the baseline data stable or otherwise acceptable?

3. Do the results show convincing contrast across the baseline, experimental, and other conditions?

4. Did the author describe data both qualitatively and quantitatively?

5. Were the results clinically valid?

C. In a group design study, were the group performances clearly distinguished?

    1. In small-group studies, did the author summarize individual differences in results?

    2. Did the author describe the group data qualitatively and quantitatively?

    3. What were the methods of analysis and were they appropriate?

    4. Did the author use statistical procedures correctly?

    5. Did the author give descriptive statistics in sufficient detail?

    6. Did the author report the value of inferential statistical tests and their probability levels?

    7. Were the results clinically valid?

D. Were the figures, tables, and appendixes used effectively?

E. Was the overall data presentation orderly and logical?

VI. Discussion

A. Did the author discuss the results adequately? Did the discussion section examine the meaning and implications of the results?

B. Did the author try to answer the research questions in light of the data?

C. Did the author clearly state whether the hypotheses were supported or not supported by the data?

D. Did the author relate the observations to previous findings?

E. Did the discussion examine the theoretical implications of the results?

F. Did the discussion suggest applied implications? Were the applied implications specific enough? Can a clinician implement these suggestions in clinical practice?

G. Did the discussion suggest additional research questions?

H. Did the discussion summarize the problems and limitations of the study?

I. Did the author avoid excessive speculation, fruitless debates, and questionable attempts to explain the results?

J. Did the author accept negative findings?

VII. Reference List

A. Did the author follow the selected format in arranging the references? Was the reference list accurate?

B. Did the author list all references cited in the text and only those cited in the text?

VIII. Appendix

A. Did the author provide needed additional materials in the appendix?

B. Was the appendix section used prudently?

C. Was the appendix necessary and sufficient?

The outline just given is not meant to be comprehensive. It is meant to alert the student to some important questions that should be answered in evaluating a research study.

Clearly, some evaluative questions, such as those concerned with the scientific importance of an investigation, are harder than others to answer. Also, it is better to do this evaluation after all other questions have been answered. Evaluating the introduction, literature review, and procedures requires conceptual as well as technical knowledge. Evaluating the discussion section also demands broad scholarship in the subject matter. Evaluation of data presentation, reference, and appendixes requires knowledge of the accepted format, such as that of the American Psychological Association (APA).

As noted before, evaluation is a judgmental process. Though it may be difficult, the student should not hesitate in making judgments and checking them with those of others who are more knowledgeable.

EVALUATION OF TREATMENT RESEARCH: A HIERARCHY OF EVIDENCE

Evaluation of treatment research is a special concern for all practitioners. The outline of evaluation given in the previous section applies to all research, including treatment research. Nonetheless, a more focused approach to evaluating treatment research is helpful. The clinician needs to make a quick judgment regarding whether the evidence offered in a favor of a treatment procedure is acceptable and whether the evidence has any generality. To facilitate this kind of judgment, I have designed a treatment evidence hierarchy that may be used in a convenient manner to evaluate treatment research (Hegde, 1998b, 2001). This evidential hierarchy is based on the classification of treatment research described in Chapter 4: (a) uncontrolled unreplicated, (b) uncontrolled directly replicated, (c) uncontrolled systematically replicated, (d) controlled unreplicated, (e) controlled directly replicated, and (f) controlled systematically replicated. Each of these six types of treatment research produces a level or hierarchy of evidence for efficacy, generality, or both.

A clinician who comes across a treatment research study should classify it into one of these six types of research. The clinician can then determine the hierarchical level of evidence, the degree of efficacy demonstrated, and the extent of generality that may be claimed. However, the clinician is likely to encounter one serious problem in applying this evidential hierarchy to treatment research: Many articles and oral presentations on treatment procedures may not be based on any kind of empirical research. In that case, it is best described as *expert advocacy*, not treatment research. The treatment procedure that is based on expert advocacy, not empirical research, should be greeted with cool skepticism until some kind of empirical evidence is marshaled in its favor.

Techniques based on expert advocacy should not be used in routine practice unless there is no technique that has evidence in its favor. This is certainly not the case with most adult and child language disorders, speech disorders, and fluency problems. The clinician should deem it unethical to select a procedure based exclusively on expert advocacy when techniques with research evidence are available.

When a treatment procedure has undergone some level of empirical investigation, the clinician can apply the following hierarchy to classify the level of evidence and the extent of generality. In most cases, the clinician can find that evidence in favor of certain treatment procedures has reached a fairly high level in the hierarchy. Generally speaking, the clinician might also prefer a technique that has reached a higher level of evidential hierarchy compared to one that is placed at a lower level.

Level 1: Uncontrolled Unreplicated

This initial level of evidence for a treatment procedure is produced by a case study. There were not controls to show that the method, not something else, produced the changes in the clients who received a treatment.

- **Evidence:** Documented improvement in routine treatment or teaching; children have learned skills under this method; clients have improved with the technique

- **Design Strategy:** Preexperimental: Group designs (e.g., one-shot group, one-group pretest–posttest); single-subject designs (*AB* design)

- **Replication:** None (good potential)

- **Evaluation:** Improvement may be claimed but not effectiveness; evidence is correlational, but better than mere expert advocacy

- **Recommendation:** The technique may be used with caution, claiming only improvement and keeping an eye for replications and controlled evaluations

Level 2: Uncontrolled Directly Replicated

This second level of evidence is produced by an investigator who repeated his or her own case study. The same improvement has been documented a second time.

- **Evidence:** Uncontrolled treatment; improvement obtained by the same clinician with different clients
- **Design Strategy:** Preexperimental
- **Replication:** Direct; no change in methods, settings, or clinicians
- **Evaluation:** Replicated improvement; still no evidence of effectiveness; good candidate for experimentation
- **Recommendation:** Use the technique with caution, claiming only improvement and watching for systematic replications and controlled research

Level 3: Uncontrolled Systematically Replicated

This level of evidence is produced by other investigators who applied a technique in different settings with different clients, possibly with some procedural modifications, obtaining similar degree of improvement.

- **Evidence:** Improvement documented by other clinicians in other settings, possibly with methodological changes
- **Design Strategy:** Preexperimental
- **Replication:** Systematic; varied settings, clinicians, and clients
- **Evaluation:** Still, only improvement is demonstrated; however, an excellent candidate for experimentation
- **Recommendation:** Use it with caution, claiming only improvement and watching for further replications and controlled evaluations

Level 4: Controlled Unreplicated

This is the beginning of controlled evidence for a treatment method. An experimental design has been used to rule out extraneous variables, thus establishing a cause–effect relation between the treatment and the changes it produced.

- **Evidence:** Treatment is demonstrated to be effective
- **Design Strategy:** Group (e.g., pretest–posttest control group; posttest-only control group); single-subject (e.g., *ABA*, *ABAB*, multiple baseline designs)
- **Replication:** None (good potential)

- **Evaluation:** Cause–effect relation has been demonstrated; treatment is shown to be effective; however, generality has not been established yet
- **Recommendation:** Use the technique with a greater degree of confidence; still be cautious because the effects have not been replicated; watch for replications

Level 5: Controlled Directly Replicated

At this level, data for generality of a treatment procedure begins to emerge because the same investigator has repeated an experimental study on a treatment procedure.

- **Evidence:** Treatment effects demonstrated when the method is repeated under the original conditions
- **Design Strategy:** Group and single-subject experimental designs
- **Replication:** Direct; replicated by the same investigator in the same setting without procedural modifications
- **Evaluation:** Treatment is not only effective but seems to have some generality as shown by the successful replication
- **Recommendation:** Use the technique with a greater degree of confidence, watching for systematic replications that may produce supportive or contradictory evidence

Level 6: Controlled Systematically Replicated

This is the highest level of evidence for effectiveness of a technique. Repeated studies have shown that the method (with or without modifications) is effective and that different clinicians in different settings can get the same or similar results.

- **Evidence:** Effectiveness as well as generality across settings, clients, and settings have been demonstrated.
- **Design Strategy:** Experimental group and single-subject designs
- **Replication:** Replicated by different investigators in different settings with methodologic modifications
- **Evaluation:** Replicated cause–effect relations; good generality
- **Recommendation:** Select this technique as the best of the available alternatives that have not reached this level of evidence; if multiple techniques have reached this level of evidence, select the one that is easier to use, socially more acceptable, or more efficient (takes less time to produce the same level of effect)

To achieve a more thorough evaluation of treatment research, the clinician should combine the outline of evaluation given in the previous section with this treatment research evidence hierarchy. In combination, the two sets of guidelines will provide a comprehensive method of evaluating treatment research evidence.

EVALUATION AND APPRECIATION OF RESEARCH

Clearly, the theme of this chapter is critical evaluation of research reports. Without counteracting that theme, I also should like to state that one should learn to appreciate research. A critical consumer of research is not necessarily the one who is always looking for the perfect study. Students working on research projects often think that their studies should be perfect in all respects. It is good to remember that a perfect study is more easily designed than conducted. Studies designed by even the best researchers are not likely to be perfect.

Because all studies tend to have some limitations, it is necessary to weigh those limitations against the strengths of a given study. In some cases, the conceptual or methodological limitations of a study can be so serious as to render the data worthless. A student should recognize such limitations. On the other hand, the limitations of other studies may be such that the results are still meaningful within those limitations. A student should recognize this as well.

The results of scientific studies on given issues can be arranged on a hierarchy of broad patterns and rough stages of progression. Some studies are uncontrolled, some have a certain degree of control, and others are more tightly controlled. The results of each of those studies should be evaluated in light of their limitations. For example, the results of a one-group pretest–posttest study or an *AB* single-subject study may indicate that a given treatment was followed by notable changes in certain client behaviors. That there was no control in the study is certainly a serious limitation, but the results may still be considered worthwhile. A conclusion that the treatment is worthy of further experimental manipulation is favorable as well as acceptable. On the other hand, an evaluation that the treatment and the changes in the client behaviors were causally related is favorable but not acceptable. The judgment that the results do not mean anything is unfavorable as well as questionable.

It may be helpful to distinguish serious *errors* in the design and implementation of a study from design *limitations* and acceptable compromises that are a part of any research study. Only serious errors in the design of a study invalidate the results. On the other hand, design limitations and acceptable compromises set limits within which meaningfulness of results can be interpreted.

It is possible to retain a critical outlook on research while maintaining a certain degree of enthusiasm for research. A critical outlook is not the same as a cynical outlook. After all, one who reads and evaluates research regularly should find some research interesting and stimulating. If not, there is no guarantee that that person will continue to read and evaluate research reports.

SUMMARY

- Professionals are consumers of research. To provide good service, professionals should be knowledgeable and critical consumers of research.

- To evaluate research, professionals should have the technical knowledge of the field, the methods of research, and experience in reading and evaluating research reports.

- Research evaluation is of two kinds:
  - Internal consistency evaluation includes a critical analysis of the methods and procedures of the study and whether they were appropriate to answer the question investigated.
  - External relevance evaluation includes a critical examination of the importance of the study and its implications for the discipline. The overall significance of the study and the generality of the results are assessed in external relevance evaluation.

- It is best to use a prepared outline in evaluating research studies.

- Treatment research may be evaluated for six levels of evidential hierarchy:
  - Uncontrolled unreplicated
  - Uncontrolled directly replicated
  - Uncontrolled systematically replicated
  - Controlled replicated
  - Controlled directly replicated
  - Controlled systematically replicated

- It is important to evaluate as well as appreciate research.

STUDY GUIDE

1. What is the difference between *understanding* and *evaluating* scientific reports?

2. Why should clinicians who are not expected to do research understand the research methods and concepts of science?

3. What kinds of difficulties do you, as a graduate student, face in understanding research articles? What can you do to overcome those difficulties?

4. What are Sidman's three criteria by which scientific studies are evaluated?

5. What is internal consistency evaluation? How is it done?

6. What is external relevance evaluation? How is it done?

7. Are there objective rules by which scientists can determine the scientific importance of data?

8. What is a treatment research evidence hierarchy? Describe it.

9. Select a journal report that you understand well. Make sure the report is of an empirical investigation (not a review or theoretical article). Using the outline of evaluation given in this chapter, evaluate the report. Have your instructor or someone knowledgeable take a look at your evaluation.

10. Select an article that reports on a treatment or teaching method. Evaluate it according to the guidelines given, combined with the treatment levels hierarchy and determine the level of evidence it offers. Make a recommendation about the use of the method and justify your recommendation.

Chapter 16

◆◆◆◆◆◆◆◆◆◆◆◆◆◆◆◆◆◆◆◆◆◆◆◆◆◆◆◆◆◆◆◆◆

Ethics of Research

- Fraud in Scientific Research
- Effects of Science on Society
- Ethical Justification of Treatment Evaluation
- Protection of Human Participants
- Ethical Issues with Treatment Research Methods
- Consequences of Ethical Constraints
- Protection of Animal Subjects
- Dissemination of Research Findings
- Summary
- Study Guide

Historically, the practice of science has raised many ethical issues because science is both a personal activity and a social activity. Science is powerful: It can produce beneficial as well as harmful effects for people. It can improve lives and living conditions. It can cure diseases. It can also create devastating effects on lives, as do weapons of mass destruction. Therefore, the effects of science may be desirable or undesirable. The products of science can be beneficial when responsible individuals and agencies use them, but science can be dangerous in the hands of wrong people. Therefore, it is no surprise that such a powerful enterprise should operate under ethical constraints. Such constraints are welcomed by both scientists and nonscientists so that the practice of science does not adversely affect individuals and society.

Scientists consider research to be an ethical activity. Scientists seek knowledge, try to solve practical problems, design new methods of treating diseases and disorders, and try to develop new technological solutions that benefit humankind. But they also have the responsibility of doing all of this in an honest, responsible, open, and ethically justifiable manner.

Clinical research in medicine and human service professions raises some additional ethical issues. Treatment-related research can sometimes pose a dilemma concerning the client's right to receive prompt and appropriate treatment and the profession's need to evaluate the effectiveness of new treatment procedures. Our discussion of ethical issues will consider the problems involved in clinical as well as nonclinical research.

In this chapter, I shall address eight fundamental ethical issues that affect research: (a) fraud in scientific research, (b) the effects of science on society, (c) the ethics of treatment evaluation, (d) the protection of human participants, (e) the consequences of ethical constraints, (f) ethical issues with treatment research methods, (g) the ethical issues relative to animal subjects, and (h) the dissemination of research findings.

FRAUD IN SCIENTIFIC RESEARCH

Scientists produce data and evidence about the behavior of natural phenomena. These data and evidence constitute knowledge of those phenomena. Normally, the reliability and validity of this knowledge are judged on methodological grounds. The results of scientific observation and experimentation are tentatively accepted when the methods and procedures were appropriate and used correctly. Typically, faulty methods and procedures of research studies are the main source of questionable data. Data produced by defective methods may reflect on the competence of scientists who produce it but not their ethical conduct.

There is another source of questionable data, which is more difficult to determine—the personal conduct of scientists themselves. Both the scientific and the general community believe, most appropriately, that scientists are people with integrity. The observations scientists report are normally not suspected on personal grounds because it is believed that (a) the data and evidence scientists report are a product of honest work, (b) the methods and procedures were indeed implemented the way they were described in the report, and (c) the reported quantitative values were observed and recorded during the study, as described procedurally.

A majority of scientists report only the findings of work they have done. Studies may have methodological limitations, but scientists try to implement the selected procedures in the best possible manner. They record the quantitative values of the studied variables as truthfully as they can. Scientific misconduct or fraudulent research lack these qualities. A panel on scientific responsibility and the conduct of research formed by the National Academy of Sciences, National Academy of Engineering, and the Institute of Medicine defined misconduct in science as "fabrication, falsification, or plagiarism, in proposing, performing, or reporting research. Misconduct in science does not include errors of judgment; errors in the recording, selection, or analysis of data; differences in opinions involving the interpretation of data; or misconduct unrelated to the research process" (Panel on Scientific Responsibility and the Conduct of Research, 1992, p. 5).

The history of science has documented several instances of fraudulent conduct by scientists in almost all disciplines. It is known that in 1912, an archaeologist reported the discovery of a human skull and jaw bone so different from the known forms of historic and prehistoric skulls that it forced scientists to think of a different evolutionary sequence. The skull came to be known as the "Piltdown man" because it was discovered in Piltdown Common, England (B. G. Campbell, 1976). However, during the 1950s, it became clear that a human skull and an ape jaw were used to construct the new find.

One of the better-known cases of possible fraud is that of the famous British psychologist Cyril Burt, who claimed that intelligence is mostly inherited. His evidence was that identical twins reared in different environments are still very similar in their intelligence as measured by standardized tests (Burt, 1972). His work had a significant effect on the practice of education and on the study of intelligence and inheritance of behavioral traits. Because of his published contributions to science, Burt was widely recognized as an international authority on the genetics of intelligence. He received numerous prestigious awards and was knighted by the British government.

A shocked scientific community learned in 1976, mainly through the popular press, that Burt may have falsified much of his data on identical twins and heritability of intelligence (Devlin, 1976; Gillie, 1976; Wade, 1976). The number of identical twin pairs he actually studied became questionable. The existence of several sets of identical twins Burt is supposed to have studied could not be documented. Whether he indeed had some of the research assistants mentioned in his publications also was questioned (Kamin, 1974). Because of these accusations, Burt's data have generally been excluded from any scientific discussion of heritability of intelligence. Nonetheless, some experts believe that although Burt was somewhat careless in reporting empirical data, the accusations against him may be false and may have been engineered by overzealous researchers who believe that intelligence is largely determined by environmental influences (Jensen, 1992). Many other kinds of research fraud that are not as well publicized have been documented (Miller & Hersen, 1992).

Plagiaristic practice of scientists is another serious problem. A review of misconduct in science conducted by the National Science Foundation found 20 allegations of plagiarism and nine allegations of data fabrication in a total of 41 allegations (Panel on Scientific Responsibility and the Conduct of Research, 1992). Some scientists and professionals who plagiarize others' writings and publish them in their own name seem to survive surprisingly well. For instance, a medical scientist, Elias A. K. Alsabti, had plagiarized already published articles and republished them under his own name. Nonetheless, he was successful in obtaining positions in at least seven universities and hospitals although at each institution his actions were either suspicious or were documented to be plagiaristic. When he was asked to leave one institution, he easily and quickly found a position in another (Miller, 1992).

Although outright fraud based on wholly cooked-up data is not discovered frequently, data distortions, partial fabrications of evidence, selective suppression or deletion of data, deceptive data analysis, deceptive reporting of data, and such other forms of fraud may be more common than thought. In addition, inappropriate protection offered to human participants, inhumane treatment of animal subjects, and misuse of research funds also are parts of unacceptable research practices (Miers, 1998). In a survey of medical fraud, 51% of reporting biostatisticians closely associated with medical treatment evaluation studies in multiple countries knew of at least one fraudulent research study (Ranstam et al., 2000). It has been suggested that the incidence of fraud may be higher in epidemiological research (Ranstam et al., 2000). In another survey, 32% of scientists suspected fraudulent practices by their colleagues (Tangney, 1987). Medical ethicists and researchers believe that the true extent of fraud in research is unknown (Miller & Hersen, 1992; Ranstam et al., 2000).

Institutional procedures to deal with research fraud did not exist prior to the 1980s (Miers, 1998; Miller & Hersen, 1992). Since then, there has been an increase in reports of scientific misconduct. One paper cites an average of two reports per month of potential misconduct received by a large federal agency that supports biomedical and behavioral research: National Institutes of Health (Miers, 1998). Various procedures to deal with research fraud now exist in most if not all universities, research institutions, and government agencies that support research (Panel on Scientific Responsibility and the Conduct of Research, 1992, 1993).

There may be actual or perceived pressure to produce certain kinds of data. Some scientists who are well known for their theories may be especially under this kind of pressure. It is not uncommon that a particular laboratory typically produces data that are consistent with one view, whereas another laboratory equally typically produces contradictory data on the same issue. It is believed that some hired research assistants are prone to distort the data they collect on behalf of professors and scientists whose theories are widely accepted (Diener & Crandall, 1978; Shaughnessy & Zechmeister, 1985).

As I discussed in Chapter 3, a scientist's public position in the form of theories and hypotheses can create pressure to uphold those positions regardless of the actual data. Instead of contradicting his or her previously stated positions, the scientist may resort to distortions in observations and interpretations of data. One way of avoiding the personally troublesome situation of having to contradict oneself is to refrain from prematurely committing oneself to a particular view.

Many scientists will not hesitate to reverse themselves or modify their positions in light of new data. Scientists are expected to say only what their data suggest, and those who do so are exemplary and should be emulated by students and other scientists.

A commitment to a view or a philosophy cannot be avoided forever, however. Accumulated experimental data have theoretical as well as philosophical implications, and they cannot and should not be ignored. Commitment to a particular view only after replicated experimental data have accumulated can reduce the chances of having to contradict oneself.

In some cases, particular views and experimental data can be questioned inappropriately. In such cases, defense of those views and data is appropriate. A scientist has every right to defend his or her position and point out the inappropriateness of apparently contradictory positions.

As noted in Chapter 3, the tendency to value data and evidence more than a particular point of view is a characteristic of all good scientists. Within the best traditions of science, scientists do not try to *prove* or *disprove* any particular view. Instead, they seek truth. It is only as a by-product of this search that a particular view gets either supported or rejected.

EFFECTS OF SCIENCE ON SOCIETY

The effects of science and research on society are also an ethical issue. Generally speaking, scientific research is for the good of society, but like all desirable ventures, it can produce some bad side effects. Such bad effects have become increasingly clear in the natural sciences.

Atomic research has vastly increased our knowledge of the physical world and has produced various kinds of benefits, including improved medical treatment procedures, but it also has increased the chances of the annihilation of humankind. Genetic research has helped us better understand the mysteries of life, with many desirable effects on society, but it also has raised the prospects of new and dangerous forms of life being inadvertently created. The chemical sciences have formulated new chemicals that are effective in treating various diseases, killing pests, and destroying crop-threatening weeds, but they also have adversely affected life by chemically polluting the world. Ethical issues such as these are complex, and the risk–benefit ratio should be weighed carefully and objectively. Unfortunately, objectivity in this case is more easily preached than practiced.

Scientists face a tremendous challenge in this case. On one hand, they are asked to solve a variety of problems so that life can be prolonged and its quality improved. On the other hand, they are asked to accomplish it in such a manner that no undesirable side effects emerge.

Regardless of such societal demands, scientists are committed to increasing their knowledge and improving the quality of life with the least amount of risk to society. They have an obligation to assess the long-term and short-term risks of their research efforts and devise methods to eliminate or reduce those risks. Conducting atomic explosions in underground sites and developing chemicals that devour other kinds of deadly chemical wastes illustrate this kind of scientific effort.

ETHICAL JUSTIFICATION OF TREATMENT EVALUATION

A special concern of clinical researchers is the effects of experimentation on clients who seek professional services. The concern is serious in the evaluation of treatment; the ethical dilemma may be real. An ethical dilemma is whether to experiment or not experiment with different treatment procedures. It is sometimes suggested that clients should be treated—not experimented on. This suggestion implies that experimental treatments are somehow more detrimental to clients than nonexperimental treatments.

A closer examination of the issue reveals that the distinction between experimental and nonexperimental treatments may be less meaningful than that between effective and ineffective (or dangerous) treatments. It is the ineffective or dangerous treatment that is detrimental to clients regardless of whether it is considered experimental or routine. It is the practice of ineffective or dangerous treatment procedures that is unethical.

When is a treatment experimental? This question is easily answered when a clinician calls a treatment experimental. The clinician then systematically collects data, uses certain control procedures, and thus tries to evaluate the effects of a particular treatment procedure. The effects may be positive, and the clients may have benefited just as much as those under an equally effective but routine treatment procedure. Nonetheless, what about the use of a treatment procedure whose effects have never been experimentally evaluated? Is this an experiment? Most people tend to think that as long as a procedure is more or less routine—and is not called "experimental" by the clinicians who use it—it is not experimental. Even more important, when the treatment procedure is not clearly defined, the goals are subjectively stated, and the improvement criteria are not specified, most people do not consider that treatment experimental. This assumption has created a false issue of ethics in treatment research.

In speech–language pathology, the practice of many treatment procedures is not based on experimental evaluations. Apparently, the practice of those procedures is based on clinical traditions and experiences. The trial-and-error approach of many clinicians may constitute an endless series of errors. When a clinical hunch is wrong, nothing better may be available, and therefore, the same ineffective practice may be perpetuated. Presumably, ineffective procedures continue to be used because the clinician either does not know that the technique does not help clients, or cannot implement a better procedure. Oddly enough, not many ethical concerns are raised about this kind of clinical practice.

Another kind of clinical practice is also oblivious of ethical concerns—a practice based on complex, impressive, but nevertheless speculative theories. Such theories are a collection of unverified hypotheses but are not recognized as such. Theories of this kind are sometimes so prestigious that in the judgment of many clinicians, a treatment procedure that is supported by a theory *ought* to work, even though there is no controlled evidence in its favor. Conversely, clinicians may believe that a treatment procedure that works well but is not a part of an accepted theory should be discarded. Unfortunately, this practice jeopardizes both service and knowledge.

It is when clinicians wish to determine the effects of treatment objectively that ethical concerns seem to be pressing. Addressing this issue, Barlow et al. (1984) stated that "if the intervention is poorly specified; goals are unclear; and if measures are weak, infrequent, or nonexistent, then there is *less* of an ethical worry. Our own cultural ambivalence about science has turned vice into virtue, sloppiness into safety" (p. 285).

The ethics of treatment evaluation involve at least three related issues. The first is whether treatment evaluation is necessary. The second is whether treatment evaluation is ethically justified. The third is whether treatment and treatment research are different kinds of activities. I shall briefly address these three issues.

Is Treatment Evaluation Necessary?

Whether treatment evaluation is necessary may not sound like an ethical issue, but it is at the heart of ethical controversy. Those who question the ethics of treatment evaluation imply that it is not necessary. When the necessity of researching treatment of a disorder is questioned, three assumptions may be implied. The first assumption is that an effective procedure to treat that disorder already exists and that the effects are objectively documented. The second assumption is that there is no room to improve the efficacy of the proven procedure. The third assumption is that there is no need to find a more effective procedure. In many cases, these assumptions may be wrong.

First, many diseases and disorders do not have treatments demonstrated to be effective. Second, the efficacy of effective treatments that do exist for certain disorders can perhaps be improved by controlled research. In the case of communicative disorders, few people assert that the field has perfectly effective treatment procedures that cannot be improved on. Third, even if there are effective procedures, it is possible to develop more effective procedures because no treatment research has reached its pinnacle. In the end, there is no choice but to experiment because clinicians (a) need effective procedures, (b) need to know that the procedures they are using are effective, (c) need to improve the efficacy of effective procedures, and (d) need to develop more effective procedures.

Is Treatment Evaluation Ethically Justified?

If it is concluded that treatment evaluation is necessary and that such treatment evaluation is no more harmful to clients than unverified procedures (which might actually be ineffective or dangerous), the second issue—whether treatment evaluation is ethically justified—appears in a different light. Obviously, treatment evaluation is justified. Indeed, systematic and objective evaluation of treatment procedures is one of the ethical responsibilities of clinical professions. Continued practice of treatment procedures whose effects are not objectively documented is unethical. Whether a treatment is old or new and whether it is practiced by a few or by many are not issues of consequence. Procedures that have been used widely and for a long time may still be ineffective and hence detrimental to clients. Therefore, it is a pseudoquestion to ask whether clinicians should experiment with their treatment procedures.

Some scientists assume that experiments that produce no effects or negative effects are of greater ethical concern than those that produce positive effects. Therefore, when treatments are evaluated and the results are nonexistent or negative, the clients may be said to have been used as "guinea pigs." However, the same procedure, used routinely, may not raise the same ethical question. Experiments showing that certain procedures are not useful or even harmful may prevent the widespread use of such procedures. Because negative evidence prevents continued damage to clients, studies that produce it should be welcome. Therefore, the outcome of an experimental treatment is never a basis on which to judge the ethics of clinical experimentation. Efforts at empirical determination of ineffectiveness or the positive or negative effects of treatment procedures is a necessary and ethical activity of clinicians. The effectiveness of a technique is known only when that technique is evaluated. As pointed out by Barlow et al. (1984, p. 287), systematic "evaluation [of a treatment] is not what makes it experimental. It just keeps us from fooling ourselves when it is."

Are Controlled Evaluations Different from Routine Treatment?

The third issue, whether routine treatment and controlled treatment evaluations are different kinds of activities, has been discussed occasionally (Siegel & Spradlin, 1985). If treatment evaluation is inherently different from treatment, then is there a justification for subjecting clients who need treatment to something other than treatment?

There is no question that in some specific respects, controlled evaluation of treatment is different from routine treatment. The crucial difference is that routine treatment does not use control procedures whereas treatment evaluation does. The group design approach uses no-treatment control groups, a placebo control group, or a standard treatment. Single-subject designs use treatment withdrawal or reversal, multiple baselines, alternating treatments, changing criterion, and so forth. Nonetheless, the difference between controlled treatment evaluations and routine treatments does not lead to the conclusion that treatment evaluation is unjustified. Before a procedure is used as routine treatment, it should undergo treatment evaluation so that people are not regularly offered an ineffective or harmful treatment. Therefore, treatment and treatment evaluation ought to be different, and both are necessary.

The discussion so far is not intended to suggest that there are no ethical problems in conducting treatment research. There are several problems, but they arise only because of the necessity of experimental treatment evaluations. In other words, whether clinicians should experimentally evaluate their procedures is not an ethically or otherwise valid question. The answer to that question is *yes*, and therefore there are ethical concerns. Several of these ethical concerns associated with treatment research are addressed in the remainder of this chapter.

In evaluating treatment effects, the researcher should take precautions to reduce the risk, if any, to the participants. In fact, steps to reduce the risks to human participants should be taken in all kinds of research, not just clinical treatment research.

PROTECTION OF HUMAN PARTICIPANTS

In this section, I shall address the issue of protection of human participants in general and, when appropriate, point out special ethical considerations relative to clinical treatment research.

Responsible scientists have always been concerned with the welfare of individuals who serve as participants in various medical, biological, behavioral, and other kinds of experiments. Scientists have known that the need to produce knowledge that will benefit humankind should be balanced with the risks that such an enterprise might pose to the human participants.

Nonetheless, abuses of human participants have occurred, especially in such institutional settings as general and mental hospitals, prisons, and military research installations (Brody, 1998; Metz & Folkins, 1985).

Human subject protection policies were not widely enforced until the U.S. Congress passed the National Research Act, which was signed into law in 1974, although several ethical guidelines were published much earlier. An early set of ethical guidelines for research are known as the Nuremberg Code published in 1949 (see Brody, 1998, for a report) after the famous Nuremberg trial in which it was revealed that Nazi physicians had conducted unconscionable and incredibly cruel experiments on Jewish people in concentration camps. The Nuremberg Code recognized for the first time that human participation in experiments should be voluntary and that the risks should be minimal (Brody, 1998). Then in 1964, the World Medical Association adopted what is known as the Helsinki Declaration on Research Ethics. The Helsinki Declaration was based on the Nuremberg Code but it further elaborated the risks and benefits of human participation in clinical research as well as basic biomedical research. The World Medical Association (2000) has periodically revised the Helsinki Declaration.

It soon became evident that abuse of human participants was not limited to an aberrant era of the Nazis. In 1966, Beecher published an article in which he made reference to 50 unethical experiments performed on human beings in post–World War II United States. He gave details on 22 of them. He cited a placebo controlled trial that evaluated the effects of the drug chloramphenicol against a placebo in patients who had typhoid fever. In this study, the patients in the placebo control group continued to receive a placebo even beyond the point where the effectiveness of the drug was clear in the experimental group, leading to a very high death rate among patients who took the placebo.

Testing potential toxicity of new drugs on institutionalized people has been an especially alarming abuse of research participants. In one experiment, toxicity of a drug on the liver was tested with healthy institutionalized people without their consent. When the participants developed hepatic dysfunction because of toxicity, their livers were biopsied to confirm the damage. Incredibly, when they got better, a few of them were given the same drug again to replicate the toxicity effects. In another experiment, institutionalized children with mental retardation were injected with isolated strains of hepatitis virus to understand the course of the disease (Beecher, 1966; Brody, 1998). Such instances as injecting cancer cells to unsuspecting patients hospitalized for various diseases also have been documented (Katz, 1972).

Unethical experiments on minority groups constitute another group of abusive studies. In one such experiment, known as the Tuskegee syphilis study, poor rural African Americans who had syphilis were initially enrolled in an observational study that began in the 1930s to understand the natural course of the disease (Jones, 1981). The study was continued until the early 1970s, although by that time penicillin was well established as the most effective treatment for syphilis. No informed consent was obtained from the patients, and they were strongly persuaded from seeking treatment that had become available. Similar abuse of human participants has been documented in most other countries (Brody, 1998).

The National Research Act of 1974 has significantly reduced abusive experiments in the United States. The act established the National Commission for the Protection of Human Subjects of Biomedical and Behavioral Research, which in 1979 issued general guidelines on human participant protection in a document known as the Belmont Report (1979). The specific rules and regulations that were subsequently issued by the U.S. Department of Health and Human Services and the Food and Drug Administration are based on the Belmont Report. These federal guidelines on ethical research practices are periodically revised, and all researchers are expected to follow the latest set of guidelines.

Most scientific and professional organizations such as the American Speech-Language-Hearing Association (2002) and the American Psychological Association (1992, 2002) have published guidelines on research ethics and human participant and animal subject protection. Furthermore, almost all universities and hospitals have their own additional guidelines. All of these guidelines are consistent with those issued by the federal agencies. Once again, researchers are expected to follow the current guidelines in their institution.

The most salient feature of the human participant protection procedures is the review of research proposals by an institutional review board (IRB). Most colleges and universities have multiple IRBs functioning at the level of the department and at the level of the school in which the department is housed. Usually, there is also a university-wide IRB that receives reports from IRBs at the lower levels.

It is now standard practice to submit all research procedures to one of these IRBs, also known as human subjects committees. These committees or boards review proposals to determine whether the proposed studies pose any risk to the participants and if so what steps should be taken to reduce that risk. The human subjects committee may also deny approval to carry out a study on the basis of unacceptable risks to the participants, but this is rare.

Because human participant protection procedures apply only to individuals who participate in research and not to routine clinical or educational procedures, a clear understanding of the legal concept of research is necessary. According to the regulations, any systematic investigation designed to develop or contribute to generalizable knowledge is research. If the clinician's purpose is to treat a client without an attempt to contribute knowledge that others may use, then the clinician is not doing research. In such cases, new treatment procedures may be used without institutional review of the procedures. However, if the clinician plans to publish the outcomes of a treatment procedure performed under controlled or uncontrolled conditions, then the study is research, and the proposal should be reviewed by an IRB.

All theses and dissertation proposals are routinely submitted to an IRB. A clinician who is not sure whether an undertaking contains an element of research or is simply a routine clinical procedure should submit a written description of the activities to an IRB for review and advice.

Institutional review boards should have at least five individuals. The federal regulations also stipulate that IRBs should contain at least one person who is not a scientist and one person who is not affiliated with the institution where the research will be conducted. (One person can satisfy both requirements.) Most college and university IRBs that review in-house proposals that do not receive federal funds do not recruit members from outside the university. Proposals that do not involve risks to participants may be reviewed only by one or two members of a university department's review committee, with a report of this action being made to a higher, fully constituted IRB. When risks are involved, such expeditious reviews are not allowed. In fact, studies that pose risks may be reviewed by multiple IRBs within an institution. The author of a research proposal may be asked to speak to the committee but does not take part in the review process. The major concerns of an IRB in reviewing research proposals include the risk–benefit ratio, informed consent, and the privacy of the participants.

Risk–Benefit Ratio

It is assumed that participation in any kind of research may involve risk to the participants. Some of the risks may be psychological. For example, research involving the experimental evaluation of the effects of shock or white noise on stuttering may create emotional stress or anxiety in participants. Procedures also may create physical harm or injury. For example, in medical research, new medical or surgical treatment procedures may pose significant risks to the lives of the patients. Certain other procedures may cause social embarrassment; for example, a study may be designed to evaluate the maintenance of target behaviors in natural settings. A person who stutters may have his or her treated fluency monitored in a supermarket, where the client may be forced to speak in difficult situations.

In this case, the IRB's tasks are to determine (a) whether the study poses risks to participants, and if so, (b) whether such risk is minimal, and if not, (c) how to handle the unacceptable level of risk. Risks are judged to be minimal when the expected level of risk does not exceed the level experienced in daily life situations. As a rough guideline, the amount of risk (stress) experienced while taking ordinary psychological or physical tests is considered minimal. In the case of research that poses minimal risk, an IRB may give quick approval to the study.

When the risk is judged to be more than minimal, the IRB does not necessarily deny permission to conduct the study. Instead, it reviews the procedures set forth by the investigator to handle that risk. The IRB may suggest modifications in the procedure. The intensity of potentially damaging experimental stimuli such as shock and noise may be limited. The participants may be allowed to determine the intensity levels presented to them. People who stutter may not be taken to social situations to test their fluency until after they have demonstrated fluency in more controlled, less embarrassing situations.

Potential risks to certain populations, such as children, are usually viewed conservatively. Whether the participants are children or adults, an IRB may suggest less stressful methods of data collection or, when this is not possible, require constant and professional monitoring of the participants' reactions to the experimental procedures. For example, the IRB may require the presence of a physician or a clinical psychologist if the experimental procedures are thought to cause physical or psychological stress. The IRB may also require that the experiment be terminated if participants show unacceptable levels of emotional reactions.

The IRBs evaluate not only the potential risks, but also the potential scientific benefits. It is important to realize that the scientific benefit, not the benefit to the participant, is what is evaluated. Other factors being equal, a research study that provides no benefits to the participants may be approved when the study is expected to generate scientific information. However, in this context, IRBs face a difficult task because they are generally not expected to evaluate the methodological or theoretical soundness of the studies they review. When it is considered appropriate, an IRB may seek an independent evaluation of the proposal's scientific merits from qualified scientists.

The federal regulations and the guidelines of professional organizations and universities are not designed to prevent all research studies that pose risks to human participants. Rather, they are intended to make sure that adequate protective measures are taken when there is risk. Many research studies that do pose various levels of risk to the participants are considered valuable because they produce scientific knowledge and eventual benefit to people. It may be noted that many people volunteer for risky experiments that may eventually benefit society. Those who volunteer for experimental medical or surgical treatments such as new drug evaluations, organ transplants, and artificial heart surgeries comprise a case in point.

Most research studies in speech–language pathology and audiology involve only a minimal risk to participants, and many clinical treatment studies actually improve the client's clinical conditions. Nonetheless, it is important to test established procedures for their experimentally demonstrated effects. Also, as new treatment procedures are developed, a cautious approach is needed. New procedures should be put to experimental tests with appropriate safeguards for the participants.

Informed Consent

A person's informed consent to participate voluntarily in research is one of the most important ethical principles of research. Informed consent involves three components. First, the participants should fully understand the procedures of the study. Second, they should freely and voluntarily consent to participate in the study. Third, the participants should be free to withdraw from the study at any time with no negative consequence to them.

Potential participants should not be contacted until after the approval of the IRB. This is because the method of participant contact itself may involve some coercion, and no person should be recruited by even the most subtle forms of coercion. For example, an instructor may ask his students to participate in an experiment in such a way as to imply that a lack of participation may have punitive consequences. A clinician may ask clients to participate in an experimental treatment while giving the impression that no other treatment is available. Therefore, an IRB should screen the proposed method of contacting and recruiting participants.

In obtaining informed consent from potential participants, the researcher should fully describe the procedures and purposes of the study. The individuals should know what is expected of them, what kinds of stimulus conditions they will be exposed to, what kinds of responses they will be asked to make, and how long they need to participate in the study. They should understand the risks and benefits of participation. In clinical treatment research, they should fully understand the procedure of the treatment being evaluated. Availability of alternative treatment procedures should be specified to the participants. When the risk is more than minimal, the possibilities of compensation also should be described. The potential participants should be informed of the names of persons (other than the author) they may contact about the research. The potential participants should understand that participation is entirely voluntary and that they are free to withdraw from the study at any stage with no penalty or prejudice. Finally, the individuals contacted should be told whether and to what extent their anonymity will be protected during and after the study.

The potential participants should have all the information in writing, usually called the informed consent form. They usually sign their name on the same document to indicate their full understanding of the procedures, risks, and benefits, and to indicate their willingness to participate in the study. The writing should be simple and nontechnical so that the individuals can understand the full implications of their participation. When the participants are children, parents give informed consent. Children 7 to 18 years old may also sign the informed consent form along with their parents. The children should be informed at a level appropriate for them to understand the procedures. Special efforts are needed to make sure that individuals with communicative disabilities understand the procedures of a study before deciding to participate.

Privacy of the Participants

The privacy of the participants of research studies is another important ethical issue. Clinicians know that the privacy or confidentiality of clients is an important professional issue regardless of research concerns; likewise, research investigators should take every possible step to protect the privacy of their participants.

Most research studies are published in one form or another. Publication will include descriptions of participants. Therefore, the participants should give informed consent to such publication. The typical procedure is to inform the participants that their confidentiality will be protected when the studies are published. In most cases, the participants' names and other identifying data will not be published.

Participant identity may be revealed in certain kinds of publications. For example, the picture of a client may be a part of a research article showing various physical characteristics of a genetic syndrome. In such cases, the clients, their guardians, or both should give explicit written permission to publish pictures. Similar permission should be obtained when an audiotape or a videotape is expected to be published in some form. Most speech and hearing centers routinely obtain such permission from the clients, their guardians, or both. This procedure facilitates the future research use of client information.

Throughout the study, information obtained about individuals, their families, institutions, and organizations should be kept strictly confidential. The participants should be informed of the procedures by which the confidentiality of the participants and institutions will be maintained. An investigator may propose, for example, that the individuals will be coded and the names of the participants will not be used in any stage of data analysis. Access to confidential information about individuals may be restricted. Only the principal investigator may know the names of the participants. An IRB may find that the safeguards need improvements and make suggestions to that effect. Eventually, the potential participants or their guardians judge for themselves whether the proposed methods of protecting confidentiality are acceptable.

The ethical issues discussed in this chapter are not always amenable to objective and unambiguous resolution. The regulations and guidelines recognize the difficulty involved in assessing the risk–benefit ratio, the need for deception, and the possibilities of the invasion of privacy of research participants. The investigator and the IRB make the best possible judgments, taking all of the important factors into consideration.

As I have noted, IRBs are responsible for making sure that individuals who serve as participants in research studies are treated fairly and honestly. However, the presence of such boards and committees does not reduce the responsibility of the investigator. It is the investigator who is ultimately responsible for his or her conduct in the course of research investigations, and the IRBs have to trust the authors in following the approved procedures.

When a violation occurs, the IRB does not have the power to take punitive steps against the investigator; the authorities of the institution investigate violations and take appropriate actions.

ETHICAL ISSUES WITH TREATMENT RESEARCH METHODS

The ethical restraints imposed on the research community have produced many beneficial effects for individuals who participate in experiments as well as society at large. Such restraints may have prevented many abusive research efforts. Nonetheless, there still are some ethical problems with certain accepted research practices. Some of these problems may be inevitable and an acceptable price to pay for scientific knowledge; others may be solved or their effects reduced by making methodological changes in investigation.

This section describes a few current research practices that do not violate existing laws and guidelines on human biomedical and behavioral research but nonetheless raise certain ethical issues. The major research practices that raise ethical concerns include informed consent, the no-treatment control groups, placebo control groups, randomization, treatment withdrawal or reversal, and general methods of participant recruitment.

Ethical Concerns with Informed Consent Procedures

As noted in this chapter, human participant protection is a phenomenon of the latter half of the 20th century. It is now a standard research practice to obtain informed consent from participants who agree to participate in a research study. This means that the participants understand the nature, procedure, and purpose of the study and that they fully understand the risks and benefits of participation. After fully understanding the study and its procedures, potential participants give their voluntary consent. The participants' signature on the informed consent form fulfills the legal obligation of this aspect of human participant protection procedure.

In recent years, questions have been raised about the effectiveness and empirical validity of most informed consent procedures used in medical treatment research. There is evidence that many patients may not fully understand the nature of randomized clinical trials (RCTs). People whose educational level is low may find the informed consent procedure especially daunting. The concept of randomization has been especially difficult for many people to grasp; for example, sometimes even after giving informed consent to participate in RCTs, participants still expect to receive the treatment they want. In some cases, less than half the participants may grasp the concept of randomization of treatment allocation (Snowdon, Garcia, & Elbourne, 1997).

Conditions under which informed consent is sometimes sought also bring into question the degree to which consent is truly "informed and voluntary." In some studies, an informed consent is sought from people who are distressed about their own or their family member's acute and rapidly deteriorating disease. Family members who face a life-or-death situation may be asked to give informed consent for a new treatment study. The validity of informed consent sought from parents for entering their newborn baby into RCTs has come under heavy criticism. Emotionally distraught parents, having just learned that their newborn has a serious, possibly life-threatening health problem, may be asked to make certain quick judgments about entering or not entering an RCT. Most parents of sick children, it has been observed, will give consent to any kind of procedure that may offer even a faint chance for their children's survival (McIntosh, 1993; Snowdon, Garcia, & Elbourne, 1997). Validity of informed consent obtained under stressful conditions from people with limited education may be highly questionable. In fact, an editorial in *Lancet*, one of the world's leading medical journals, concluded that "informed consent from poorly educated parents entering a complex trial in stressful conditions is a sham" ("Your Baby Is in a Trial," 1995, p. 806). For these and other reasons, some investigators wonder whether informed consent is just a myth (Silverman, 1989).

Besides raising ethical concerns, informed consent has permanently changed the nature of data collected in RCTs. This issue of the effects of informed consent on data and their interpretation will be addressed in a later section.

Ethical Concerns with No-Treatment Control Groups

As described in Chapters 4 and 8, RCTs and any kind of treatment research that uses a group design for treatment evaluation may use a control group that receives no treatment until the end of the study. Some studies have long durations, months or even several years. Therefore, participants in the no-treatment control group may go without a much-needed treatment for a long time. Provided the participants understand that they may not receive treatment when they agree to participate, the use of such no-treatment control groups are acceptable under most governmental and institutional research guidelines, although some international guidelines are more restrictive than those in the United States (Brody, 1998). Nonetheless, many medical researchers have raised valid ethical issues with this accepted research practice.

Most RCTs in medicine employ multiple physicians as principal investigators who are responsible to recruit patients to the trial. In recent years, there has been significant difficulty in recruiting patients to RCTs in medicine. Many eligible patients are unwilling to participate in clinical trials. One reason they do not want to participate in a randomized clinical trial involving a no-treatment control group and one experimental group that receives a treatment is that they would have a 50% chance of receiving no treatment. When they realize that they only have a 50% chance of receiving treatment for their disease in a study, they seek treatment outside the scope of the study. In essence, the patients opt out of the study so their disease may be treated immediately.

Even those patients who agree to participate in a study involving a no-treatment control group may drop out of the study as their clinical condition worsens or when they find out that those in the experimental group are getting better with treatment. In one study in speech–language pathology, parents of control group children who stuttered demanded treatment for their children when they learned that fluency of children in the experimental group had improved (Onslow, Andrews, & Lincoln, 1994). When control group participants demand the experimental or some other treatment, the investigators have no choice but to offer it.

Those who stay with the study and receive no treatment may be frustrated with their participation or distressed about not getting treatment. From a legal standpoint, the investigators may not be concerned because the participants have agreed to participate on their own accord (the validity of this claim will be addressed in a later section). From an ethical standpoint, the matter may be serious. For example, a postrandomization study of patient reactions to random assignment has revealed that patients may be "heartbroken" to find that they are not allocated to the treatment group (Snowdon, Garcia, & Elbourne, 1997).

There is evidence that many physicians and surgeons are reluctant to enter their patients into RCTs because of the uncertainty involved in the trials, that is, the possibility that treatment will be denied to their sick patients. Many practitioners think that their primary responsibility is to their individual patients, not to the aggregate of patients with which the trials are concerned (Taylor, 1985). Pediatricians may be especially reluctant to enter sick children under their care into randomized experiments (Morris, Zaritsky, & LeFever, 2000). Generally, physicians who do not enter their eligible patients into randomized trials cite their ethical commitment to providing the best possible care for their patients. They see a conflict between this commitment and the denial of treatment to control groups in clinical trials. Other reasons for practitioners' reluctance to enter their patients into trials involve the informed consent procedure, addressed previously.

Treatment denial to a control group is acceptable when no treatment for a disorder or disease is available and the treatment being evaluated is the only potential recourse. Recognizing this, many RCTs in medicine use control groups that receive an existing or standard treatment while the experimental group receives the new treatment under investigation. From a scientific standpoint, it is better to compare a new treatment with no treatment; however, comparing the effects of a new treatment against those of an existing treatment is an ethically justified compromise.

In most experiments, control conditions used with the single-subject designs are just as effective as control groups without the ethical issues associated with those groups. One of the ethical guidelines researchers follow is that a risky procedure is justified only when there are no alternative methods of securing valid data: Single-subject designs offer alternative procedures that avoid control groups who do not receive treatment for extended durations.

Ethical Concerns with Placebo Control Groups

In RCTs, a control group may receive a placebo, described in Chapter 4. The placebo control groups were designed when it was found that many patients feel better when they take something that is thought to be medicine, even though it has no medicinal properties (such as a sugar or lactose pill). The placebo effect suggested that some of the effects of a new medication (actually, any medication) may be due to this placebo effect. In scientific experiments on treatment effects, investigators believe that they have to demonstrate that the effects of a medicine exceeded that of the presumed placebo effect.

As pointed out in Chapter 4, the presence and the extent of the placebo effect have been debated in medical literature. Our concern here is not whether the placebo effect is real, but what ethical problems the widely used placebo control groups pose for both the investigators and participants.

Participants who are members of a placebo control group in RCTs receive an inert material or a lactose tablet that looks exactly like the drug whose effect is under investigation. In a single-blind study, the participants who receive a placebo do not know that fact. In a double-blind study, neither the participants nor the immediate investigators who administer the placebo (as well as the medicine) and measure the effects know that fact.

Patients who receive a placebo, like those who receive no treatment, go without much-needed treatment. Beyond that, those who receive a placebo in a single- or double-blind study tend to believe that they are being treated; that is the essence of the placebo concept. That they have given informed consent has no effect on this hope or expectation. As noted before, patients in a no-treatment control group may be heartbroken to know that they are not getting treatment in an RCT; this applies to placebo control group participants as well, except that for a while, they are fooled into thinking that they are getting real medicine. Consequently, patients may think that RCTs that involve either no treatment or placebo are a gamble, and many who participate in such experiments have much uneasiness about them (Madden, 1994).

In surgical treatment evaluation, a placebo is less commonly used, but when it is used, it raises the most serious ethical concerns. Placebos in surgical treatment studies involve performing sham surgical procedures to make the patients think that they have been operated on to treat a condition. For instance, in a randomized placebo-controlled evaluation of the effects of intracerebral transplantations of fetal mesencephalic tissue in patients with Parkinson's disease, a hole was drilled into the skull of the placebo control group patients to simulate the surgical treatment procedure (Dekkers & Boer, 2001). Patients randomly assigned to placebo control groups in all surgical treatment evaluation studies undergo such sham surgery which exposes them to unnecessary risks of injury, infection, surgical accidents, and other unexpected negative consequences.

From an ethical standpoint, one could argue that the administration of a placebo is a misleading aspect of RCTs. It is especially so in studies in which the participants are blinded; in such cases, the participants are given a worthless treatment, and to compound the ethical problems, this fact is concealed from them. In light of the controversy about its very existence, the ethical problems of placebo administration may outweigh its presumed advantages. That the patients have given informed consent to be randomized in a study that uses a control group does not remove these ethical concerns (Rothman & Michels, 1994). In fact, the revised Declaration of Helsinki issued by World Medical Association (2000) states that placebo-controlled clinical trials are unethical when a new treatment can be compared against standard treatments.

Ethically, no-treatment control groups may fare slightly better than placebo control groups. Minimally, patients participating in no-treatment control groups are not fooled into thinking that they are receiving treatment. Physically, patients in both the types of control groups may suffer serious consequences of denied treatment, including deterioration in symptoms, reduced effectiveness of subsequent treatment because of more advanced disease, and possibly death. Participants in placebo-controlled experiments involving medicine may fare slightly better than those in experiments involving surgical treatment. Setting aside the serious consequences of not treating a disease, placebo in medical research is at least a harmless lactose tablet; placebo in surgical treatment research is an invasive procedure, offering only risks, no benefits.

Ethical Concerns with Randomization

Theoretically, randomization, as described in Chapter 4, should be done at two levels. First, potential participants should be randomly selected from a population to which the conclusions are eventually extended. Second, the randomly drawn sample of participants should be once again randomly assigned to treatment and control groups. Thus, random drawing and random assignment are the two requirements that might assure statistical generality. In practice, though, participants are rarely drawn randomly from a population. Only those who give consent to participate in a study are randomly assigned to treatment and experimental groups.

Statisticians and others argue that randomization is the essential element of objective treatment evaluation—an argument rejected by those who advocate the single-subject approach. The central ethical issue with randomization is that people are assigned to one of the several groups including one that receives a less effective treatment, a more effective treatment, no treatment, or a placebo treatment. It is true that patients or their families (in the case of children) will have given informed consent. As discussed before, informed consent may or may not be truly informed and valid in the case of all participants, and even when it is, the participants will have hopes of receiving a treatment or a more effective treatment. In many desperate conditions, people volunteer in the hopes of beating the odds of randomization in favor of receiving a beneficial treatment. But when they find out that they have been assigned to a less effective treatment or to a placebo, many refuse further participation; those who continue their participation resent randomization. A study of the reactions of parents who had entered their babies into a randomized clinical trial showed that most parents had strong negative reactions to the random method of allocating treatment. The parents thought that was against the basic tenet of making treatment decisions based on the clinical condition of a patient (Snowdon, Garcia, & Elbourne, 1997).

Many practicing physicians and surgeons are reluctant to enter their eligible patients to RCTs because they believe that random allocation of treatment is inherently against their ethical responsibility of treating their patients with the best possible care (Taylor, 1985; Verdu-Pascal & Castello-Ponce, 2001). Research scientists, however, argue that when it is not known what the best possible treatment is, it needs to be discovered by experimentation. When, in scientists' judgment, randomization is the only way to generate valid scientific data on different treatment options, they see no compelling ethical dilemmas. No one, of course, would argue against the ethical need for treatment evaluation. However, arguments can be made that randomization is neither needed nor justified in all cases of treatment evaluation. Single-subject designs are applicable in most cases where randomized group designs are used; these designs can generate scientifically valid data to help choose the best possible treatment without the ethical concerns of randomization of treatment allocation.

Ethical Concerns with Treatment Withdrawal or Reversal

Concerns raised so far apply to group designs with random selection and assignment of participants to different treatments, placebo treatment, or no treatment. Most single-subject designs avoid those procedures and thus the ethical concerns associated with them. The *ABA* and *ABAB* designs, however, do pose some ethical concerns because of treatment withdrawal and reversal associated with them. These concerns were discussed in detail in Chapter 9 and are only briefly reviewed in this chapter.

In the *ABA* design, the participants derive only a temporary benefit. If the treatment is effective, it will be evident in the experimental (*B*) condition. Whether effective or not, the treatment is finally withdrawn in the final *A* condition. In the case where the treatment has been effective, the clinical problem is allowed to return to its baseline level in the withdrawal condition. This return to baseline creates ethical problems. For the clients and the family, it is illogical to reverse the beneficial effects of a treatment. Although the clients and their families will have given informed consent, anecdotally, some fail to appreciate the need for this type of research. And they may be correct because there are alternatives—such as multiple baseline designs.

Treatment reversal, essentially the same as withdrawal in its final effect (which is to recover the baseline), can cause ethical problems and participant rejection, similar to those caused by randomization. In some cases, reversal may be more distressing than withdrawal. In behavioral treatment research, when the treatment is withdrawn, the client is simply engaged in conversation, play, and such other activities. Therefore, withdrawal looks natural to consumers. The reversal, however, does not look natural to them. In reversal, an incompatible behavior may be taught, and in many cases, the incompatible behavior is the very undesirable behavior that was reduced under treatment. For instance, differential reinforcement may reduce errors of articulation in the *B* condition and the same differential reinforcement technique may be used to increase the errors in the reversal condition.

As pointed out in Chapter 9, some research questions are best served by the reversal design. In all other cases, it may be preferable to avoid the reversal as a control mechanism.

The *ABAB* design also may contain either a reversal or withdrawal condition and poses similar ethical problems. These problems are somewhat muted because those conditions are temporary, the effective treatment is reinstated, and the participants end the experiment with accrued benefit from the experiment. One might still consider multiple baseline designs as ethically more attractive alternatives because these designs do not involve treatment withdrawal or reversal. The *ABAB* design is more powerful in demonstrating the cause–effect relations, however.

Ethical Concerns with Participant Recruitment

Participant recruitment procedures, even when they do not explicitly violate existing ethical guidelines on research, can still pose ethical problems. Participant recruitment is typically difficult for treatment research. Most investigators try to do their best in recruiting participants who are appropriate for their studies. Investigators try to balance participants of different characteristics. Nonetheless, practical difficulties in recruiting participants with expected characteristics can create certain ethical problems.

One of the problems faced by speech–language pathologists and perhaps psychologists as well is the repeated use of the same participants in multiple experiments. Psychology students are often recruited for participation in experimental studies that faculty members conduct, and the same students may be repeatedly used in multiple experiments. The students' experience in one experiment may influence their performance in the other. In communicative disorders, the same few individuals that are seeking treatment for months and years may be used as participants in multiple treatment efficacy studies. This is likely to happen in cases of aphasia, developmental disabilities, stuttering, autism, hearing impairment, and other conditions that require long-term treatment. In all such cases, the results may be somewhat ambiguous because the experimental design used may make no allowance for analyzing the effects of prior participation in studies. Minimally, the investigator should give the study participation history of all the participants in research submitted for publication.

Another problem in participant recruitment may involve subtle forms of coercion. In spite of an investigator's best effort to avoid any hint of coercion, people in certain positions may feel an obligation to participate in an experimental study. Students, for example, when asked to consider participation in an experiment may feel obligated to participate, in spite of the faculty member's insistence that the participation is entirely voluntary. Clinicians who are providing treatment or those who are supervising clinical practicum in university clinics and, in turn, request participation of clients also may exert subtle forms of coercion.

There may be no effective solution to the problem of subtle coercion that people who are asked to participate in experimental research may feel. Recognizing this potential problem, however, is the ethical responsibility of all investigators who will then take all steps necessary to minimize such coercion. Investigators who work hard to earn a reputation for not taking punitive measures and not showing subtle, unpleasant reactions to nonparticipants will have done their best to minimize ethical concerns of this kind.

All treatment researchers know that there are participants who are difficult to recruit. Generally, people belonging to minority groups, people belonging to lower socioeconomic classes, and people who live far from urban research centers may be difficult to recruit for experimental studies. Medical treatment research sometimes tend to oversample men at the cost of women. People living near a university often are easily recruited by university-based researchers. These practical exigencies, however, create ethical dilemmas because they exclude a significant portion of people from participating in treatment evaluation studies. On the other hand, the conclusions of the very studies in which they do not participate are frequently extended to unrepresented members of the population. This is unacceptable both scientifically and ethically; all investigators have an ethical responsibility to recruit a diverse set of people, representative of the group to whom the conclusions of a study are meant to be generalized.

While nonparticipation of people who are economically or otherwise disadvantaged is a serious problem, overrepresentation of disadvantaged people in certain kinds of studies is an equally serious problem. There is some evidence that in studies on new and risky treatment for serious diseases, disadvantaged people (relatively poor, less educated, and without health insurance) may be overrepresented. On the other hand, studies on disease prevention include a disproportional number of healthy, more affluent, and educated people (Gorkin et al., 1996; McKee et al., 1999). Such imbalances in recruiting participants is an ethical issue because the burden of evaluating the unproven and potentially risky techniques may fall on the shoulders of the disadvantaged while deriving long-term benefits from disease prevention research may be the privilege of the affluent. From a scientific standpoint, both are biased samples that limit generality, which is a separate but equally troubling issue.

CONSEQUENCES OF ETHICAL CONSTRAINTS

Ethical constraints on research, especially the procedures designed to protect human participants are necessary. No one argues that the restrictions should be relaxed to make it easier to conduct treatment and other kinds of experimental research. On the contrary, even tighter restrictions on treatment research practice may need to be imposed because of the repeated research fraud and persistent ethical concerns with currently accepted treatment evaluation procedures described previously. Nonetheless, it is necessary to discuss some unexpected or unwanted consequences that ethical restraints have on the conduct of all research, especially on treatment research.

The data that treatment research generates under current ethical guidelines are inherently different from those that could be generated under a different set of circumstances. In making appropriate interpretations of treatment data, one needs to consider the conditions under which they were collected. Failure to consider the effects of ethical restraints on data collection may lead to questionable conclusions. Even more important, in the era of informed consent and voluntary participation in treatment research, certain standard methods of treatment research may be questionable. This section addresses the consequences of informed consent and voluntary participation and the participants' autonomy in the research process. These factors have decidedly changed the nature of treatment research evidence and have serious consequences for data interpretation.

Effects of Informed Consent and Voluntary Participation

Participation without the informed consent of individuals is a serious ethical breach that is no longer expected to happen. On the other hand, informed consent and voluntary participation have changed the way the participants are supposed to be recruited randomly; that is, the requirements of informed consent can create problems for many research studies. A troubling problem is the scientific consequence of informing the participants about certain procedures and their expected effects.

The ethical problems associated with informed consent were previously discussed. This section covers the effects that informed consent has on the nature and quality of data. The biasing effects of full disclosure and the de facto self-selection of participants are both examined.

Biasing Effects of Informed Consent

When participants are given the full details regarding the purposes and procedures of certain treatment techniques, a biasing effect may be created. This effect may then confound the effects of the treatment itself. For example, if people who stutter are told that the purpose of the experiment is to decrease their stuttering with a verbal "no" every time they stutter, some participants may monitor their stuttering more carefully. Such monitoring may produce its own effect on the frequency of stuttering.

A verbal conditioning study has documented the effects of disclosing the purpose of an experiment to the participants (Resnick & Schwartz, 1973). In this study, one group of participants was told that the purpose of the study was to increase a certain class of verbal behaviors by verbal reinforcers, which was the actual purpose of the study. Another group was simply told that the purpose was to study certain aspects of communication. The group that was informed of the actual purpose of the experiment did not show an increase in behaviors that were followed by the experimenter's verbal stimuli, whereas the group that was not informed showed the typical increase.

There are also research questions that cannot be answered unless the purposes of a study are concealed. For example, if a psychologist studies anger in a contrived laboratory situation, telling the potential participants about the purpose and the procedure of the study may make it subsequently impossible to evoke anger. Similarly, if a psychologist studies the conditions under which people express surprise, full disclosure of the stimuli to be used in evoking surprise will leave nothing to study.

Many researchers in the past have not fully disclosed the purpose and the procedures of their studies to the participants. This has raised the ethical question of deception (Kelman, 1972; Milgram, 1977). Deception may be mild or extreme. A general description of the purpose and procedure may be provided while some crucial information is withheld from the participants. Deception may also involve total misrepresentation of the purposes of the study. The acceptability of a certain degree of deception or misrepresentation that does not create additional risks to the participants and that is considered absolutely essential to the study is debatable. One extreme position would consider any level of deception unethical and unacceptable and the other extreme position may allow it. Generally speaking, ethical standards of research require full disclosure.

Aspects of a study may be concealed only when the study itself does not produce any negative effects for the participants and there is no other way of studying that phenomenon (such as in a study on surprising conditions or stimuli). In such cases, participants who are not informed should be debriefed as soon as their participation is over. In debriefing, the participants are given a full description of the actual purposes and procedures of the study with an explanation as to why the information was withheld from them until the end of their participation. This is done to avoid any potential negative effects of the experimental procedures and the deception. For example, individuals who were made to experience anxiety, anger, or some other strong emotion in front of an audience may feel better when they find out the true nature of the experiment.

Effects of Participants' Autonomy

The most serious consequence for data generation is caused by the participants' autonomy, granted under all ethical guidelines on research. Unlike in the preinformed consent era, all participants now participate on their own accord. As noted before in this chapter, the participants may withdraw from any study at any time without negative consequence to them. In treatment studies, they may demand a treatment they are not assigned to, may demand treatment when they are assigned to a no-treatment or placebo control group, may request modification in their existing treatment plan, and so forth. These requirements, whose necessity and validity are not in question, produce profound consequences for treatment research, especially for RCTs.

The inevitable consequence of participant autonomy is that in all RCTs, participants are self-selected. Participant autonomy and randomization are contradictory terms. It is well documented that potential and eligible participants freely exercise their autonomy, as they should. In fact, 50% or more of eligible patients refuse to participate in RCTs because of the fear of randomization (Blichert-Toft, Mouridsen, & Andersen, 1996; Snowdon, Garcia, & Elbourne, 1997). When participants retain the right to agree or refuse to participate, when they may drop out of the study at any time, when they are allowed to demand and get the treatment they were not assigned to, then there is essentially no random selection or random assignment of participants. Therefore, the participant autonomy renders randomization of RCTs meaningless. In RCTs, who gets into the study, who gets what treatment, who gets no treatment, and who gets the placebo is supposedly determined by randomization. But none of this holds good when patients "vote with their feet" (Silverman & Altman, 1996, p. 171) in all RCTs.

Feinstein (1970), a distinguished medical researcher, is among the very few who recognize that participant autonomy negates randomization. The general problem of participant autonomy, however, has been widely recognized by medical experts who call this a *nonconsenting bias* (Marcus, 1997) or *volunteer bias* (Edlund, Craig, & Richardson, 1985). Because of participant autonomy, the participants who eventually complete a randomized clinical trial may not represent the population of patients who have the same disorder or disease. Consequently, the results of a study cannot be extended; in other words, because of participant autonomy, the RCTs cannot claim statistical generality. Unfortunately, most of them do so anyway. For example, medical researchers continue to insist on RCTs because they allow statistical generality.

What is suggested here should be clear to the reader: Informed consent of participants is more valuable than the method of randomization. If ethically justified informed consent has a negative consequence for randomization, then the researchers should reconsider the theory, method, and value of randomization. Because researchers do need to keep informed consent, they may have to give up some of the cherished, but rarely realized, benefits of randomization.

PROTECTION OF ANIMAL SUBJECTS

This chapter has concentrated on the ethical treatment of human participants because of the preponderance of research involving human participants in clinical disciplines and education. However, ethical guidelines also should be followed when animal subjects are used in research.

Animals are frequently used in laboratory and field experiments. Research studies in medicine, biology, ethology, psychology, and pharmaceutics involve animals. Most new drugs are first used with animal subjects. New surgical procedures often are experimentally performed on animals. When the effects of new chemicals (other than drugs) are studied, once again animals are the primary subjects. In behavioral and psychological research, animals with normal neurophysiological structures and those with altered structures (e.g., induced brain lesions) have been subjected to various stimuli. Any new research on the brain that involves an invasive procedure is first tried out on animals. Monkeys, rats, mice, cats, dogs, and fish often are used in these experiments.

In communicative disorders, the use of animal subjects is limited. However, there are special problems in studies using animals. In the study of the evolution and functioning of phonation, various species of animals are studied. Some of these studies may involve surgical procedures to analyze the structures of phonatory mechanisms. Research on subhuman language or communication systems has involved animals, especially chimpanzees that have been taught various forms of nonverbal communication.

Animals probably are more frequently used in the study of audition. Chinchillas, for example, have been used frequently in the study of hearing because their auditory mechanism is similar to that of humans. Other animals used in auditory research include gerbils, cats, monkeys, guinea pigs, rats, mice, and birds. By using animals to study the electrical responses of cochlea, scientists have helped develop and refine cochlear implants for people who are deaf. Much of our knowledge of noise-induced hearing loss is derived from experimental research with animal subjects. Research on ototoxicity frequently involves animal subjects (Folkins, Gorga, Luschei, Vetter, & Watson, 1993).

The appropriateness of using animals in potentially dangerous experiments has been an issue in recent years (Folkins et al., 1993; Rosenfeld, 1981). Advocates of animal rights have argued that many scientific experiments in which animals are subjected to painful procedures are unethical and should be banned. Those who justify the use of animal experiments remind us that many life-saving drugs, vaccines, and surgical procedures would not have been developed without animal experimentation.

In spite of the controversy, animals will continue to be used as subjects in scientific experiments. Therefore, the need to follow ethical guidelines in the care of laboratory animals is clear. There are various local, state, and federal laws pertaining to the use of animals in scientific research. Among others, the American Psychological Association (2002), National Institutes of Health (1991), and National Research Council (1988) have published guidelines on the care and use of animals in research laboratories. These guidelines are periodically revised, and new federal guidelines are published in the *Federal Register*. Researchers should consult the current guidelines and adhere to them.

The guidelines suggest that the acquisition, care, use, and disposal of animals should follow federal, state, and local laws. The guidelines specify that those who engage in animal experimentation receive special training in the care of animal subjects. The experimenters are expected to minimize discomfort, illness, deprivation, stress, and pain due to the experimental procedures. Before animals are subjected to such procedures, scientists should consider alternative methods that are less painful or stressful. Radical procedures should be justified in terms of the scientific, educational, or applied benefit. Animals should be anesthetized before they are subjected to surgical procedures. Animals should be housed in comfortable and clean settings in which they are properly fed. While in the custody of scientists, animals should receive humane care. All institutions and laboratories that use animals in research should have an institutional animal care and use committee to review policies and procedures and to ensure that the animal subjects are used according to established guidelines (Folkins et al., 1993).

DISSEMINATION OF RESEARCH FINDINGS

The worth of a piece of research is judged by other scientists, and when possible, by society at large. However, people—including scientists—can make this judgment only when research findings are disseminated. Therefore, dissemination of research findings is an ethical responsibility of researchers.

One can argue that if research findings are never going to be published, any amount of risk that the participants experience is unacceptable. Even when no risk is involved, efforts are involved. As participants, individuals give their time for research. Many experience inconvenience because of their participation in research. Individuals are expected to volunteer for research on the assumption that they contribute to the advancement of scientific knowledge. Unpublished results, unfortunately, do not advance scientific knowledge.

The information generated by scientific studies should receive the widest possible dissemination and the most appropriate dissemination. A majority of scientific studies are appropriately first published in scientific journals. When certain findings are technical and subject to misunderstanding by the general public, it may not be desirable to publish those findings in popular media. When it is judged that the findings of a treatment study are highly tentative, it may not be appropriate to disseminate them to potential clients who may be candidates for that or similar treatment. Most scientists prefer that the initial findings be published in a scientific or professional journal so that other experts can evaluate those findings and, if possible, replicate them. Scientists typically react negatively to publications of "new" and "revolutionary" scientific findings and clinical treatment procedures in popular media. Scientifically well-established findings, of course, should receive the widest possible dissemination. Such findings may be published in popular sources as well as in professional journals.

In conclusion, when scientists pay due attention to the ethical principles that govern research and publication, a responsible practice of science emerges. Ethical principles are meant to reduce the undesirable side effects of scientific research and thereby increase the potential of benefit to humankind. Every researcher should be fully knowledgeable in ethical principles so that the practice of science will be as responsible as its products are enlightening.

SUMMARY

- The practice of science is an ethical activity. It is presumed that scientists report only what they observed and studied and that no data are falsified or fabricated. However, cases of scientific fraud are periodically reported.

- Scientists seek to produce positive effects, but negative effects may be associated with many desirable effects of science. The effects of science on society is an ethical issue.

- In clinical sciences, an important ethical issue is that of treatment evaluation. It is the ethical responsibility of clinical scientists and professionals to evaluate the effects of their treatment procedures and other services; however, they need to do this in an ethically justifiable manner.

- All researchers should follow established procedures of protecting human participants and animal subjects in research. The human participant protection procedures involve such issues as the risk–benefit ratio, informed consent of participants, and the protection of participants' privacy.

- There are ethical concerns with treatment research methods: Informed consent may not fully accomplish its objectives; no-treatment and placebo control procedures pose special ethical dilemmas; randomization may be both unethical and ineffective; some participant recruitment strategies may be questionable.

- Ethical constraints, though necessary, have certain consequences for study design and data interpretation. Informed consent and participant autonomy essentially negate randomization because under these rules all participants are self-selected.

- An ethical responsibility of researchers is to disseminate research findings. Such dissemination justifies research and the acceptable risk and inconvenience the participants may have faced.

STUDY GUIDE

1. What are the sources of questionable data?

2. How are theories and hypotheses related to the questions of reliability and validity of data?

3. Describe some of the undesirable side effects of science and technology. What steps do you suggest to counteract them?

4. What is an apparent ethical dilemma of clinical experimentation?

5. When is a treatment experimental?

6. What are some of the false questions relative to the ethics of clinical experimentation?

7. Is the question, "Should we experiment with treatment procedures?" ethically or otherwise valid? Justify your answer.

8. Should one experiment with an untested treatment procedure that has been used widely over a number of years? Why or why not?

9. Does the practice of a treatment procedure, when it is not called "experimental," raise ethical questions? Under what conditions are such questions likely to be raised?

10. What is "research" according to the National Research Act?

11. What is an institutional review board?

12. How is the membership of an institutional review board constituted?

13. What are the major concerns of an institutional review board?

14. What is a risk–benefit ratio? How is it determined? In this process, whose risk and whose benefits are evaluated?

15. Does the presence of risk to the participants automatically mean that a study cannot be conducted? Justify your answer.

16. What are the three components of informed consent?

17. Can you contact potential participants before obtaining permission from an institutional review board? Justify your answer.

18. You wish to evaluate a stuttering treatment program using one of the group designs. Describe the procedures for obtaining informed consent from your participants.

19. What procedures would you use in protecting the privacy of your clients who participate in research studies?

20. What are the ethical concerns with informed consent procedures?

21. Summarize the ethical concerns with no-treatment and placebo control groups. What solutions would you offer?

22. What ethical consequences does randomization have on data?

23. What are the negative consequences of treatment withdrawal or reversal? How are these consequences handled?

24. Describe the major ethical problems with participant recruitment.

25. Describe the various consequences of ethical constraints on data and their interpretation.

References

◆◆◆◆◆◆◆◆◆◆◆◆◆◆◆◆◆◆◆◆◆◆◆◆◆◆◆◆◆◆◆◆◆◆◆◆◆

Agency for Health Care Policy and Research. (1994). *Distinguishing between efficacy and effectiveness.* Rockville, MD: Author.

Allport, G. D. (1962). The general and the unique in the psychological sciences. *Journal of Personality, 30,* 405–422.

Altman, J. (1974). Observational study of behavior: Sampling methods. *Behavior, 7,* 227–267.

American Psychological Association. (1992). Ethical principles of psychologists and code of conduct. *American Psychologist, 47,* 1597–1611.

American Psychological Association. (2001). *Publication manual of the American Psychological Association* (5th ed.). Washington, DC: Author.

American Psychological Association. (2002). *Guidelines in the ethical conduct in the care and use of animals.* Retrieved August 10, 2002, from http://www.apa.org/science.anguide.htm

American Speech-Language-Hearing Association. (2002). *Ethics in research and professional practice.* Retrieved August 10, 2002, from http://www.asha.org

Attanasio, J. (1986). Therapy and research: Response to Siegel and Spradlin. *Journal of Speech and Hearing Disorders, 51,* 378.

Bachrach, A. J. (1969). *Psychological research: An introduction.* New York: Random House.

Baer, D. M., Wolf, M. M., & Risley, T. R. (1968). Some current dimensions of applied behavior analysis. *Journal of Applied Behavior Analysis, 10,* 117–119.

Baken, R., & Orlikoff, R. (2000). *Clinical measurement of speech and voice* (2nd ed.). Albany, NY: Singular Thomson Learning.

Baker, S. (1981). *The practical stylist* (2nd ed.). New York: Harper & Row.

Bannister, D. (1966). Psychology as an exercise in paradox. *Bulletin of British Psychological Society, 19,* 21–26.

Barlow, D. H., & Hayes, S. C. (1979). Alternating treatments design: One strategy for comparing the effects of two treatments in a single subject. *Journal of Applied Behavior Analysis, 12,* 199–210.

Barlow, D. H., Hayes, S. C., & Nelson, R. O. (1984). *The scientist practitioner: Research and accountability in clinical and educational settings.* New York: Pergamon.

Barlow, D. H., & Hersen, M. (1984). *Single case experimental designs* (2nd ed.). New York: Pergamon.

Bates, J. D. (1980). *Writing with precision.* Washington, DC: Acropolis.

Batten, M. (1968). *Discovery by chance: Science and the unexpected.* New York: Funk & Wagnall.

Battle, D. E. (2002). *Communication disorders in multicultural populations* (3rd ed.). Boston: Butterworth-Heinemann.

Beecher, H. K. (1955). The powerful placebo. *Journal of the American Medical Association, 159,* 1602–1606.

Beecher, H. K. (1966). Ethics and clinical research. *New England Journal of Medicine, 274,* 1354–1360.

Blichert-Toft, M., Mouridsen, H., & Andersen, K. W. (1996). Clinical trials. *Seminar in Surgical Oncology, 12*(1), 32–38.

Bloodstein, O. (1995). *Handbook on stuttering* (5th ed.). San Diego, CA: Singular.

Bolgar, H. (1965). The case study method. In B. B. Wolman (Ed.), *Handbook of clinical psychology* (pp. 28–39). New York: McGraw-Hill.

Borden, G. J., Harris, K. S., & Raphael, L. J. (2003). *Speech science primer: Physiology, acoustics, and perception of speech* (4th ed.). Philadelphia: Lippincott, Williams & Wilkins.

Boring, E. (1950). *A history of experimental psychology* (2nd ed.). New York: Appleton-Century-Crofts.

Box, J. F. (1978). *R. A. Fisher: The life of a scientist.* New York: Wiley.

Branch, M. N. (1991). Behavioral pharmacology. In I. H. Iversen & K. A. Lattal (Eds.), *Experimental analysis of behavior: Part 2* (pp. 21–77). Amsterdam: Elsevier.

Brody, B. A. (1998). *The ethics of biomedical research: An international perspective.* New York: Oxford University Press.

Brown, R. (1973). *A first language: The early stages.* Cambridge, MA: Harvard University Press.

Browning, R. M. (1967). A same-subject design for simultaneous comparison of three reinforcement contingencies. *Behavior Research and Therapy, 5,* 237–243.

Bryson-Brockmann, W., & Roll, D. (1996). Single-case experimental designs in medical education: An innovative research method. *Academic Medicine, 7*(1), 78–85.

Burt, C. (1972). Inheritance of general intelligence. *American Psychologist, 27,* 175–190.

Byar, D. P., & Piantadosi, S. (1985). Factorial designs for randomized clinical trials. *Cancer Treatment Reports, 69*(10), 1055–1063.

Calvin, W. H., & Ojemann, G. A. (1980). *Inside the brain.* New York: New American Library.

Campbell, B. G. (1976). *Humankind emerging.* Boston: Little, Brown.

Campbell, D. T., & Stanley, J. C. (1966). *Experimental and quasi-experimental designs for research.* Chicago: Rand McNally.

Campbell, N. (1952). *What is science?* New York: Dover.

Cannon, W. (1945). *The way of an investigator.* New York: Norton.

Capelli, R. (1985). *An experimental analysis of morphologic acquisition.* Unpublished master's thesis, California State University, Fresno, CA.

Chomsky, N. (1957). *Syntactic structures.* The Hague: Mouton.

Christensen, L. B. (1980). *Experimental methodology* (2nd ed.). Boston: Allyn & Bacon.

Clatterbaugh, K. (1999). *The causation debate in modern philosophy 1637–1739.* New York: Routledge.

Cochran, W. C. (1980). Fisher and the analysis of variance. In S. Fienberg, J. Gani, J. Kiefer, & K. Krickeberg (Eds.), *R. A. Fisher: An appreciation* (pp. 17–34). New York: Springer-Verlag.

Coleman, T. J. (2000). *Clinical management of communication disorders in culturally diverse children.* Boston: Allyn & Bacon.

Cook, T. D., & Campbell, D. T. (1979). *Quasi-experimental design: Design and analysis issues for field settings.* Chicago: Rand McNally.

Cudahy, E. (1988). *Introduction to instrumentation in speech and hearing.* Baltimore: Williams & Wilkins.

Curtis, J. F., & Schultz, M. C. (1986). *Basic laboratory instrumentation for speech and hearing.* Boston: Little, Brown.

De Cesari, R. (1985). *Experimental training of grammatic morphemes: Effects on the order of acquisition.* Unpublished master's thesis, California State University, Fresno, CA.

Dekkers, W., & Boer, G. (2001). Sham neurosurgery in patients with Parkinson's disease: Is it morally acceptable? *Journal of Medical Ethics, 27*(3), 151–156.

Devlin, T. (1976, October 25). Theories of IQ pioneer completely discredited. *London Times.*

Diener, E., & Crandall, R. (1978). *Ethics in social and behavioral research*. Chicago: University of Chicago.

Donabedian, A. (1980). *Explorations in quality assessment and monitoring: Volume I. The definition of quality and approaches to assessment*. Ann Arbor, MI: Health Administration Press.

Dukes, W. F. (1965). *N* = 1. *Psychological Bulletin, 64*, 74–79.

Eddington, E. S. (1967). Statistical inference from *N* = 1 experiments. *Journal of Psychology, 65*, 195–199.

Edlund, M. J., Craig, T. J., & Richardson, M. A. (1985). Informed consent as a form of volunteer bias. *American Journal of Psychiatry, 142*, 624–627.

Education for All Handicapped Children Act of 1975, 20 U.S.C. § 1400 *et seq.*

Edwards, A. L. (1960). *Experimental design in psychological research* (Rev. ed.). New York: Holt, Rinehart & Winston.

Feinstein, A. R. (1970). Statistics versus science in the design of experiments. *Clinical Pharmacology and Therapeutics, 11*, 282–292.

Feinstein, A. R. (1995). Meta-analysis: Statistical alchemy for the 21st century. *Journal of Clinical Epidemiology, 48*, 71–97.

Ferster, C. B., & Skinner, B. F. (1957). *Schedules of reinforcement*. New York: Appleton-Century-Crofts.

Finn, R. (1999). *Cancer clinical trials*. Sebastopol, CA: O'Reilly.

Fisher, R. A. (1925). *Statistical methods for research workers*. London: Oliver & Boyd.

Fisher, R. A. (1942). *Design of experiments*. London: Oliver & Boyd.

Fisher, R. (1951). *The design of experiments* (6th ed.). New York: Hefner.

Fisher, R. A. (1956). *Statistical methods and scientific inference*. London: Oliver & Boyd.

Flower, R. M. (1983). Keynote address: Looking backwards and looking forward: Some views through a four-decade window. In N. S. Rees & T. L. Snope (Eds.), *Proceedings of the 1983 national conference on undergraduate, graduate, and continuing education* (Rep. No. 13, pp. 9–15). Washington, DC: American Speech-Language-Hearing Association.

Folkins, J. W., Gorga, M. P., Luschei, E. S., Vetter, D. K., & Watson, C. S. (1993). The use of nonhuman animals in speech, language, and hearing research. *Asha, 35*, 57–65.

Follett, W. (1998). *Modern American usage: A guide* (1st rev. ed.). New York: Hill & Wang.

Frattali, C. (Ed.). (1998). *Measuring outcomes in speech-language pathology*. New York: Thieme.

Freedman, L. S., & Green, S. B. (1990). Statistical designs for investigating several interventions in the same study: Methods for cancer prevention trials. *Journal of National Cancer Institute, 82*, 910–914.

Freud, S. (1944). *New introductory lectures on psychoanalysis*. New York: Norton.

Gadlin, H., & Ingle, G. (1975). Through the one-way mirror: The limits of experimental self-reflection. *American Psychologist, 30*, 1003–1009.

Gillie, O. (1976, October 24). Crucial data was faked by eminent psychologist. *Sunday London Times.*

Gittleman-Foster, N. (1983). *Observer reliability in the measurement of dysfluencies with trained and untrained observers*. Unpublished master's thesis, California State University, Fresno, CA.

Glass, G. V., Wilson, V. L., & Gottman, J. M. (1974). *Design and analysis of time-series experiments*. Boulder, CO: Associated University Press.

Goodman, N. (1967). The epistemological argument. *Synthese, 17*, 23–28.

Gorkin, L., Schron, E. B., Handshaw, K., Shea, S., Kinney, M. R., Branyon, M., et al. (1996). Clinical trial enrollers vs. nonenrollers: The Cardiac Arrhythmia Suppression Trial (CAST) Recruitment and Enrollment Assessment in Clinical Trials (REACT) project. *Controlled Clinical Trials, 17*(1), 46–59.

Gotzsche, P. C., & Olsen, O. (2000). Is screening for breast cancer with mammography justifiable? *Lancet, 355,* 129–134.

Grmek, M. D. (1981). A plea for freeing the history of scientific discoveries from myth. In M. D. Grinek, R. S. Cohen, & G. Cymino (Eds.), *On scientific discovery* (pp. 9–42). London: Reidel.

Hacking, I. (1975). *The emergence of probability.* New York: Cambridge University Press.

Hald, A. (1998). *A history of mathematical statistics from 1750 to 1930.* New York: Wiley.

Hargis, C. H. (1984). *English syntax: An outline for clinicians and teachers of language handicapped children* (2nd ed.). Springfield, IL: Thomas.

Hartman, D. P., & Hall, R. V. (1976). The changing criterion design. *Journal of Applied Behavior Analysis, 9,* 537–532.

Hayes, S. C. (1981). Single-case experimental design and empirical clinical practice. *Journal of Consulting and Clinical Psychology, 49,* 193–211.

Hegde, M. N. (1980a). Issues in the study and explanation of language behavior. *Journal of Psycholinguistic Research, 9,* 1–22.

Hegde, M. N. (1980b). An experimental-clinical analysis of grammatical and behavioral distinctions between verbal auxiliary and copula. *Journal of Speech and Hearing Research, 23,* 864–877.

Hegde, M. N. (1998a). *Treatment procedures in communicative disorders* (3rd ed.). Austin, TX: PRO-ED.

Hegde, M. N. (1998b, April). *Treatment research: Market-driven or science-driven?* Paper presented at the Treatment Efficacy Research Conference, Vanderbilt University, Nashville, TN.

Hegde, M. N. (2001, November). *Treatment research: Designs and evaluative criteria.* A symposium presented at the Annual Convention of the American Speech-Language-Hearing Association, New Orleans, LA.

Hegde, M. N. (2003). *A coursebook on scientific and professional writing* (3rd ed.). Albany, NY: Singular Thomson Learning.

Hegde, M. N., Noll, M. J., & Pecora, R. (1978). A study of some factors affecting generalization of language training. *Journal of Speech and Hearing Disorders, 44,* 301–320.

Heise, D. R. (1975). *Causal analysis.* New York: Wiley

Hennekens, C. H., & Buring, J. E. (1987). *Epidemiology in medicine.* Boston: Little, Brown.

Hicks, P. L. (1998). Outcomes measurements requirements. In C. Frattali (Ed.), *Measuring outcomes in speech-language pathology* (pp. 28–49). New York: Thieme.

Higgins, S. T., & Hughes, J. R. (1998). Human behavioral pharmacology: An overview of laboratory methods. In K. A. Lattal & M. Perone (Eds.), *Handbook of research methods in human operant behavior* (pp. 579–618). New York: Plenum Press.

Hill, G., Forbes, W., Kozak, J., & McNeill, I. (2000). Likelihood and clinical trials. *Journal of Clinical Epidemiology, 53*(3), 223–227.

Hoagwood, K., Hibbs, E., Brent, D., & Jensen, P. J. (1995). Efficacy and effectiveness in studies of child and adolescent psychotherapy. *Journal of Consulting and Clinical Psychology, 63,* 683–687.

Homer, R. D., & Baer, D. M. (1978). Multiple probe technique: A variation of the multiple baseline. *Journal of Applied Behavior Analysis, 11,* 189–196.

Hrobjartsson, A., & Gotzsche, P. C. (2001). Is the placebo powerless?—An analysis of clinical trials comparing placebo with no treatment. *The New England Journal of Medicine, 344,* 1594–1602.

Huck, W. S., Cormier, W. H., & Bounds, W. G., Jr. (1974). *Reading statistics and research.* New York: Harper & Row.

Individuals with Disabilities Education Act of 1990, 20 U.S.C. § 1400 *et seq.*

Jensen, A. (1992). Scientific fraud or false accusations? The case of Cyril Burt. In D. J. Miller & M. Hersen (Eds.), *Research fraud in the behavioral and biomedical sciences* (pp. 97–124). New York: Wiley.

Johnson, W. (1955). A study of the onset and development of stuttering. In W. Johnson & R. R. Leutenegger (Eds.), *Stuttering in children and adults* (pp. 37–73). Minneapolis: University of Minnesota.

Johnson, W., & Associates (1959). *The onset of stuttering.* Minneapolis: University of Minnesota.

Johnston, J. M., & Pennypacker, H. S. (1993). *Strategies and tactics of human behavioral research* (2nd ed.). Hillsdale, NJ: Erlbaum.

Jones, J. (1981). *Bad blood.* New York: Free Press.

Kamhi, A. G., Pollock, K. E., & Harris, J. L. (1996). *Communication development and disorders in African American children.* Baltimore: Brookes.

Kamin, L. J. (1974). *The science and politics of I.Q.* Hillsdale, NJ: Erlbaum.

Kane, T. S. (1988). *The new Oxford guide to writing.* New York: Oxford University Press.

Kaptchuk, T. J. (1998). Powerful placebo: The dark side of the randomized controlled trial. *Lancet, 451,* 1722–1725.

Kaptchuk, T. (2001). The double-blind, randomized placebo-controlled trial: Gold standard or golden calf? *Journal of Clinical Epidemiology, 54,* 541–549.

Katz, J. (1972). *Experiments with human beings.* New York: Russell Sage Foundation.

Kayser, H. (1998). *Bilingual speech–language pathology: An Hispanic focus.* San Diego, CA: Singular.

Kazdin, A. E. (1982). *Single-case research designs: Methods for clinical and applied settings.* New York: Oxford University.

Kazdin, A. E. (1998). Drawing valid inferences from case studies. In A. E. Kazdin (Ed.), *Methodological issues and strategies in clinical research* (2nd ed., pp. 403–417). Washington, DC: American Psychological Association.

Kelman, H. C. (1972). Human use of human subjects: The problem of deception in social psychological experiments. *Psychological Bulletin, 67,* 1–11.

Kendall, P., Flannery-Schroeder, E. C., & Norton-Ford, J. (1999). Therapy outcome research methods. In P. C. Kendall, J. N. Butcher, & G. N. Holmbeck (Eds.), *Research methods in clinical psychology* (2nd ed., pp. 330–363). New York: Wiley.

Kendall, P., & Norton-Ford, J. (1982). Therapy outcome research methods. In P. Kendall & J. Butcher (Eds.), *Handbook of research methods in clinical psychology* (pp. 429–460). New York: Wiley.

Kent, R. D. (1983). Issue IX: Role of research: How can we improve the role of research and educate speech–language pathologists and audiologists to be competent users of research? In N. S. Rees & T. L. Snope (Eds.), *Proceedings of the 1983 national conference on undergraduate, graduate, and continuing education* (Rep. No. 13, pp. 76–86). Washington, DC: American Speech-Language-Hearing Association.

Kent, R. D. (1985). Science and the clinician: The practice of science and the science of practice. In R. D. Kent (Ed.), *Application of research to assessment and therapy. Seminars in Speech and Language, 6,* 1–12.

Kerlinger, F. N. (1986). *Foundations of behavioral research* (3rd. ed.). New York: Holt, Rinehart & Winston.

Kienle, G. S., & Kiene, H. (1997). The powerful placebo effect: Fact or fiction? *Journal of Clinical Epidemiology, 50,* 1311–1318.

Kirszner, L. G., & Mandell, S. R. (1992). *The Holt handbook* (3rd ed.). New York: Holt, Rinehart & Winston.

Lee, B. S. (1950). Effects of delayed speech feedback. *Journal of the Acoustical Society of America, 22,* 824–826.

Lee, B.S. (1951). Artificial stutter. *Journal of Speech and Hearing Disorders, 16*, 53–55.

Lee, J. J., Lieberman, R., Sloand, J. A., Piantadosi, S., & Lipman, S. M. (2001). Design considerations for efficient prostate cancer chemoprevention trials. *Urology, 57*(4) (Suppl. 1), 2005–2012.

Madden, M. (1994). What women affected by breast cancer think about research and randomization: A report of the SSRU pilot study. In P. Aldersen (Ed.), *Breast cancer, random control trials, and consent* (pp. 62–76). London: SSRU.

Marcus, S. M. (1997). Assessing non-consent bias with parallel randomized and nonrandomized clinical trials. *Journal of Clinical Epidemiology, 50*(7), 823–828.

Marvel, M. K., & Amodei, N. (1992). Single-subject experimental designs: A practical research alternative for practicing physicians. *The Family Practice Research Journal, 12*(2), 109–121.

McCall, W. A. (1923). *How to experiment in education.* New York: Macmillan.

McIntosh, N. (1993). Strengthen ethical committee's role. *British Medical Journal, 307*, 1496.

McKee, M., Gritton, A., Black, N., McPherson, K., Sanderson, C., & Bain, C. (1999). Interpreting the evidence: Choosing between randomized and non-randomized studies. *British Medical Journal, 319*, 312–315.

McKim, W. A. (1986). *Drugs and behavior: An introduction to behavioral pharmacology.* Englewood Cliffs, NJ: Prentice Hall.

McLaughlin, S. (1998). *Introduction to language development.* San Diego, CA: Singular.

McReynolds, L. V., & Engmann, D. L. (1974). An experimental analysis of the relationship between subject noun and object noun phrases. In L. V. McReynolds (Ed.), *Developing systematic procedures for training children's language* (Monograph No. 18, pp. 30–46). Rockville Pike, MD: American Speech-Language-Hearing Association.

McWhorter, K. T. (1993). *The writer's express.* Boston, MA: Houghton Mifflin.

Meinert, C. L. (1986). *Clinical trials: Design, conduct, and analysis.* New York: Oxford University Press.

Metz, D. E., & Folkins, J. W. (1985). Protection of human subjects in speech and hearing research. *Asha, 27*, 25–29.

Miers, M. (1998). Current NIH perspectives on misconduct in science. In A. E. Kazdin (Ed.), *Methodological issues and strategies in clinical research* (2nd ed., pp. 787–694). Washington, DC: American Psychological Association.

Milgram, S. (1977, October). Subject reaction: The neglected factor in the ethics of experimentation. *Hastings Center Report.*

Miller, D. J. (1992). Plagiarism: The case of Elias A. K. Alsabati. In D. J. Miller & M. Hersen (Eds.), *Research fraud in the behavioral and biomedical sciences* (pp. 80–96). New York: Wiley.

Miller, D. J., & Hersen, M. (Eds.). (1992). *Research fraud in the behavioral and biomedical sciences.* New York: Wiley.

Morris, A. D., Zaritsky, A. L., & LeFever, G. (2000). Evaluation of ethical conflicts associated with randomized, controlled trials in critically ill children. *Critical Care Medicine, 28*(4), 1152–1156.

Morris, W., & Morris, M. (1985). *Harper dictionary of contemporary usage* (2nd ed.). New York: Harper.

National Commission for the Protection of Human Subjects of Biomedical and Behavioral Research. (1979). *The Belmont report: Ethical principles and guidelines for the protection of human subjects for research.* Washington, DC: U.S. Department of Health, Education, and Welfare.

National Institutes of Health. (1991). *Preparation and maintenance of higher animals during neuroscience experimentation: Report of a National Institutes of Health workshop* (NIH Publication No. 91-3207). Bethesda, MD: Author.

National Research Council. (1988). *Use of laboratory animals in biomedical and behavioral research*. Washington, DC: National Academy Press.

Newman, E. (1976). *A civil tongue*. New York: Warner.

Newsom, C., Favell, J. E., & Rincover, A. (1983). Side effects of punishment. In S. Axelrod & J. Apsche (Eds.), *The effects of punishment on human behavior* (pp. 285–316). New York: Academic Press.

Olswang, L. B., Thompson, C. K., Warren, S. F., & Minghetti, N. J. (Eds.). (1990). *Treatment efficacy research in communication disorders*. Washington, DC: American Speech-Language-Hearing Foundation.

Onslow, M., Andrews, C., & Lincoln, M. (1994). A control/experimental trial of an operant treatment for early stuttering. *Journal of Speech and Hearing Research, 37*, 1244–1259.

Panel on Scientific Responsibility and the Conduct of Research. (1992). *Responsible science: Ensuring the integrity of the research process* (Vol. 1). Washington, DC: National Academy Press.

Panel on Scientific Responsibility and the Conduct of Research. (1993). *Responsible science: Ensuring the integrity of the research process* (Vol. 2). Washington, DC: National Academy Press.

Payne, J. C. (1997). *Adult neurogenic language disorders: Assessment and treatment*. San Diego, CA: Singular.

Perkins, W. H. (1985). From clinical dispenser to clinical scientist. *Seminars in Speech and Language, 6*, 13–21.

Piaget, J. (1952). *The origins of intelligence in children*. New York: International University Press.

Piaget, J. (1959). *The language and thought of the child*. London: Routledge & Kegan Paul.

Pocock, S. J. (1983). *Clinical trials: A practical approach*. New York: Wiley.

Pringle, M., & Churchill, R. (1995). Randomized controlled trials in general practice: Gold standard or fool's gold? *British Medical Journal, 311*, 1382–1383.

Randal, J. (1998). How RCTs came to their own. *Journal of the National Cancer Research Institute, 90*, 1257–1258.

Ranstam, J., Buyse, M., George, S. L., Evans, S., Geller, N. L., Sherrer, B., et al. (2000). Fraud in medical research: An international survey of biostatisticians. *Controlled Clinical Trials, 21*(5), 415–427.

Resnick, J. H., & Schwartz, T. (1973). Ethical standards as an independent variable in psychological research. *American Psychologist, 28*, 134–139.

Robertson, S. C., & Colburn, A. P. (1997). Outcomes research for rehabilitation: Issues and solutions. *Journal of Rehabilitation Outcomes Measurement, 1*(5), 15–23.

Roseberry-McKibbin, C., & Hegde, M. N. (2000). *An advanced review of speech–language pathology*. Austin, TX: PRO-ED.

Rosenfeld, A. (1981). Animal rights vs. human health. *Science, 18*, 22.

Rothman, K. J., & Greenland, S. (1998a). Causation and causal inference. In K. J. Rothman & S. Greenland (Eds.), *Modern epidemiology* (2nd ed., pp. 7–28). Philadelphia: Lippincott Williams & Wilkins.

Rothman, K. J., & Greenland, S. (1998b). *Modern epidemiology* (2nd ed.). Philadelphia: Lippincott Williams & Wilkins.

Rothman, K. J., & Michels, K. B. (1994). The continued unethical use of placebo controls. *New England Journal of Medicine, 331*, 394–398.

Ruben, D. (1990). *Explaining explanation*. New York: Routledge.

Rusch, F. R., & Kazdin, A. E. (1981). Toward a methodology of withdrawal designs for the assessment of response maintenance. *Journal of Applied Behavior Analysis, 14*, 131–140.

Seymour, C. M., & Nober, E. H. (1998). *Introduction to communication disorders: A multicultural approach*. Boston: Butterworth-Heinemann.

Shapiro, D. A., & Shapiro, D. (1983). Comparative therapy outcome research: Methodological implications of meta-analysis. *Journal of Consulting and Clinical Psychology, 51,* 42–53.

Shapiro, M. B. (1961). The single case in fundamental clinical psychological research. *British Journal of Medical Psychology, 34,* 255–262.

Shaughnessy, J. J., & Zechmeister, E. B. (1985). *Research methods in psychology*. New York: Knopf.

Sidman, M. (1960). *Tactics of scientific research*. New York: Basic Books.

Siegel, G. M. (1987). The limits of science in communication disorders. *Journal of Speech and Hearing Disorders, 52,* 306–312.

Siegel, G. M., & Spradlin, J. E. (1985). Therapy and research. *Journal of Speech and Hearing Disorders, 50,* 226–230.

Silverman, F. H. (1998). *Fundamentals of electronics for speech-language pathologists and audiologists*. Englewood Cliffs, NJ: Prentice Hall.

Silverman, W. A. (1989). The myth of informed consent: In daily practice and in clinical trials. *Journal of Medical Ethics, 15*(1), 6–11.

Silverman, W. A., & Altman, D. G. (1996). Patients' preferences and randomized trials. *Lancet, 347,* 171–174.

Sinclair, W. J. (1901). *Semmelweis: His life and his doctrine*. Manchester, England: Manchester University Press.

Skinner, B. F. (1953). *Science and human behavior*. New York: Free Press.

Skinner, B. F. (1956). A case history in scientific method. *American Psychologist, 11,* 221–233.

Skinner, B. F. (1966). Operant behavior. In W. K. Honig (Ed.), *Operant behavior: Areas of research and application* (pp. 12–32). New York: Appleton-Century-Crofts.

Skinner, B. F. (1969). *Contingencies of reinforcement: A theoretical analysis*. New York: Appleton-Century-Crofts.

Skinner, B. F. (1972). *Cumulative record: A selection of papers* (3rd ed.). New York: Appleton-Century-Crofts.

Skinner, B. F. (1974). *About behaviorism*. New York: Knopf.

Smith, B., & Sechrest, L. (1998). Treatment of aptitude X treatment interactions. In A. E. Kazdin (Ed.), *Methodological issues and strategies in clinical research* (2nd ed., pp. 495–520). Washington, DC: American Psychological Association.

Snowdon, C., Garcia, J., & Elbourne, D. (1997). Making sense of randomization: Responses of parents of critically ill babies to random allocation of treatment in a clinical trial. *Social Sciences and Medicine, 45,* 1337–1355.

Solomon, R. L. (1949). An extension of control group design. *Psychological Bulletin, 46,* 137–150.

Stevens, S. (1951). Mathematics, measurement, and psychophysics. In S. Stevens (Ed.), *Handbook of experimental psychology* (pp. 1–49). New York: Wiley.

Streng, A. H. (1972). *Syntax, speech, and hearing*. New York: Grune & Stratton.

Strunk, W., Jr., & White, E. B. (1979). *The elements of style* (3rd ed.). New York: Macmillan.

Tangney, J. P. (1987). Fraud will out—or will it? *New Scientist, 115,* 62–63.

Taylor, K. M. (1985). The doctor's dilemma: Physician participation in randomized clinical trials. *Cancer Treatment Report 69,* 1095–1100.

Tomarken, A. J. (1999). Methodological issues in psychophysiological research. In P. C. Kendall, J. N. Butcher, & G. N. Holmbeck (Eds.), *Handbook of research methods in clinical psychology* (2nd ed., pp. 251–276). New York: Wiley.

Tucker, D. J., & Berry, G. (1980). Teaching severely multihandicapped students to put on their own hearing aids. *Journal of Applied Behavior Analysis, 13,* 65–75.

Ulman, J. D., & Sulzer-Azaroff, B. (1975). Multielement baseline design in educational research. In E. Ramp & G. Semb (Eds.), *Behavior analysis: Areas of research and application* (pp. 377–391). Englewood Cliffs, NJ: Prentice Hall.

Valsiner, J. (Ed.). (1986a). *The individual subject and scientific psychology.* New York: Plenum Press.

Valsiner, J. (1986b). Different perspectives on individual-based generalizations in psychology. In J. Valsiner (Ed.), *The individual subject and scientific psychology* (pp. 391–404). New York: Plenum Press.

Verdu-Pascal, F., & Castello-Ponce, A. (2001). Randomized clinical trials: A source of ethical dilemmas. *Medical Ethics, 27*(3), 177–178.

Wade, N. (1976). IQ and heredity: Suspicion of fraud beclouds classic experiment. *Science, 194,* 916–919.

Watson, J. B., & Rayner, R. (1920). Conditioned emotional reactions. *Journal of Experimental Psychology, 3,* 1–14.

Wilson, B. (1987). Single-case experimental designs in neuropsychological rehabilitation. *Journal of Clinical and Experimental Neuropsychology, 9,* 527–544.

Wilson, D. (1976). *In search of penicillin.* New York: Knopf.

Wilson, F. (1985). *Explanation, causation, and deduction.* Boston: Reidel.

World Medical Association. (2000). Declaration of Helsinki (Rev. ed.). Retrieved July 30, 2002, from www.wma.net/e/policy/17-c_e.html

Yates, B. T. (1998). Toward the incorporation of costs, cost-effectiveness analysis, and cost benefits analysis into clinical research. In A. E. Kazdin (Ed.), *Methodological issues and strategies in clinical research* (2nd ed., pp. 577–593). Washington, DC: American Psychological Association.

Young, M. A. (1969a). Observer agreement: Cumulative effects of rating many samples. *Journal of Speech and Hearing Research, 12,* 135–143.

Young, M. A. (1969b). Observer agreement: Cumulative effects of repeated ratings of the same samples and knowledge of results. *Journal of Speech and Hearing Research, 12,* 144–155.

Young, M. A. (1975). Observer agreement for marking moments of stuttering. *Journal of Speech and Hearing Research, 18,* 530–540.

Your baby is in a trial. (1995). *Lancet, 345,* 805–806.

Zinsser, W. (1990). *On writing well: An informal guide to writing nonfiction* (4th ed.). New York: Harper & Row.

Author Index

Subject Index

◆◆◆◆◆◆◆◆◆◆◆◆◆◆◆◆◆◆◆◆◆◆◆◆◆◆◆◆◆